CULTURAL PSYCHIATRY
WITH CHILDREN, ADOLESCENTS, AND FAMILIES

CULTURAL PSYCHIATRY WITH CHILDREN, ADOLESCENTS, AND FAMILIES

Edited by

Ranna Parekh, M.D., M.P.H.

Cheryl S. Al-Mateen, M.D.

Maria Jose Lisotto, M.D.

R. Dakota Carter, M.D., Ed.D.

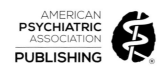

AMERICAN
PSYCHIATRIC
ASSOCIATION
PUBLISHING

If you wish to buy 50 or more copies of the same title, please go to www.appi.org/specialdiscounts for more information.

Copyright © 2021 American Psychiatric Association Publishing

ALL RIGHTS RESERVED

First Edition

Manufactured in the United States of America on acid-free paper
24 23 22 21 20   5 4 3 2 1

American Psychiatric Association Publishing
800 Maine Avenue SW
Suite 900
Washington, DC 20024-2812
www.appi.org

Library of Congress Cataloging-in-Publication Data
Names: Parekh, Ranna, editor. | Al-Mateen, Cheryl S., editor. | Lisotto, Maria Jose, editor. | Carter, R. Dakota, editor.
Title: Cultural psychiatry with children, adolescents, and families / edited by Ranna Parekh, Cheryl S. Al-Mateen, Maria Jose Lisotto, R. Dakota Carter.
Identifiers: LCCN 2020044378 (print) | LCCN 2020044379 (ebook) | ISBN 9781615373338 (paperback ; alk. paper) | ISBN 9781615373710 (ebook)
Subjects: MESH: Ethnopsychology—methods | Mental Health | Family—psychology | Infant | Child | Adolescent
Classification: LCC RC455.4.E8 (print) | LCC RC455.4.E8 (ebook) | NLM WM 31 | DDC 362.196/890089—dc23
LC record available at https://lccn.loc.gov/2020044378
LC ebook record available at https://lccn.loc.gov/2020044379

British Library Cataloguing in Publication Data
A CIP record is available from the British Library.

Contents

Part I
Race and Ethnicity

Part II
Cultural Concepts

Part III
External Influences

Part IV
Developmental Stages, Family, and Clinical Implications

Part V
Applied Concepts

Contributors

Balkozar Adam, M.D.
Clinical Professor, Department of Psychiatry, University of Missouri, Columbia, Missouri

Cheryl S. Al-Mateen, M.D., FAACAP, DFAPA
Professor, Departments of Psychiatry and Pediatrics, Virginia Commonwealth University School of Medicine, Richmond, Virginia

Joy K.L. Andrade, M.D.
General Psychiatrist and Child-Adolescent Psychiatrist; Assistant Professor, Department of Psychiatry, John A. Burns School of Medicine, University of Hawai'i at Mānoa, Honolulu, Hawaii

Maria Baez, M.D.
Assistant Clinical Professor of Psychiatry, Department of Child and Adolescent Psychiatry, Hassenfeld Children's Hospital at New York University Langone; Department of Child and Adolescent Psychiatry, Bellevue Hospital, New York, New York

Joseph T. Bell, M.D.
Medical Director and Pediatrician, Pembroke Pediatrics, Lumberton, North Carolina

Delores S. Bigfoot, Ph.D.
Professor, Department of Pediatrics, University of Oklahoma Health Sciences Center, Oklahoma City, Oklahoma

L. Lee Carlisle, M.D., DFAACAP
Associate Professor, Department of Psychiatry and Behavioral Sciences, University of Washington School of Medicine; Attending Physician, Seattle Children's Hospital, Seattle, Washington

R. Dakota Carter, M.D., Ed.D.
Child, Adolescent, and Adult Psychiatrist; Chief Medical Officer, Highlands Behavioral Health System, Denver, Colorado

Aisha Sanober Chachar, MBBS, FCPS
Adult, Child, and Adolescent Psychiatrist; Medical Director, Alleviate Addiction Suffering Trust and AAS Recovery Center, Karachi, Pakistan

Janet C. Chen, M.D.
Chief of Child and Adolescent Ambulatory Services and Assistant Professor of Clinical Psychiatry, Weill Cornell Medicine, New York, New York

Jang E. Cho, M.D.
Child and Adolescent Psychiatrist, Cultivate Psychiatry, Yakima, Washington

Shaylin P.Y.K. Chock, M.D.
General Psychiatrist, Child-Adolescent Psychiatrist, and Forensic Psychiatrist; Assistant Professor, Department of Psychiatry, John A. Burns School of Medicine, University of Hawai'i at Mānoa, Honolulu, Hawaii

Lisa M. Cullins, M.D.
Attending Physician, Emotion and Development Branch, National Institute of Mental Health, National Institutes of Health, Bethesda, Maryland

Rebecca Susan Daily, M.D., DFAPA, DFAACAP
Child, Adolescent, and Adult Psychiatrist and Co-Chair, Native American Child Committee, American Academy of Child and Adolescent Psychiatry, Crestview Hills, Kentucky

Ludmila De Faria, M.D.
Associate Professor, Department of Psychiatry, University of Florida; Director, Transitional Age Youth/Young Adult Clinic, Gainesville, Florida

Mary Lynn Dell, M.D., D.Min.
Medical Director, Psychiatry and Behavioral Health, Children's Hospital New Orleans; Department of Psychiatry, Louisiana State University and Tulane University, New Orleans, Louisiana

Lisa R. Fortuna, M.D., M.P.H.
Chief of Psychiatry, Zuckerberg San Francisco General Hospital; Vice-Chair of Psychiatry, University of California San Francisco, Zuckerberg San Francisco General Hospital and Trauma Center, San Francisco, California

Brittnie Fowler, M.D.
Child and Adolescent Psychiatry Fellow, Tulane University School of Medicine, New Orleans, Louisiana

Stefanie Gillson, M.D.
Resident Physician, Yale Psychiatry, Yale University, New Haven, Connecticut

Schuyler W. Henderson, M.D., M.P.H.
Associate Professor of Clinical Psychiatry, Department of Child and Adolescent Psychiatry, Hassenfeld Children's Hospital at New York University Langone; Department of Child and Adolescent Psychiatry, Bellevue Hospital, New York, New York

Pratik Jain, M.D.
Child and Adolescent Psychiatrist; Forensic Fellow, Yale Law and Psychiatry, New Haven, Connecticut

Aron Janssen, M.D.
Associate Professor of Psychiatry and Vice Chair of Child and Adolescent Psychiatry, Ann and Robert H. Lurie Children's Hospital, Chicago, Illinois

Kathryn L. Jones, M.D., Ph.D.
Assistant Professor, Virginia Commonwealth University School of Medicine, Richmond, Virginia

Debra E. Koss, M.D., FAACAP, DFAPA
Clinical Assistant Professor, Department of Psychiatry, Rutgers-Robert Wood Johnson Medical School, Piscataway, New Jersey; President, New Jersey Psychiatric Association; Member, APA Council on Advocacy and Government Relations; Co-chair, AACAP Advocacy Committee

Annie S. Li, M.D.
Director, Children's Comprehensive Psychiatry Emergency Program, Bellevue Hospital Center; Clinical Assistant Professor of Clinical and Adolescent Psychiatry, NYU Langone, New York, New York

Maria Jose Lisotto, M.D.
Child and Adolescent Psychiatrist, Cambridge Health Alliance; Instructor, Department of Psychiatry, Harvard Medical School, Cambridge, Massachusetts

Richard Livingston, M.D., DFAACAP
Co-chair, Native American Child Committee, American Academy of Child and Adolescent Psychiatry; Professor, Department of Psychiatry, University of Arkansas, Little Rock, Arkansas

Amalia Londoño Tobón, M.D.
Adult and Child Psychiatrist; Postdoctoral Clinical and Research Fellow in Perinatal Mental Health, Brown University Department of Psychiatry and Human Behavior, Providence, Rhode Island

Omar M. Mahmood, Ph.D.
Acting Clinical Director of Psychology, Sidra Medicine, Doha, Qatar; Assistant Professor of Psychology in Clinical Psychiatry, Weill Cornell Medical College, New York, New York

Andrés Martin, M.D., M.P.H.
Riva Ariella Ritvo Professor, Child Study Center, Yale School of Medicine, New Haven, Connecticut

Courtney L. McMickens, M.D., M.P.H., M.H.S.
Psychiatrist, Cityblock Health, Inc., Brooklyn, New York

Ayesha Irshad Mian, M.D., DFAACAP, SFHEA
Former and Founding Dean of Students, Associate Professor and immediate past Chair, Department of Psychiatry, Aga Khan University, Karachi, Pakistan

Jessica Moore, M.D.
Assistant Professor, Department of Psychiatry, University of Texas Southwestern Medical Center, Dallas, Texas

Phillip Murray, M.D., M.P.H.
Assistant Clinical Professor of Psychiatry, Atrium Health, Carolinas Health System, Charlotte, North Carolina

Wanjikū F.M. Njoroge, M.D.
Assistant Professor of Psychiatry, University of Pennsylvania Perelman School of Medicine; Program Director, Child and Adolescent Psychiatry Fellowship Program, Children's Hospital of Philadelphia; Medical Director, Young Child Clinic, Department of Child and Adolescent Psychiatry and Behavioral Sciences, Children's Hospital of Philadelphia; Faculty, PolicyLab, Children's Hospital of Philadelphia, Philadelphia, Pennsylvania

Auralyd Padilla, M.D.
Senior Associate Training Director, Assistant Professor of Psychiatry, University of Massachusetts Medical School, Worcester, Massachusetts

Ranna Parekh, M.D., M.P.H., DFAPA
Chief Diversity and Inclusion Officer, American College of Cardiology, Washington, D.C.; Former Deputy Medical Director and Director of Diversity and Health Equity, American Psychiatric Association; Consultant Psychiatrist, Massachusetts General Hospital, Boston, Massachusetts

Sejal Patel, M.P.H.
Senior Program Manager, American Psychiatric Association, Washington, D.C.

John Sargent, M.D.
Professor of Psychiatry and Pediatrics, Department of Psychiatry, Tufts Medical Center, Tufts University School of Medicine, Boston, Massachusetts

Neha Sharma, D.O.
Assistant Professor, Department of Psychiatry, Tufts Medical Center, Tufts University School of Medicine, Boston, Massachusetts

Jonathan J. Shepherd, M.D., FAPA, DFAACAP
Chief Medical Director, Hope Health Systems, Inc., Woodlawn, Maryland; President, Board of Directors, Black Mental Health Alliance, Inc., Baltimore, Maryland

Suzan Song, M.D., M.P.H., Ph.D.
Director, Division of Child/Adolescent and Family Psychiatry, and Associate Professor, George Washington University Medical Center, Washington, D.C.

Sarah Y. Vinson, M.D.
Founder, Lorio Psych Group; Associate Clinical Professor of Psychiatry and Pediatrics, Morehouse School of Medicine, Atlanta, Georgia

Collin Weintraub, B.S.
Medical Student, Virginia Commonwealth University School of Medicine, Richmond, Virginia

Kamille Wiliams, M.D.
Psychiatry Resident, Morehouse School of Medicine, Atlanta, Georgia

Disclosure of Interests

The following contributors to this book have indicated a financial interest in or other affiliation with a commercial supporter, a manufacturer of a commercial product, a provider of a commercial service, a nongovernmental organization, and/or a government agency, as listed below:

Cheryl S. Al-Mateen, M.D., FAACAP, DFAPA *Royalties:* Springer

Mary Lynn Dell, M.D., D.Min. *Royalties:* Oxford University Press and Abingdon Press

Sarah Y. Vinson, M.D. Executive Editor, *Ourselves Black* online and print magazine; Owner, Lorio Psych Group (clinical and consultation practice)

The following contributors have indicated that they have no financial interests or other affiliations that represent or could appear to represent a competing interferes with their contributions to this book:

Balkozar Adam, M.D.; Maria Baez, M.D.; L. Lee Carlisle, M.D., DFAACAP; R. Dakota Carter, M.D., Ed.D.; Janet C. Chen, M.D.; Jang E. Cho, M.D.; Lisa M. Cullins, M.D.; Ludmila De Faria, M.D.; Brittnie Fowler, M.D.; Schuyler W. Henderson, M.D., M.P.H.; Aron Janssen, M.D.; Annie S. Li, M.D.; Maria Jose Lisotto, M.D.; Courtney L. McMickens, M.D., M.P.H., M.H.S.; Phillip Murray, M.D., M.P.H.; Wanjikũ F. M. Njoroge, M.D.; Ranna Parekh, M.D., M.P.H., DFAPA; Neha Sharma, D.O.; Suzan Song, M.D., M.P.H., Ph.D.

Foreword

IT is an honor to be asked to contribute to an academic volume designed to improve mental health systems, deliver improved and higher-quality care, and identify and offer effective solutions for the continued health and mental health disparities present in our health care system today. I am especially honored to have been invited to write the foreword for this one, *Cultural Psychiatry With Children, Adolescents, and Families*, which is edited by four psychiatrists accomplished in their respective fields. These coeditors have assembled a group of knowledgeable clinicians, educators, and researchers and have woven the intersection of science, clinical care, cultural influence, and needs of populations that have unique issues or that receive care in special settings into an accessible volume to assist clinicians in providing the best possible care to children and adolescents with mental illness and their families. This volume goes beyond earlier works that identified the issues, and in some cases proposed solutions, only some of which have been implemented.

To better understand the sociocultural context for what is presented, we must start with the work done to address cultural issues in children's mental health service systems, starting with the 1989 National Institute of Mental Health's Child and Adolescent Service System Program's Minority Initiative Resource Committee monograph "Towards a Culturally Competent System of Care" (Cross et al. 1989). This monograph helped us understand that when racial and ethnic minority children are involved, cultural issues must be factored into every aspect of the care being provided, from the initial presentation through the diagnostic assessment period, and must be incorporated into development of the treatment plan.

In 2000, the "Report of the Surgeon General's Conference on Children's Mental Health: A National Action Agenda" (U.S. Department of Health and Human Services 2000) stated that African American and Hispanic children are identified and referred for mental health treatment at the same rates as other children but are much less likely to actually receive specialty mental health services or psychotropic medications. This report was followed by another surgeon general's report specifically addressing the importance of understanding mental illness across the life span in the context of race, culture, and ethnicity (U.S. Department of Health and Human Services 2001). Examples such as these make it clear that when primary health care, schools, child welfare services, and the mental health system fail to identify and provide culturally appropriate services, children will fall through the cracks and often end up in restrictive out-of-home placement, presenting challenges to normal child development.

To address those challenges, this volume starts with a review of the issues unique to racial and ethnic minority groups and goes further by introducing issues of intersectionality (e.g., gender identity, sexuality, spirituality, the impact of family values and culture). In other chapters, the authors explore the role of social determinants of health on child development (Chapter 10), the complex needs of immigrant and refugee populations (Chapters 11 and 12), and special issues of culture and mental health across the life span from infants to college-age students (Chapters 17 and 20). Chapter 19 on the impact of early life microaggressions is especially important for clinicians treating children and adolescents as we come to understand more about microaggressions as some of the adverse childhood experiences that significantly impact overall health and psychological well-being in adulthood. The chapters on the influence of media and technology (Chapters 14 and 15) are followed by one highlighting the workforce needs and clinical challenges seen in rural areas (Chapter 16), which represent another diverse and underserved population. Finally, the volume concludes with the presentation of several cases of patients with a combination of characteristics from sections of the book to demonstrate the use of the DSM-5 Cultural Formulation Interview as the basis for the cultural formulation of each case (American Psychiatric Association 2013a, 2013b).

Cultural Psychiatry With Children, Adolescents, and Families is a timely addition to the growing body of science and clinical practice references needed to address the challenging environments in which children, adolescents, and their families endeavor to survive. Drs. Parekh, Al-Mateen, Lisotto, and Carter are to be commended because they have created a volume that gives me hope that with its use, mental health services for children, adolescents, and their families will be improved significantly and these youth will be able to thrive, leading to positive health and life outcomes.

Altha J. Stewart, M.D.
Senior Associate Dean for Community Health Engagement
Chief, Social and Community Psychiatry
Director, Center for Health in Justice Involved Youth
University of Tennessee Health Science Center
145th President, American Psychiatric Association
Memphis, Tennessee

References

American Psychiatric Association: Cultural concepts in DSM-5. Arlington, VA, American Psychiatric Association, 2013a. Available at: www.psychiatry.org/File%20Library/Psychiatrists/Practice/DSM/APA_DSM_Cultural-Concepts-in-DSM-5.pdf. Accessed April 24, 2020.

American Psychiatric Association: Cultural Formulation Interview (CFI), in Diagnostic and Statistical Manual of Mental Disorders, Fifth Edition. Arlington, VA, American Psychiatric Association, 2013b, pp 750–757

Cross TL, Dennis KW, Isaacs MR: Towards a Culturally Competent System of Care: A Monograph on Effective Services for Minority Children Who Are Severely Emotionally Disturbed. Washington, DC, CASSP Technical Assistance Center, Georgetown University Child Development Center, March 1989.

U.S. Department of Health and Human Services: Report of the Surgeon General's Conference on Children's Mental Health: A National Action Agenda. Washington, DC, U.S. Department of Health and Human Services, 2000. Available at: www.ncbi.nlm.nih.gov/books/NBK44233. Accessed: April 24, 2020.

U.S. Department of Health and Human Services: Mental Health: Culture, Race, and Ethnicity—A Supplement to Mental Health: A Report of the Surgeon General. Rockville, MD, Substance Abuse and Mental Health Services Administration, 2001

CHAPTER 1
Introduction to Cultural Psychiatry

Cheryl S. Al-Mateen, M.D., FAACAP, DFAPA
Ranna Parekh, M.D., M.P.H., DFAPA
Maria Jose Lisotto, M.D.
R. Dakota Carter, M.D., Ed.D.

Editors' Aim

This volume is designed for health providers of all disciplines caring for the mental health of children, adolescents, and families in a variety of clinical settings in the United States. Of note, many of the concepts discussed apply globally as well. Because of rapidly changing demographics, "minority" youth since 2018 represent the majority in the United States, with 50.1% of children younger than age 15 identifying as nonwhite (Frey 2019). U.S. mental health has become synonymous with cultural mental health for children and adolescents (Figure 1–1).

Additionally, today's attention to mental health and escalating rates of suicide, substance use, and mood disorders permeate every aspect of health care and delivery systems. In this book, the editors and authors aim to provide history, theory, and evidence-based practice to the various dimensions influencing mental health in children, adolescents, transitional age youth (TAY), and families. Although there are numerous volumes dedicated to cultural aspects of mental health, there are few textbooks focused on the role of culture in the mental health assessment, diagnosis, and care of children, adolescents, and their families. In this volume, we emphasize the importance of the DSM-5 Cultural Formulation Interview (CFI) and Outline for Cultural Formulation (OCF; American Psychiatric Association 2013) when caring for youth, similar to care of adults. These instruments are perhaps even more relevant in populations where psychosocial development is in

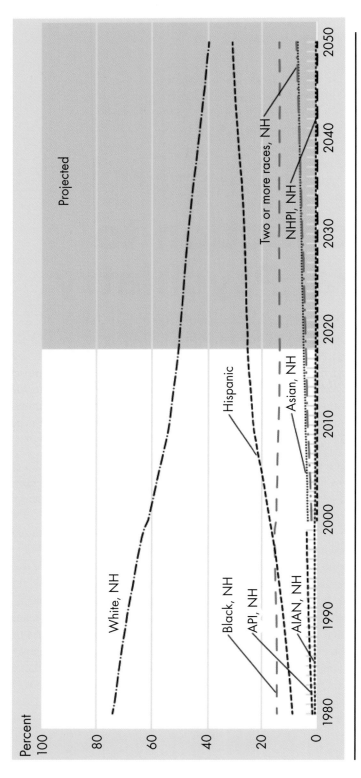

FIGURE 1–1.   Indicator POP3: percentage of children ages 0–17 in the United States by race and Hispanic origin, 1980–2018 and projected 2019–2050.

Note.   AIAN=American Indian and Alaskan Native; API=Asian and Pacific Islander; NH=non-Hispanic origin; NHPI=Native Hawaiian and Other Pacific Islander. Each group represents the non-Hispanic population, with the exception of the Hispanic category itself. Persons of Hispanic origin may be of any race.

Source.   U.S. Census Bureau, Population Division. Reprinted from ChildStats.gov: Forum on Child and Family Statistics. 2019. Available at: www.childstats.gov/americaschildren/demo.asp. Accessed December 26, 2019.

flux and family compositions are diverse. The editors hope that this volume will serve as a companion to the indispensable *Clinical Manual of Cultural Psychiatry,* 2nd Edition (Lim 2015) for those clinicians working with children, adolescents, TAY, and families.

What Is Cultural Psychiatry?

Social psychiatry began in the late 1700s and early 1800s with a focus on delivering humanistic care to psychiatrically hospitalized patients (Westermeyer 2018). The focus was "psychiatry as related to social institutions" (Westermeyer 2018, p. 133). Cultural psychiatry began during the mid-1800s when social psychiatrists started considering the effects of cultural influences on psychiatric disorders (Westermeyer 2018). Early reports focused on unusual clinical syndromes from non-Western countries and relegated cultural concepts to exotic or isolated groups (Ton and Lim 2015).

By the mid-1900s, psychiatrists and other professionals with training in sociology and cultural anthropology expanded the perspective. During the 1980s, there were studies of child and adolescent refugees paralleling the studies of adults, as well as cross-cultural aspects of assessing children and their families, child abuse, and the impact of war (Westermeyer 2018). Westermeyer noted that "cultural psychiatry has focused on the psychology of the patient and the clinician as culturally derived or influenced, and the assessment and care of patients from cultural backgrounds notably different from those of their clinicians" (Westermeyer 2018, p. 137). This has included understanding psychopathology related to immigration, translation of psychiatric scales and instruments, use of interpreters, understanding the patient's world view, and appreciating the impact of cultural aspects of transference and countertransference as well as similarities and differences in psychopharmacology (Ton and Lim 2015; Westermeyer 2018). Currently, social and cultural psychiatry overlap and contribute to each other. We think this is seen most clearly in the need for child and adolescent mental health professionals to be knowledgeable about social determinants of mental health, including the multiple systems (e.g., education, social services, juvenile justice) that impact our patients on a daily basis; patients' and families' social identities; cultural norms; and cultural expectations, as well as how these factors interact with one another.

Fundamental Concepts in Cultural Psychiatry

Three critical concepts are frequently discussed in this volume: culture, mental health, and psychological development. *Culture* is defined as the "integrated pattern of human behavior that includes thoughts, communications, actions, customs, beliefs, values, and institutions of a racial, ethnic, religious or social group" (Cross et al. 1989, p. iv). The World Health Organization defines health as "a state of complete physical, mental and social well-being and not merely the absence of disease or infirmity" (World Health Organization 2003, p. 7).

Mental health is further defined as

> a state of well-being whereby individuals recognize their abilities, are able to cope with the normal stresses of life, work productively and fruitfully, and make a contribution to their communities....

TABLE 1–1. Core terms related to mental health disparities and health equity

Health inequality or difference is the "difference in health status or in the distribution of health determinants between different population groups."[a]

Health disparity is "a particular health difference that is closely linked with social, economic, and/or environmental disadvantage. Health disparities adversely affect groups…who have systematically experienced greater obstacles to health based on their racial and/or ethnic group; religion; socioeconomic status; gender; age; mental health; cognitive, sensory or physical disability; sexual orientation or gender identity; geographic location; or other characteristics historically linked to discrimination or exclusion."[a]

Health care disparity relates to "differences in the quality of healthcare that are not due to access, clinical need, patient preferences, or appropriateness of the intervention. "these differences would include the roles of bias, discrimination, and stereotyping at the individual (provider and patient), institutional, and health system levels."[b]

Health equity is attaining the highest level of health for all people. It requires "valuing everyone equally with focused and ongoing societal efforts to address avoidable inequalities, historical and contemporary injustices, and the elimination of health and healthcare disparities."[a]

Social determinants of health are "the conditions in which people are born, grow, live, work and age, and the systems put in place to deal with illness. These circumstances are shaped by the distribution of money, power and resources at global, national and local levels. The social determinants of health are mostly responsible for health inequities—the unfair and avoidable differences in health status seen within and between countries"[c]

[a]National Partnership for Action to End Health Disparities 2011, p. 9.
[b]Smedley et al. 2003.
[c]World Health Organization 2020.

> The risk is higher among the poor, homeless, the unemployed, persons with low education, victims of violence, migrants and refugees, indigenous populations, children and adolescents, abused women and the neglected elderly. (World Health Organization 2003, p. 7)

As providers caring for children and adolescents, we understand that *psychological development* is a lifelong process: "the development of human beings' cognitive, emotional, intellectual, and social capabilities and functioning over the course of the life span, from infancy through old age" (Encyclopædia Britannica 2019). The understanding of development within the context of culture is critical for those working with patients of any age when it comes to understanding the meaning of their presenting complaints, behaviors, and psychopathology (Guerra et al. 2019; Rey et al. 2015; Sroufe 2009).

Health and mental health disparities (see Table 1–1 for definitions) exist within the United States (Smedley et al. 2003; U.S. Department of Health and Human Services 2001) as well as globally (Kakuma et al. 2011). Recommendations for alleviating these disparities include promoting evidence-based guidelines and increasing the numbers of minority health care providers, as well as providing access to interpreters in health care settings, maximizing the use of primary care practice capabilities, increasing awareness of disparities, and developing the ability to provide *culturally competent* care to patients (Smedley et al. 2003).

Culturally competent care can be understood as one's ability to interact effectively with patients of different cultures. Multiple authors have described the components of culturally competent care (Table 1–2). Culturally competent psychiatric care was initially meant to improve the psychiatric treatment of immigrant and minority individuals (Qureshi et al. 2008). We now

TABLE 1–2. Components of culturally competent health care

System of care[a]

A set of behaviors, knowledge, attitudes, and policies that come together in a system or organization or among professionals that enables effective work in cross-cultural situations[a]

Individual practitioners[b]

Capacity for cultural self-awareness without letting it have undue influence on attitudes toward people from other backgrounds

Acceptance of and respect for cultural differences

Developing knowledge and understanding about the patient's culture

Adapting clinical care to fit the cultural context of the patient and family to ensure that quality care is delivered

The system[c]

Values and respects diversity

Has ability and willingness to assess its own culture

Is aware of the dynamics of cultural differences between the system and a population group

Institutionalizes the recognition and use of cultural knowledge

Adapts to diversity

[a]Adapted from Cross et al. 1989, p. 28.
[b]Adapted from Cross et al. 1989, pp. 47–50.
[b]Adapted from Betancourt et al. 2003; Cross et al. 1989, pp. 34–36; Substance Abuse and Mental Health Services Administration 2016.

know that there are cultural differences within the majority population. We also realize that cultural competence is not an achievable end point—one cannot know everything about all cultures. A complementary concept is that of *cultural humility,* defined as the "ability to maintain an interpersonal stance that is other-oriented…in relation to aspects of cultural identity that are most important to the person" (Hook et al. 2013, p. 354). *Cultural curiosity* recognizes that cultures are constantly changing and that there is a need for lifelong learning, as in other aspects of health care (Hook et al. 2013; Mikhaylov 2016; Tervalon and Murray-Garcia 1998).

Betancourt (2003) noted that

> when sociocultural differences between patient and provider aren't appreciated, explored, understood or communicated in the medical encounter, patient dissatisfaction, poor adherence, and poorer health outcomes result…. Historical factors for patient mistrust, provider bias, and their impacts…have also been documented. (p. 560)

Betancourt elaborated that approaches to enhance clinician attitudes, knowledge, and skills must be addressed by providing needed education to health care professionals. Topics that should be covered are found in Table 1–3. Attitudes include an appreciation of the impact of sociocultural factors on values, beliefs, and concepts about help-seeking with regard to mental health, including stigma. Also included are concepts of racism, sexism, and other forms of implicit bias. The mental health clinician and patient bring their own attitudes and experiences to the clinical encounter. These should be recognized, appreciated, and fully considered so that the interaction is effective and of benefit to the patient. Cross et al. (1989) also elucidated the continuum of cultural competence (see this volume, Chapter 13, "The Global State of Child and Adolescent Mental Health," Table 13–6).

TABLE 1-3. Topics for clinician education in cross-cultural mental health care in children and adolescents

Attitudes	Knowledge	Skills and tools
Self-awareness	Cultural identity	Interviewing skills
Implicit bias	Idioms of distress	Patient-centered care
Explicit bias (racism and other -isms)	Cultural syndromes	Culturally diverse toys, books, artwork, and magazines in your office and waiting room
Cultural humility	Acculturation	
Cultural competency	Cultural explanations of perceived causes	Interpreters and cultural brokers
Self-reflection	Mental health disparities	Paperwork in multiple languages
Awareness of the impact of sociocultural factors on a patient's health values, beliefs, and behaviors	Historical trauma	DSM-5 Outline for Cultural Formulation
	Social determinants of health	DSM-5 Cultural Formulation Interview
	Evidence-based guidelines and treatments	Practice Parameter for Cultural Competence in Child and Adolescent Psychiatric Practice (Pumariega et al. 2013)
		Knowledge of culturally specific evidence-based treatments

Source. Adapted from Betancourt 2003.

Knowledge includes an understanding of cross-cultural issues, including incidence and prevalence, that relate to mental health disparities. It also includes pertinent cultural information, such as historical trauma, that may impact health behaviors. It is important to not inadvertently encourage development of stereotypes or simplistic assumptions in providing such knowledge (Kleinman and Benson 2006). Rather, clinicians should strive for what Lo and Fung (2003) describe as a generic cultural competence, which involves knowledge and skills that are effective in any cross-cultural encounter and specific skills that are useful for a particular ethnocultural community.

Skills and tools help the clinician to elicit and appreciate patients' social contexts and conceptualization of their illness while engaging patients in shared decision-making. The Practice Parameter for Cultural Competence in Child and Adolescent Psychiatric Practice (Pumariega et al. 2013) is one such tool, with 13 principles to guide child and adolescent mental health professionals in their work with diverse children and families (Table 1–4). Ecklund and Johnson (2007) also provide guidelines on cultural competence with young patients (Table 1–5).

Use of Interpreters

One critical skill when it comes to mental health care is the ability to access interpreter services during clinical encounters with the identified patient and his or her caregivers. Given the complex communicative demands associated with mental health care, it would be unthinkable to care for patients, let alone children and adolescents, without sharing a common language. This entails not only actual language skills such as knowledge of vocabulary, grammar, and syntax

TABLE 1–4. AACAP practice parameters for work with diverse children and families

Identify and address barriers that may prevent diverse individuals from obtaining mental health services

Conduct the evaluation in the language in which the child and family are proficient

Understand the impact of dual language competence on the child's adaptation and functioning

Be cognizant of your own cultural biases and address them

Apply knowledge of cultural differences in development, idioms of distress, and symptomatic presentation to clinical formulation and diagnosis

Assess for history of immigration-related loss or trauma and community trauma and address them in treatment

Evaluate and address acculturation stress and intergenerational acculturation family conflict

Make a special effort to include family members and key members of traditional extended families in assessment, treatment planning, and treatment

Evaluate and utilize the child and family's cultural strengths in treatment interventions

Treat the child and family in familiar settings within their community when possible

Support parents to develop appropriate behavioral management skills compatible with their cultural values and beliefs

Use evidence-based psychological and pharmacological interventions specific to the child and family's ethnic/racial population

Identify ethnopharmacological factors that may influence the child's response to medications, including side effects

Abbreviation. AACAP=American Academy of Child and Adolescent Psychiatry.
Source. Adapted from Pumariega et al. 2013.

TABLE 1–5. Cultural competence with child patients

Be culture affirmative, not culture tolerant—have genuine respect

Be aware of the complexity of cultural identity (intersectionality)

Avoid assumptions based on a patient's apparent culture; develop an individualized conceptualization instead

Avoid cultural biases, positive or negative; work to develop an accurate understanding of risks and protective factors of cultural experiences and context

Integrate cultural assessment throughout the intake processes

Quickly address any cultural discomfort, including your own, when it is present

Be sensitive to the cumulative effects of oppression, prejudice, and racism in the life of the patient that may affect therapeutic rapport

Source. Adapted from Ecklund and Johnson 2007.

but also cultural assumptions and expectations, idioms, and cultural expressions of distress, which become accessible only through interpreter services unless the provider is well versed and proficient in the patient's language.

Interpreters are the bridge across the communicative abysm between mental health providers and children, adolescents, TAY, and families who either speak a different language from the clinician or are deaf or hard of hearing. During psychiatric clinical encounters, patients are expected to share very personal and sensitive information; if providers are not able to grasp the full extent and the subtle meanings behind what is shared, especially when a patient is underage, it would be impossible for the provider to accurately diagnose and treat the patient.

Patients with limited English proficiency or English as a second language struggle even more when it comes to mental health visits. Communication of abstract concepts such as emotions and psychiatric symptoms in a language other than one's mother tongue is extremely challenging, especially during times of internal distress (Bauer and Alegría 2010; Eneriz-Wiemer et al. 2014). Access to culturally affirmative and linguistically accessible mental health services is a fundamental right for all individuals, and interpreters are key when it comes to ensuring effective and culturally tailored care during psychiatric clinical encounters.

For many persons with profound hearing loss whose primary language is American Sign Language, deafness is a culture rather than a disability, and they use the capitalized term Deaf. Individuals who are Deaf or deaf (including individuals who are hard of hearing or deaf-blind) are entitled to accessible mental health services in their language (National Association of the Deaf 2008), pursuant to the Americans with Disabilities Act of 1990 (Americans with Disabilities Act. 42 U.S.C. §§ 12101 et seq.) and the Rehabilitation Act of 1973 (Rehabilitation Act of 1973. 29 U.S.C. §§ 791 et seq.), both of which require equal access to services for people with disabilities. There is a specialized training and certification for interpreters with mental health expertise (National Association of the Deaf 2020a). On-site interpreters or medical staff fluent in sign language should be the primary method by which health care providers and patients communicate; only when qualified on-site interpreters are unavailable in urgent matters should providers use video remote interpreting (VRI) services to "fill the gap" (National Association of the Deaf 2020b).

Figure 1–2 illustrates the therapeutic triad model, which not only underscores the importance of incorporating interpreters as essential team members but also identifies the critical role that interpreters play when it comes to connecting clinician and patient through verbal communication and contextualization of nonverbal communication. As shown in Figure 1–2, spoken language interpreters should be positioned with the clinician and patient in an equilateral triangle "so that each individual can have a clear view of the others in order to effectively communicate and receive nonverbal communication" (Ton and Lim 2015, p. 30). In contrast, however, a sign language interpreter should sit closer to the clinician in a more acute isosceles triangle so that the patient can easily see both the interpreter's hands and the clinician's facial expressions simultaneously (Figure 1–3).

Use of a Cultural Broker or Cultural Consultant

An additional skill is the use of a cultural broker or cultural consultant (Ton and Lim 2015). Although an interpreter may fulfill this role with the permission of the patient, a clinician can identify colleagues in mental health or primary care from the same cultural group who can provide general information about attitudes and/or perspectives that are relevant for the care of patients. Colleagues can provide clinicians a greater cultural context in order to better understand the clinical work as well as additional aspects of the family's culture that would be relevant to diagnosis and treatment. Religious or cultural leaders with cultural expertise can also fill this need (Singh et al. 1999; Ton and Lim 2015). When gathering this information from individuals outside the treatment team, it is important to maintain the patient's anonymity and confidentiality.

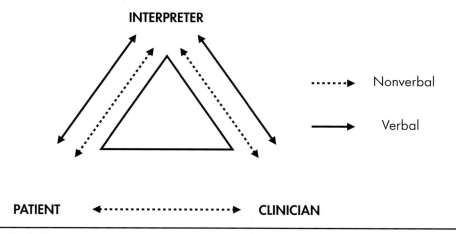

FIGURE 1–2. Therapeutic triad model.

Source. Reprinted from Ton H, Lim RF: Assessment of culturally diverse individuals: introduction and foundations, in *Clinical Manual of Cultural Psychiatry,* 2nd Edition. Edited by Lim RF. Arlington, VA, American Psychiatric Publishing, 2015, p. 31. Copyright © American Psychiatric Publishing 2015. Used with permission.

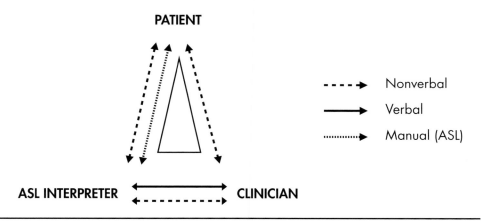

FIGURE 1–3. Therapeutic triad model with an American Sign Language (ASL) interpreter.

Source. Adapted from Ton and Lim 2015. Used with permission.

Bias and Microaggressions

The Institute of Medicine identified health care provider bias, stereotyping, and clinical uncertainty as factors that may contribute to health care disparities (Smedley et al. 2003). Research shows that unconscious or implicit biases can lead to differential patient treatment based on race, gender, weight, age, language, income, sexual orientation, disability, and insurance status (Smedley et al. 2003). Racial bias and discrimination can be subtle and difficult to recognize, especially for nonminority individuals. These types of subtle racism can be a form of *microaggression*, defined as a "comment or action that subtly and often unconsciously or unintentionally expresses a prejudiced attitude toward a member of a marginalized group (such as a racial minority)" (Merriam-Webster 2020). For more detailed discussion, see Chapter 19, "Microaggressions."

The American Academy of Pediatrics (AAP), the primary professional home to most U.S. pediatricians, published the policy statement *The Impact of Racism on Child and Adolescent Health* in August 2019 (Trent et al. 2019). The American Academy of Child and Adolescent Psychiatry (AACAP) has endorsed this statement. Both AACAP and the American Psychiatric Association (APA) have noted that racism is a social determinant of health with significant impacts on the health of children, adolescents, and emerging adults. Racism, which is mediated through implicit and explicit biases, institutional structures, and interpersonal relationships, undermines health equity of youth and their families (Trent et al. 2019, p. 2).

In this book, several authors reveal the impacts of minority stress and the influence various demographic criteria can impose on those communities because of negative experiences directed at them. Various theoretical concepts capture the conflict between environmental and dominant cultures and minority group members (Meyer 1995; Mirowsky and Ross 1989; Pearlin 1999). The minority stress theory captures the notion that members of subsets of the population, usually representing diverse communities, may have higher rates of stress and negative health outcomes compared with a majority peer group. These outcomes are highly correlated to negative experiences that minority group members have on the basis of their identity. These experiences are related to discrimination, prejudice, stigma, marginalization, and microaggressions that are additive and harmful to the group experiencing it (Meyer 2003). The minority stress model is intended to capture the lived experiences of minority group members, and it can also offer solutions. The model helps practitioners identify significant community needs and the conscious choices that can be made to rectify the negative influences leading to disparities and poor health outcomes.

Acculturation

Acculturation is the process through which cultures come together. This includes migration experiences, as well as becoming involved with increasingly diverse individuals through other experiences such as moving or going away to college (Berry 1998) (Figure 1–4). For further discussion, see Chapter 9, "Diverse Families and Family Treatment," and Chapter 20, "Cultural Aspects of College Mental Health."

Cultural Formulation

The OCF was introduced in DSM-IV as a supplement to the five axes and to mitigate difficulties encountered in cross-cultural encounters (American Psychiatric Association 1994) and was accompanied by a Glossary of Culture-Bound Syndromes. The OCF was created through clinical ethnographic research and social theory to enrich appreciation of the sociocultural context (Lewis-Fernandez et al. 2016). The resulting ethnography provides a more personal account than the clinician might otherwise obtain (Kleinman and Benson 2006). DSM-IV also listed specific culture, age, and gender features in the comments for various diagnoses.

		Identification with cultural group/heritage culture	
		Strong	**Weak**
Identification with majority/host culture	**Strong**	Acculturated Integrated bicultural	Assimilated
	Weak	Separated dissociated	Marginalized

FIGURE 1–4. **Acculturation.**

Source. Adapted from Berry 1998; Kim et al. 2018.

In DSM-5, culture-related diagnostic issues are provided for all diagnoses (Table 1–6). DSM-5 also includes a section on cultural formulation that contains the OCF (Table 1–7), the CFI, and cultural concepts of distress. For detailed discussion of these tools, see Chapter 21, "DSM-5 Outline for Cultural Formulation and Cultural Formulation Interview," and the appendces in this book. The Appendix to DSM-5 also includes a Glossary of Cultural Concepts of Distress, which describes "some common cultural syndromes, idioms of distress, and causal explanations" (American Psychiatric Association 2013, p. 14) (see Appendix C).

Members of a particular culture may label an experience by using cultural explanations or perceived causes. For example, mental health professionals in the United States use the term *depression* to describe a specific clinical syndrome that meets specific DSM criteria. However, an individual may use the same term to describe symptoms that may meet criteria for a different clinical syndrome. For this reason, it is helpful to have patients describe to you what they mean when they use a clinical term. At the time of this writing, members of the lay public frequently use the term *bipolar* to describe anyone with "mood swings" and "unpredictable behaviors." Further questioning may reveal that these individuals are describing a personality disorder, normal adolescence, or genuine mood symptoms.

Providers caring for youth and families should possess cross-cultural skills because expressions for psychological or emotional distress can differ across cultures. *Idioms of distress* are linguistic or somatic patterns of experiencing and expressing illness, affliction, or general stress (Kirmayer 2001) that can be mistaken for mental disorders. Common idioms of distress include "I've got problems with my nerves" or "my heart is telling me." Some people might say "I'm depressed" to describe an emotional state of acute sadness, while others might experience such symptoms as somatization, anger, irritability, or "falling out" (a sudden collapse that may or may not be preceded by dizziness). Some complex expressions of distress unique to a given culture will be discussed more in depth in various chapters of this book.

TABLE 1–6.   Cultural issues in DSM-5

Culture-related diagnostic issues

Each diagnosis includes cultural and socioeconomic factors, recognizing that "[i]deas that appear to be delusional in one culture…may be commonly held in another…. The assessment of affect requires sensitivity to differences in styles of emotional expression, eye contact, and body language, which vary across cultures. If the assessment is conducted in a language that is different from the individual's primary language, care must be taken to ensure that alogia is not related to linguistic barriers. In certain cultures, distress may take the form of hallucinations or pseudo-hallucinations and overvalued ideas that may present clinically similar to true psychosis but are normative to the patient's subgroup" (American Psychiatric Association 2013, p. 103).

Cultural concepts of distress

Cultural syndromes: clusters of symptoms and attributions that tend to co-occur among individuals in specific cultural groups, communities, or contexts and are recognized locally as coherent patterns of experience

Cultural idioms of distress: ways of expressing distress that are not specific symptoms or syndromes but provide collective, shared ways of experiencing or talking about personal or social concerns

Cultural explanations or perceived causes: labels, attributions, or features of an explanatory model that indicate culturally recognized meaning or etiology for symptoms, illness, or distress

Outline for Cultural Formulation

Cultural Formulation Interview

Topics Covered in This Volume

The practice of cultural psychiatry with children, adolescents, and transitional age youth (TAY) requires an understanding of typical development, systems of care, and families. In this volume, we include chapters on "Diverse Families and Family Treatment" (Chapter 9), "Infant Psychiatry" (Chapter 17), and "Cultural Aspects of College Mental Health" (Chapter 20) in order to broaden the clinician's understanding of the impact of culture when caring for these populations. The author of the chapter on mental health of college students discusses the complexities around TAY entering colleges and universities given their developmental stage. For health care providers caring for college-age populations, the interrelationship between culture and mental health is among the most dominant aspects of visits to counseling and student health centers.

Our patients are impacted by the micro and macro systems in which they live. These systems are covered in several chapters: "Social Determinants of Child and Adolescent Mental Health" (Chapter 10), "Adoption and Foster Care Systems" (Chapter 18), and "Microaggressions" (Chapter 19). Several chapters unpack the increasing impacts of the state of the world: "Aliens, Illegals, Deportees" (Chapter 11), "Clinical Strategies to Address the Mental Health of Forcibly Displaced Children" (Chapter 12), and "The Global State of Child and Adolescent Mental Health" (Chapter 13). Chapter 13 amplifies the concepts in Chapter 10 to the global scale. Two chapters, "Gender and Sexuality in the Twenty-First Century" (Chapter 7) and "Religion and Spirituality in Child and Adolescent Cultural Psychiatry" (Chapter 8), span both macro and micro levels.

TABLE 1–7.   Outline for Cultural Formulation

Category for assessment	Description
Cultural identity of the individual	Describe the individual's racial, ethnic, or cultural reference groups that may influence his or her relationships with others; access to resources; and developmental and current challenges, conflicts, or predicaments. For immigrants and racial or ethnic minorities, the degree and kinds of involvement with both the culture of origin and the host culture or majority culture should be noted separately. Language abilities, preferences, and patterns of use are relevant for identifying difficulties with access to care, social integration, and the need for an interpreter. Other clinically relevant aspects of identity may include religious affiliation, socioeconomic background, personal and family places of birth and growing up, migrant status, and sexual orientation.
Cultural conceptualizations of distress	Describe the cultural constructs that influence how the individual experiences, understands, and communicates his or her symptoms or problems to others. These may include cultural syndromes, idioms of distress, and explanatory models of perceived causes. The level of severity and meaning of the distressing experiences should be assessed in relation to the norms of the individual's cultural reference groups. Assessment of coping and help-seeking patterns should consider the use of professional as well as traditional, alternative, or complementary sources of care.
Psychosocial stressors and cultural features of vulnerability and resilience	Identify key stressors and supports in the individual's social environment (may include both local and distant events) and the role of religion, family, and other social networks (i.e., friends, neighbors, coworkers) in providing emotional, instrumental, and informational support. Social stressors and supports vary with cultural interpretations of events, family structure, developmental tasks, and social context. Levels of functioning, disability, and resilience should be assessed in light of the individual's cultural reference groups.
Cultural features of the relationship between the individual and the clinician	Identify differences in culture, language, and social status between an individual and clinician that may cause difficulties in communication and may influence diagnosis and treatment. Experiences of racism and discrimination in the larger society may impede establishing trust and safety in the clinical diagnostic encounter. Effects may include problems eliciting symptoms, misunderstanding of the cultural and clinical significance of symptoms and behaviors, and difficulty establishing or maintaining the rapport needed for an effective clinical alliance.

TABLE 1–7. Outline for Cultural Formulation *(continued)*

Category for assessment	Description
Overall cultural assessment	Summarize the implications of the components of the cultural formulation identified in earlier sections of the OCF for diagnosis and other clinically relevant issues or problems as well as appropriate management and treatment intervention.

Source. American Psychiatric Association: *Diagnostic and Statistical Manual of Mental Disorders*, 5th Edition. Arlington, VA, American Psychiatric Association, 2013. Copyright © 2013 American Psychiatric Association. Used with permission.

The authors of Chapter 13 report that one in five children and adolescents worldwide suffers from a mental health disorder. Furthermore, more than 50% of mental health disorders begin by age 14 and 75% by age 24 years, making the role of child and adolescent mental health professionals critical. Global mental health promotes health equity for the world's child and adolescent populations and provides possible models for services and advocacy for vulnerable U.S. youth populations.

This volume also covers community through a chapter on "Rural Psychiatry" (Chapter 16) and through chapters discussing social identities typically considered part of culture: racial and ethnic groups. Authors describe the heterogeneity as well as overarching principles within the most prevalent minority subgroups represented by the following chapters: "The Black Diaspora" (Chapter 2), "A Broad Overview of American Indian, Alaskan Native, and Native Hawaiian/Pacific Islander Cultures" (Chapter 3), "Mental Health in Asian American Populations" (Chapter 4), "Bridging the Gap in Psychiatric Care of Latinx Youth and Families" (Chapter 5), and "The Role of Culture, Stigma, and Bias on the Mental Health of Arab American Youth" (Chapter 6).

The increasing use of technology impacts not only our day-to-day lives but increasingly our culture and the provision of care itself. These concepts are broached in "Digital Media, Culture, and Child and Adolescent Mental Health" (Chapter 14) and "Culture of Technology" (Chapter 15). Children, adolescents, and families today are more likely to interact with technology and social media. However, this increased connectivity can have an immense, and not always positive, impact on the mental health of children, adolescents, and TAY. Increased connectivity and changes in technology have also expanded access to information around mental health, as well as how to access care. At the same time, global use of these devices and platforms has also led to new mental health challenges, innovative and at times even challenging interactions with communities (e.g., cyberbullying), and rapid cultural shifts related to ever-changing technology.

DSM-5 includes the OCF and the CFI, to be used by any clinician trying to deepen their understanding of the cultural aspects of the care of any patient. Both are reviewed through their application in conceptualizing complex clinical cases in Chapter 21, "DSM-5 Outline for Cultural Formulation and Cultural Formulation Interview." Although we focus on the OCF and CFI, there are multiple models for pulling cultural information together into a formulation for working with children and adolescents, including use of team-based cultural consultation service case discussion seminars (Rousseau and Guzder 2015; Sturm et al. 2017).

Given that this book is directed to mental health clinicians, we include information to discuss how to better advocate for children, adolescents, TAY, and families. Traditionally, mental health policy and regulatory issues have been a challenging quagmire for the engaged provider.

Therefore, we have included a chapter on "Advocacy" (Chapter 22) to help with these issues. Chapter 23 is a glossary explaining in more depth many of the terms used throughout this book.

Motor, language, cognitive, and social development appear to differ across cultures (Pumariega et al. 2013), as do expressions for psychological or emotional distress. As such, it is vital for mental health care professionals to understand the importance of developing a biopsychosocial or biopsychosociocultural formulation for care, as well as taking a nonjudgmental stance, coming from true clinical curiosity rather than fear.

The editors' goal is for readers to be able to think ethnographically while remaining patient centered when it comes to acknowledging and exploring each patient's culture so that patients and their family can teach providers about their own culture. We know that cultural traditions and histories inform parenting and the developmental tasks that our patients and families are traversing; we hope this book will help you contextualize culture from each of your patients and increase your understanding of cultural dynamics, intersectionality, and specific mental health needs of diverse youth populations.

It is of paramount importance that providers remain open-minded and take a nonjudgmental stance when discussing, educating others about, or learning about various aspects of culture. These topics are personal and unique and may not be completely applicable in every case. Intersectionality, a theoretical framework emphasizing the interconnected nature of social and political identities (e.g., race, ethnicity, class, gender and gender identity, sexuality) that creates overlapping and interdependent systems of discrimination or disadvantage, must also be considered. Individuality and unique experience must be queried and accounted for during interviews. Clinicians must remain open to listening to and learning from patients' experiences, understanding their own cultural identity (and possible biases), and reflecting on the impact of culture on the mental health needs of those for whom they are caring.

The coeditors and contributing authors appreciate that this compendious volume, although meant to be comprehensive, is not exhaustive. The attention to culturally informed mental health care in DSM has been leading the way for ongoing research and best evidence-based practices to follow suit. In parallel, rapidly evolving perceptions of culture and culturally informed attitudes in this era of social media continue to raise the important antennae of cultural curiosity. Hence, the coeditors strongly encourage readers to critically review chapters of this book as part of their lifelong journey toward cultural humility. This text should be used as only one important reference, which, coupled with lectures, grand rounds, articles, clinical supervision, and, above all, patient examination, will hopefully enhance the clinician's ability to provide effective and culturally sensitive care.

One final note: In order to preserve patient confidentiality, the names and identifying details have been changed in all clinical vignettes.

The Syndemic

Culture is dynamic. After the manuscript of this book was completed and submitted for publication, two major cultural phenomena occurred; the novel coronavirus SARS-CoV-2 (COVID-19) pandemic, affecting everyone worldwide, and a resurgence of the conversation around racial equality and structural racism in the United States. The COVID-19 pandemic not only has led to death, illness, and ongoing confusion about what the future holds but has also highlighted the importance of social determinants of health. For several months during 2020, thousands of people took to the streets to protest racial inequality and structural racism, leading to a resurgence of important conversations about race, inequality, the deep economic crisis, and provider burnout. These conversations have reverberated worldwide. All of the above can be summarized by the term *syndemic*, defined as "the synergistic nature of the health and social problems facing the poor and underserved" (Singer and Snipes 1992). Several authors now have included an addendum to their chapters to elaborate on these issues.

References

American Psychiatric Association: Diagnostic and Statistical Manual of Mental Disorders, 4th Edition. Washington, DC, American Psychiatric Association, 1994

American Psychiatric Association: Diagnostic and Statistical Manual of Mental Disorders, 5th Edition. Arlington, VA, American Psychiatric Association, 2013

Bauer A, Alegría M: Impact of patient language proficiency and interpreter service use on the quality of psychiatric care: a systematic review. Psychiatr Serv 61(8):765–773, 2010

Berry JW: Acculturative stress, in Readings in Ethnic Psychology. Edited by Organista PB, Chun KM, Marin G. New York, Routledge, 1998, pp 117–122

Betancourt JR: Cross-cultural medical education: conceptual approaches and frameworks for evaluation. Acad Med 78(6):560–569, 2003

Betancourt JR, Green AR, Carrillo JE, et al: Defining cultural competence: a practical framework for addressing racial/ethnic disparities in health and health care. Public Health Rep 118(4):293–302, 2003

Cross TL, Bazron BJ, Dennis KW, Isaacs MR: Towards a Culturally Competent System of Care: A Monograph on Effective Services for Minority Children Who Are Severely Emotionally Disturbed. Washington, DC, Georgetown University Child Development Center, 1989

Ecklund K, Johnson WB: Toward cultural competence in child intake assessments. Prof Psychol Res Pr 38(4):356–362, 2007

Encyclopædia Britannica: Psychological development. Chicago, IL, Britannica, March 14, 2019. Available at: www.britannica.com/science/psychological-development. Accessed April 12, 2020.

Eneriz-Wiemer M, Sanders LM, Barr DA, et al: Parental limited English proficiency and health outcomes for children with special health care needs: a systematic review. Acad Pediatr 14(2):128–136, 2014

Frey WH: Less than half of US children under 15 are white, census shows. Washington, DC, Brookings Institution, June 24, 2019. Available at: www.brookings.edu/research/less-than-half-of-us-children-under-15-are-white-census-shows. Accessed April 12, 2020.

Guerra NG, Williamson AA, Lucas-Molina B: Normal development: infancy, childhood and adolescence, in JM Rey's IACAPAP e-Textbook of Child and Adolescent Mental Health. Edited by Rey JM, Martin A. Geneva, Switzerland, International Association for Child and Adolescent Psychiatry and Allied Professions, 2019. Available at: https://iacapap.org/content/uploads/A.2.-DEVELOPMENT-072012.pdf. Accessed April 12, 2020.

Hook JN, Davis DE, Owen J, et al: Cultural humility: measuring openness to culturally diverse clients. J Counsel Psychol 60(3):353–366, 2013

Kakuma R, Minas H, van Ginneken N, et al: Human resources for mental health care: current situation and strategies for action. Lancet 378(9803):1654–1663, 2011

Kim SY, Schwartz SJ, Perreira KM, et al: Culture's influence on stressors, parental socialization, and developmental processes in the mental health of children of immigrants. Annu Rev Clin Psychol 14:343–370, 2018

Kirmayer LJ: Cultural variations in the clinical presentation of depression and anxiety: implications for diagnosis and treatment. J Clin Psychiatry 62(suppl 13):22–30, 2001

Kleinman A, Benson P: Anthropology in the clinic: the problem of cultural competency and how to fix it. PLoS Med 3(10):e294, 2006

Lewis-Fernandez R, Aggarwal NK, Kirmayer LJ: Cultural formulation before DSM-5, in Handbook on the Cultural Formulation Interview. Edited by Lewis-Fernández R, Aggarwal NK, Hinton L, et al. Arlington, VA, American Psychiatric Publishing, 2016, pp 1–26

Lim RF (ed): Clinical Manual of Cultural Psychiatry, 2nd Edition. Arlington, VA, American Psychiatric Publishing, 2015

Lo H-T, Fung KP: Culturally competent psychotherapy. Can J Psychiatry 48(3):161–170, 2003

Merriam-Webster: Microaggression. Springfield, MA, Merriam-Webster, 2020. Available at: www.merriam-webster.com/dictionary/microaggression. Accessed April 12, 2020.

Meyer IH: Minority stress and mental health in gay men. J Health Soc Behav 36:38–56, 1995

Meyer IH: Prejudice, social stress, and mental health in lesbian, gay and bisexual populations: conceptual issues and research evidence. Psychol Bull 129:674–697, 2003

Mikhaylov NS: Curiosity and its role in cross-cultural knowledge creation. Int J Emot Educ 8(1):95–108, 2016

Mirowsky J, Ross CE: Social causes of psychological distress. Hawthorne, NY, Aldine de Gruyter, 1989

National Association of the Deaf: Position statement supplement: culturally affirmative and linguistically accessible mental health services. Silver Spring, MD, National Association of the Deaf, 2008. Available at: www.nad.org/resources/health-care-and-mental-health-services/mental-health-services/culturally%20affirmative-and-linguistically%20accessible-services. Accessed April 12, 2020.

National Association of the Deaf: Position statement on mental health interpreting services with people who are deaf. Silver Spring, MD, National Association of the Deaf, 2020a. Available at: www.nad.org/about-us/position-statements/position-statement-on-mental-health-interpreting-services-with-people-who-are-deaf. Accessed April 12, 2020.

National Association of the Deaf: Video remote interpreting (VRI) in healthcare settings. Silver Spring, MD, National Association of the Deaf, 2020b. Available at: www.nad.org/uploaded-documents/advocacy-letter-healthcare-providers-VRI.pdf. Accessed April 12, 2020.

Pearlin LI: The stress process revisited: reflections on concepts and their interrelationships, in Handbook of the Sociology of Mental Health. Edited by Aneshensel CS, Phelan JC. New York, Kluwer Academic/Plenum, 1999, pp 395–415

National Partnership for Action to End Health Disparities: National Stakeholder Strategy for Achieving Health Equity. Rockville, MD, U.S. Department of Health and Human Services, Office of Minority Health, 2011

Pumariega AJ, Rothe E, Mian A, et al: Practice parameter for cultural competence in child and adolescent psychiatric practice. J Am Acad Child Adolesc Psychiatry 52(10):1101–1115, 2013

Qureshi A, Collazos F, Ramos M, et al: Cultural competency training in psychiatry. Eur Psychiatry 23:49–58, 2008

Rey JM, Assumpção FB, Bernad CA, et al: History of child psychiatry, in IACAPAP e-Textbook of Child and Adolescent Mental Health. Edited by Rey JM, Martin A. Geneva, Switzerland, International Association for Child and Adolescent Psychiatry and Allied Professions, 2015, pp 1–72

Rousseau C, Guzder J: Teaching cultural formulation. J Am Acad Child Adolesc Psychiatry 54(8):611–612, 2015

Singer M, Snipes C: Generations of suffering: experiences of a treatment program for substance abuse during pregnancy. J Health Care Poor Underserved 3(1):222–234, 1992

Singh NN, McKay JD, Singh AN: The need for cultural brokers in mental health services. J Child Fam Stud 8(1):1–10, 1999

Smedley BD, Stith AY, Nelson AR (eds): Unequal Treatment: Confronting Racial and Ethnic Disparities in Health Care. Institute of Medicine, Committee on Understanding and Eliminating Racial and Ethnic Disparities in Health Care. Washington, DC, National Academies Press, 2003

Sroufe LA: The concept of development in developmental psychopathology. Child Dev Perspect 3(3):178–183, 2009

Sturm G, Bonnet S, Coussot Y, et al: Cultural sensitive care provision in a public child and adolescent mental health centre: a case study from the Toulouse University Hospital Intercultural Consultation. Cult Med Psychiatry 41(4):630–655, 2017

Substance Abuse and Mental Health Services Administration: Improving Cultural Competence: Quick Guide for Clinicians. Publ SMA 16-4931. Rockville, MD, Center for Substance Abuse Treatment, 2016. Available at: https://store.samhsa.gov/product/Improving-Cultural-Competence/sma16-4931?referer=from_search_result. Accessed August 9, 2020.

Tervalon M, Murray-Garcia J: Cultural humility versus cultural competence: a critical distinction in defining physician training outcomes in multicultural education. J Health Care Poor Underserved 9(2):117–125, 1998

Ton H, Lim RF: Assessment of culturally diverse individuals: introduction and foundations, in Clinical Manual of Cultural Psychiatry, 2nd Edition. Edited by Lim RF. Washington, DC, American Psychiatric Publishing, 2015, pp 1–41

Trent M, Dooley DG, Dougé J: The impact of racism on child and adolescent health. Pediatrics 144(2):e20191765, 2019

U.S. Department of Health and Human Services: Mental Health: Culture, Race, and Ethnicity. A Supplement to Mental Health: A Report of the Surgeon General. Rockville, MD, Substance Abuse and Mental Health Services Administration, 2001. Available at: www.ncbi.nlm.nih.gov/books/NBK44243. Accessed April 12, 2020.

Westermeyer J: Developmental aspects of cultural psychiatry, in Textbook of Cultural Psychiatry. Edited by Bhugra D, Bhui K. New York, Cambridge University Press, 2018, pp 132–142

World Health Organization: Investing in mental health. Geneva, Switzerland, World Health Organization, 2003. Available at: https://apps.who.int/iris/bitstream/handle/10665/42823/9241562579.pdf. Accessed April 12, 2020.

World Health Organization: Social determinants of health. Geneva, Switzerland, World Health Organization, 2020. Available at: www.who.int/social_determinants/sdh_definition/en. Accessed April 11, 2020.

PART I
Race and Ethnicity

CHAPTER 2

The Black Diaspora

Cultural Psychiatry Perspectives on African American Children and Adolescents and Their Families

Lisa M. Cullins, M.D.
Jessica Moore, M.D.

CULTURAL psychiatry is the study and treatment of mental illness in individuals guided by thoughtful consideration and integration of race, ethnicity, religion, and cultural backgrounds (Caracci and Mezzich 2001). At its core, cultural psychiatry seeks to improve the efficacy of clinical services—diagnosis, care, and treatment—for people of diverse backgrounds. The Black Diaspora, by definition, is the dispersion of people of African descent, language, and culture from their country of origin to various parts of the world. However, fondly and endearingly, its connotation is a celebration of the richness and complexities of people of African descent and their culture. Each African American family has their own unique story: traditions, belief systems, and roots that extend far across the globe, shaping and forming their experiences and perspectives. In this chapter, we examine how these multigenerational experiences and perspectives interface and are intricately involved in clinical diagnosis and treatment, health-seeking behaviors, risk and protective factors, and overall mental health and well-being of African American children and adolescents and their families.

Mental illness has no boundaries and pervades all socioeconomic classes, races, and ethnicities. Although African Americans make up only 13% of the U.S. population or 38.9 million (2 million identify as Black Caribbean and 3.1 million as multiracial or multiethnic), studies have shown that African American and Black Caribbean populations have a higher prevalence of chronicity and disability associated with psychiatric disorders (Rastogi et al. 2011; Shim et al. 2009). In the National Survey of American Life, African American and Black Caribbean individuals were more likely than white individuals to have chronic major depressive disorder and with greater severity and disability (Shim et al. 2009).

Ascertaining accurate prevalence rates of psychiatric disorders can be challenging in Black populations, particularly children and adolescents, for a variety of reasons. African Americans are disproportionately represented in populations that may be missed or excluded in prevalence studies (youth who are homeless or in foster care and/or the juvenile justice systems), and consequently, rates of mental illness may be underestimated. Stigma may also prevent African Americans from disclosing mental health symptoms (Pumariega et al. 2013). Further, historical racism and human subject violations, such as the Tuskegee syphilis experiment, have left African Americans wary of participation in research across disciplines (Park 2017). Thus, there are variances in prevalence rates of psychiatric disorders in the research literature—revealing that African American youth have higher, lower, or similar rates of psychiatric symptoms compared with their white counterparts (Kann et al. 2018; U.S. Department of Health and Human Services 2001).

Risk Factors

Despite discrepancies in prevalence of psychiatric disorders, what is clear is that African American youth can be significantly impaired by psychiatric symptomatology. This is evidenced by the increasing suicide rate among African American youth (Goldston et al. 2008; U.S. Department of Health and Human Services 2001). Data from the 2017 Youth Risk Behaviors Study indicate that African American students have higher rates of suicide attempts (9.8%) compared with white students (6.1%) (Kann et al. 2018). The reasons for this increased suicide rate are multifactorial. Reports of racism and discrimination have been linked with higher suicide rates mediated by increased depression, hopelessness, and substance abuse (Goldston et al. 2008). Disparities in educational attainment, economic advancement, and social progress have also been considered vulnerabilities that may place African Americans at risk for suicide (Balis and Postolache 2008).

Numerous factors may disrupt and fracture the mental health and well-being of youth and families from the Black Diaspora. Familial instability; poverty; and employment, housing, and food insecurities are contributing risk factors for psychiatric illness. Other risk factors include compounded community trauma (i.e., witnessing violence both at home and in the community), polyvictimization, neighborhood social disorganization, repeated experiences of discrimination, and chronic exposure to racism (Matlin et al. 2011). Unfortunately, African American families are disproportionately affected by these identifiable risk factors and social determinants of health. For African Americans, the unemployment rate is 6.5% compared with 3.9% in the general population (U.S. Bureau of Labor Statistics 2018). U.S. Census data from the most recent American Community Survey (U.S. Census Bureau 2017) indicate that the poverty rate is 23.0% for African Americans compared with 13.4% for the general population. The poverty rate for African

Americans younger than age 18 is 32.8% as compared with the national rate of 18%, and African American families with children constitute 50.5% of the homeless population (U.S. Census Bureau 2017; U.S. Department of Housing and Urban Development 2018). Additionally, African American youth are disproportionately represented in populations that have high mental health needs, comprising 50%–70% of the juvenile justice system and 45%–50% of the foster care system (Alegria et al. 2011; U.S. Department of Health and Human Services 2001). In sum, African American families face educational, financial, and housing fragilities, challenges in accessing care, and other social disparities that put them at risk for increased mental health needs.

Protective Factors

Equal to the magnitude of risk factors stacked against African American and Black Caribbean children and families are their strengths and protective factors. Community connectedness is an important protective factor. Ethnic enclaves may provide mental health benefits by enhancing residents' collective identity and reducing exposure to discrimination (Matlin et al. 2011). These benefits may mitigate some of the socioeconomic disadvantages that typically characterize racially segregated communities and may facilitate psychosocial adjustment (Matlin et al. 2011). Links to church, close interpersonal relationships, and family cohesion have been found to be protective factors for African American youth. The word *church* is used broadly here to reflect and embrace the heterogeneity of religion and spirituality in the Black Diaspora. Research has suggested that religion and spirituality have a positive impact as a protective factor for suicide in particular because involvement in the church may encourage social connection, boost self-esteem, and provide meaning to one's life (Balis and Postolache 2008). Similar to the posited benefits of social and community supports, positive early teacher interactions have been found to enhance resilience and adaptability and build self-esteem, leading to the preservation of mental health and well-being even amid psychosocial stressors.

Acculturation

Notably, for Black Caribbean families, immigration and the acculturation process play a significant role in both their risk and protective factors. Although few data exist for the Black Caribbean population, immigration and acculturative stress have been well studied and may have adverse psychological impacts (Easter 2018; Guy 2001; Rothe et al. 2011a, 2011b). Less is known about protective factors. It is posited, however, that family connectedness may bolster resilience, and high levels of ethnic identification may protect individuals from negative outcomes such as depression in youth of Caribbean origin who were born in the United States (Rothe et al. 2011a; Tummala-Narra and Claudius 2013).

Disparities in Mental Health Care

Once signs and symptoms of a psychiatric disorder have been identified, African American youth and families succumb to significant health disparities at multiple stages—diagnostic, treatment and level of care, and basic access and quality of care—which leads to unmet mental health needs and poor outcomes. Clinically, it has been shown that African Americans are more likely to be diagnosed with a psychotic disorder than a mood disorder as compared with their white counterparts with similar symptom compilation (Alegria et al. 2011; Bell et al. 2015a, 2015b; Muroff et al. 2008). Once it has been determined that the child or adolescent may benefit from treatment, African American youth are more likely to be placed in settings that are more restrictive than community outpatient settings (Alegria et al. 2011; Assari and Caldwell 2017).

It has also been shown that African American youth and families confront numerous obstacles to acquiring care. They are more likely to be uninsured, and even when insurance barriers are resolved, underutilization of mental health service for African Americans continues after socioeconomic factors, psychiatric diagnosis, and actual need are all accounted for (Assari and Caldwell 2017). Last, it has been shown that African American youth and families receive suboptimal care. African Americans are less likely to receive standard treatments of care that are culturally sensitive, including psychotherapy and psychological counseling. They are also less likely to receive specialized mental health care (Jones et al. 2018; Merikangas et al. 2011; U.S. Department of Health and Human Services 2001). In particular, African Americans hailing from rural areas are less likely than their white rural counterparts to receive mental health services for mood disorders, an effect not demonstrated in urban youth (Merikangas et al. 2011). This may be mediated by stigma (see section "Stigma") and limited access to quality affordable services (Murry et al. 2011).

Compounding these health care inequities is the disproportion of underrepresented minority medical providers. Of note, African American physicians are more likely than white physicians to treat African American patients (Komaromy et al. 1996). Further, African American patients are more likely to seek care and experience a higher level of confidence and trust in their care with an African American provider (Laveist and Nuru-Jeter 2002). However, the number of underrepresented minority medical providers is astonishingly low. Currently, only 6% of medical school graduates are African American; 4.2% of psychiatrists are African American, and 2% of psychologists and 4% of social workers identify as African American (Association of American Medical Colleges 2016; U.S. Department of Health and Human Services 2001). Thus, cultural psychiatry must be approached at both the patient and the provider level.

Culture and history play an important role in the understanding and belief systems of African American and Black Caribbean youth in regard to recognizing mental illness and health-seeking behaviors. Cultural mistrust (the tendency to distrust white individuals and the majority group culture in the United States due to direct and vicarious exposure to racism) and perceived discrimination (the belief that one is being treated poorly and/or unfairly on the basis of race, ethnicity, gender, age, religion, physical appearance, sexual orientation, or other characteristics) are two sociocultural factors that impact health-seeking behaviors. Cultural mistrust can function as an adaptive mechanism by which Blacks can defend against discriminatory treatment and oppression (Dean et al. 2018). However, both cultural mistrust and perceived discrimination may have associated negative health behaviors: less trust in health care providers, early termination of treatment, delays in treatment, and poor adherence to health care (Dean et al. 2018). Further, greater perceived discrimination is related to greater anxiety and depression, more psychological distress, and less general well-being (Dean et al. 2018).

Stigma

Mental illness continues to be highly stigmatized worldwide, transcending all cultures. Mental illness may be a source of shame if it is perceived as a sign of personal weakness or shortcoming, which may ultimately discourage individuals from seeking professional help (Bailey et al. 2009, 2014). African American families attribute delay of treatment to fear that their child will be "labeled" by a diagnosis or that the diagnosis may affect the child's ability to secure employment or military assignment (Bailey et al. 2014). Thus, stigma in the African American community has been coupled with both shame and a sense of failure and fear of educational and economic disadvantage. The shame and sense of failure are complicated by both spiritual (unwavering faith) and cultural or racial (strength and resilience as a people) underpinnings and expectations.

Facilitating Treatment

When clinicians have the privilege to engage this population of youth and families, they must seize the moment because African Americans' path to treatment, as mentioned earlier, is typically riddled with many obstacles and much discouragement and disappointment. Examples of statements and questions clinicians can use to establish rapport with patients are found in Table 2–1. Key aspects of the therapeutic relationship include the following:

1. *Clinician self-awareness:* Be aware of your own biases and avoid imparting personal judgments during conversations with patients and families.
2. *Doctor-patient relationship:* A strong therapeutic rapport can be made only through a culturally sensitive lens (Barner et al. 2011). Clinicians must disarm themselves and learn from their patients. Having a clear conceptualization of the patient's belief systems and perception and understanding of illness is paramount in both establishing rapport and developing an appropriate treatment plan. Clinicians, in parallel, must also have a clear grasp of their own cultural beliefs, attitudes, and perceptions, which may vary greatly from those of their patients.
3. *Meeting the child and family where they are:* Understand the child and family's strengths and build on them. In this process, identify natural supports for the families, which may include extended family members, faith-based and community resources, encouraging teachers, mentors, and coaches. The clinician should view and include these natural supports collaboratively as part of the clinical team; because these individuals know the child and family well and promote community connectedness, they are a protective factor.
4. *Improve parent-child communication:* Help caregivers choose words to express their sentiment that their child or adolescent can comprehend and process given his or her developmental stage; help navigate with the caregiver the appropriate timing to engage in these types of conversations with the child; and, if the caregiver so chooses, facilitate the conversation in a supportive therapeutic environment.
5. *Service delivery models in natural settings:* Clinicians should make use of integrated mental health and collaborative care models. In addition to identifying and working collaboratively

with natural supports to enhance the mental health and well-being of African American youth and their families, service delivery models should be considered and developed in natural settings (e.g., school health programs, pediatric medical homes) with multilingual, multicultural staff or providers. These types of culturally sensitive service delivery models in natural settings help mitigate common systemic barriers. For instance, providing clinical services in natural settings may enhance trust at institutional and provider levels and even decrease stigma because the natural setting is a familiar place typically connected to the community. Families may simply feel more comfortable in these natural settings. Often, service delivery models in natural settings offer more flexible clinic hours and/or may simply be more convenient and easier to access for families with more restrictive work hours and limited modes of transportation.

Clinical Vignette

Timothy is a 16-year-old African American male. For most of his educational history, he has been an honor roll student, well liked by his peers and teachers. Over the summer between eighth and ninth grade, he moved with his parents and sisters into a new neighborhood following his mother's job promotion. Timothy and his family had been living with his grandmother and aunt for most of his life. Although Timothy would miss his grandmother, he and his family were excited about this new opportunity and having their own home. A few weeks prior to the start of school, Timothy began stating that he was dreading going back to school. He was a little more withdrawn, preferring to stay at home when his family went out somewhere, and seemed to be more defensive, easily frustrated, and irritable. Nonetheless, Timothy started his new school without any difficulty.

Timothy did quite well his first year in high school. He tried out for the football team and had a winning season. Academically, he maintained his grades, getting mostly As with a few Bs. He did what he was supposed to do at home, helping out when needed, and was compliant with rules and chores. After he completed the tasks that were asked of him, he preferred to spend a lot of time in his room by himself. It was not until the start of Timothy's tenth-grade year that his mother began to have some concerns. Despite a successful first year on the football team, he decided not to participate on the football team in tenth grade. His fall semester grades dropped to As, Bs, and a few Cs. When Timothy's mother asked if everything was all right, Timothy said he was "fine." He said that he just didn't want to do football this year and that he got the Cs because he had "just messed up on the test" and would be able to bring up the grades. Timothy's mother was still concerned but felt that, overall, he was doing OK and that she would just "watch and see."

Timothy began to show early signs of depression after he moved from his community of origin. Previously a vibrant, engaging young man, eager to learn, he become more withdrawn, isolative, easily frustrated, and irritable. Although he was still compliant with home rules, completing his chores, getting up on time, going to school, and doing his work, he felt anxious and dreaded going back to school. He was experiencing sleepless nights and decreased appetite, and it was becoming exceedingly difficult for him to stay focused in school or to work efficiently. He felt as if he were either "doing something bad" or "incapable of doing something great."

Timothy kept all of this to himself because he did not want to disappoint his family, especially given that it appeared that they were all doing just fine and adjusting well to the move. His sisters were making new friends. His parents were happy that they had a place they could call their own. Timothy, however, missed his old house, his grandmother, and his friends. He missed going outside and hanging out until the lights came on. In his new neighborhood, he was one of the few Black males. Although most people were nice to him, he felt out of place. One night, when Timothy was walking home in the evening from the recreation center, a police car pulled up next to him, and the officer asked if he was lost. He experienced many more similar incidents, even at school. He just kept these incidents and feelings packed inside himself, never sharing them with

TABLE 2–1. Establishing rapport and engaging families

Clinician role	Examples of statements and open-ended questions
Provide structure and framework for treatment during the initial evaluation	"My main job is to listen and learn from you so I can figure out what would be most helpful for you and your family."
Elicit information about past psychiatric history and contact with the health care and/or mental health care system	"Please tell me what your experience has been like thus far with getting help for your child."
Listen attentively and acknowledge and validate the patient and family's experiences, good or bad	"It seems that you have encountered many roadblocks and obstacles along the way. It definitely seems like it has not been easy, and I am so sorry you experienced that. But I applaud you for your perseverance and am happy that I have the opportunity to meet with you today."
Wrap up the initial evaluation and clinic visit and succinctly address the child and family's needs	"I know we have discussed a lot today. Was there anything else that you need help with? How can I be helpful?"
Meet initially with caregivers alone and support them in having a difficult conversation with their child or adolescent (e.g., pertaining to the child's safety and well-being, racism and discrimination, police brutality, community violence)	"What do you want your child to know about [issue]? Share with me why you think it is important. What are some of your concerns? Is there anything you are worried about in discussing this with your child? Tell me why you think it may be the right time to discuss it, or when would be the right time to have this conversation."
Listen attentively and acknowledge and validate the caregiver's belief that this topic area is important	"From what you have shared, I understand why this is important to you."
If there are aspects of a topic area that the clinician would like the caregiver to reconsider, explain further or explore in more depth	"I'm wondering if…." "What do you think about…?" "I'm wondering what you mean by…." "Is it is possible that…?"

his parents because he did not want to worry them. He intellectualized these occurrences, thoughts, and feelings as "this is just the way things are, and I just have to deal with it."

As time went on, Timothy's symptoms worsened. It was unclear whether protective factors had been dampened, the progression of his illness intensified, or a combination of both. One main protective factor, community connectedness, was essentially absent, and this absence may have been the primary culprit for his deterioration. Fortunately, Timothy's parents became concerned that their son was in fact suffering from depression. Their primary care provider confirmed and supported their sentiments and referred them to her child psychiatrist colleague who was integrated into her pediatric clinic. The psychiatrist recommended a combination treatment including both therapy and antidepressant medication.

Timothy found therapy to be a safe place where he could talk about everything without being judged. He shared his experiences of discrimination and racism in his new community and school and his feelings of being isolated and missing the people and social organization of his previous neighborhood. He missed his old teachers who always encouraged him. He missed his elderly neighbors shouting out to him as he walked to school to do well so he could be somebody one day. He talked about his peers and the difficulty he was having with navigating interpersonal relationships. Therapy was a time to rebuild his confidence, self-esteem, and self-worth that had eroded after the move. This process took some time because Timothy was still experiencing negative messages in his environment, but he began to feel better slowly. As his anhedonia dissipated, his grades improved, and he began to reengage in extracurricular activities.

Conclusion

Children, adolescents, and their families of the Black Diaspora have profuse cultural origins and complex identities that influence and shape health-seeking behaviors. Mental illness is abundant and present in all peoples, races, ethnicities, and cultures. When overlooked or left untreated, mental illness can threaten life trajectories of children and adolescents. With ongoing advancements in psychiatry, effective treatments are available. However, for African American youth and families in particular, significant impediments persist that continue to obstruct appropriate access and quality of care. Culturally sensitive, collaborative, and integrated service delivery models may have some promise in recalibrating the inequities of access and quality of care for this special population of youth and families.

Clinical Pearls

- Youth and families of the Black Diaspora have vast histories that shape their multigenerational experiences and perspectives, but each family has its own journey and its own unique story. Every patient encounter should be an opportunity for the clinician to hear the voices of the children, adolescents, and families they have the privilege to serve and to validate and learn from the stories they share (see Table 2–1).

- When possible, extend the multidisciplinary and collaborative clinical team to encourage teachers, faith-based and community supports, mentors, coaches, and primary care providers who know the child and family well to further enhance community connectedness with natural supports.

- Always meet the child and family where they are. Identify their understanding of illness and the meaning of the illness for the family system, as well as their treatment readiness, recognizing and building on their strengths.

Self-Assessment Questions

1. What factor mediates risk of suicide in African Americans?

    A. Depression.
    B. Hopelessness.
    C. Substance abuse.
    D. All of the above.

2. Identify a strength unique to the Black community that may serve as a protective factor for their mental health and well-being.

    A. Community connectedness.
    B. Music.
    C. Herbal remedies.
    D. None of the above.

3. What barrier might African American youth and families confront that contributes to lower utilization of mental health services?

    A. Stigma.
    B. Lack of insurance.
    C. Cultural mistrust.
    D. All of the above.

4. What specific questions will you add to your usual base of interview questions to include content from this chapter?

5. How might you adjust your current rubric for patient conceptualization to include these concepts?

6. As you reflect, how does the information in this chapter inform your future practice?

Answers

1. D
2. A
3. D

References

Alegria M, Vallas M, Pumariega A: Racial and ethnic disparities in pediatric mental health. Child Adolesc Psychiatr Clin N Am 19(4):759–774, 2011

Assari S, Caldwell CH: Mental health service utilization among Black youth: psychosocial determinants in a national sample. Children (Basel) 4(5):#40, 2017

Association of American Medical Colleges: Diversity in Medical Education: Facts and Figures 2016. Washington, DC, Association of American Medical Colleges, 2016. Available at: http://www.aamc diversityfactsandfigures2016.org/report-section/section-1. Accessed April 12, 2020.

Bailey R, Blackmon H, Stevens S: Major depressive disorder in the African American population: meeting the challenges of stigma, misdiagnosis, and treatment disparities. J Natl Med Assoc 101(1):1084–1089, 2009

Bailey RK, Jaquez-Gutierrez MC, Madhoo M: Sociocultural issues in African American and Hispanic minorities seeking care for attention-deficit/hyperactivity disorder. Prim Care Companion CNS Disord 16(4), 2014

Balis T, Postolache T: Ethnic differences in adolescent suicide in the United States. Int J Child Health Hum Dev 1(3):281–296, 2008

Barner JC, Bohman TM, Brown CM, et al: Use of complementary and alternative medicine (CAM) for treatment among African-Americans: a multivariate analysis. Res Social Adm Pharm 6(3):196–208, 2011

Bell CC, Jackson A, Bell B: Misdiagnosis of African-Americans with psychiatric issues, part I. J Natl Med Assoc 107:25–34, 2015a

Bell CC, Jackson A, Bell B: Misdiagnosis of African-Americans with psychiatric issues, part II. J Natl Med Assoc 107:35–41, 2015b

Caracci G, Mezzich JE: Culture and urban mental health. Psychiatr Clin North Am 24(3):581–593, 2001

Dean KE, Long AC, Matthews RA, et al: Willingness to seek treatment among Black students with anxiety or depression: the synergistic effect of sociocultural factors with symptom severity and intolerance of uncertainty. Behav Ther 49(5):691–701, 2018

Easter M: For Black immigrants here illegally, a battle against both fear and historic discrimination. Los Angeles Times, January 8, 2018. Available at: www.latimes.com/local/lanow/la-me-black-undocumented-20171010-story.html. Accessed April 12, 2020.

Goldston DB, Molock SD, Whitbeck LB, et al: Cultural considerations in adolescent suicide prevention and psychosocial treatment. Am Psychol 63:14–31, 2008

Guy TC: Black immigrants of the Caribbean: an invisible and forgotten community. Adult Learning 13(1):18–21, 2001

Jones AL, Cochran SD, Leibowitz A, et al: Racial, ethnic, and nativity differences in mental health visits to primary care and specialty mental health providers: analysis of the Medical Expenditures Panel Survey, 2011–2015. Healthcare (Basel) 6(2):E29, 2018

Kann L, McManus T, Harris WA, et al: Youth Risk Behavior Surveillance—United States, 2017. MMWR Surveill Summ 67(8):1–114, 2018

Komaromy M, Grumbach K, Drake M, et al: The role of Black and Hispanic physicians in providing health care for underserved populations. N Engl J Med 334(20):1305–1310, 1996

Laveist TA, Nuru-Jeter A: Is doctor-patient race concordance associated with greater satisfaction with care? J Health Soc Behav 43(3):296–306, 2002

Matlin S, Molock SD, Tebes JK: Suicidality and depression among African American adolescents: the role of family and peer support and community connectedness. Am J Orthopsychiatry 81(1):108–117, 2011

Merikangas KR, He JP, Burstein M, et al: Service utilization for lifetime mental disorders in U.S. adolescents: results of the National Comorbidity Survey—Adolescent Supplement (NCS-A). J Am Acad Child Adolesc Psychiatry 50(1):32–45, 2011

Muroff J, Edelsohn GA, Joe S, Ford BC: The role of race in diagnostic and disposition decision-making in a pediatric psychiatric emergency service (PES). Gen Hosp Psychiatry 30(3):269–276, 2008

Murry VM, Heflinger CA, Suiter SV, et al: Examining perceptions about mental health care and help-seeking among rural African American families of adolescents. J Youth Adolesc 40(9):1118–1131, 2011

Park J: Historical origins of the Tuskegee experiment: the dilemma of public health in the United States. Uisahak 26(3):545–578, 2017

Pumariega AJ, Rothe E, Mian A, et al; American Academy of Child and Adolescent Psychiatry (AACAP) Committee on Quality Issues (CQI): Practice parameter for cultural competence in child and adolescent psychiatry. J Am Acad Child Adolesc Psychiatry 52(10):1101–1115, 2013

Rastogi S, Johnson T, Hoeffel E, et al: The Black population: 2010. 2010 Census Briefs, September 2011. Available at: www.census.gov/prod/cen2010/briefs/c2010br-06.pdf. Accessed August 9, 2020.

Rothe EM, Pumariega AJ, Sabagh D: Identity and acculturation in immigrant and second generation adolescents. Adolesc Psychiatry 1(1):72–81, 2011a

Rothe EM, Tzuang D, Pumariega AJ: Acculturation, development, and adaptation. Child Adolesc Psychiatr Clin N Am 19:681–696, 2011b

Shim RS, Compton MT, Rust G, et al: Race ethnicity as a predictor of attitudes toward mental health treatment seeking. Psychiatr Serv 60(10):1336–1341, 2009

Tummala-Narra P, Claudius M: Perceived discrimination and depressive symptoms among immigrant-origin adolescents. Cultur Divers Ethnic Minor Psychol 19(3):257–269, 2013

U.S. Bureau of Labor Statistics: Labor force characteristics by race and ethnicity, 2017. Rep 1076. Washington, DC, U.S. Bureau of Labor Statistics, August 2018. Available at: www.bls.gov/opub/reports/race-and-ethnicity/2017/pdf/home.pdf. Accessed April 12, 2020.

U.S. Census Bureau: American Community Survey 2017 ACS 1-year estimates selected population profiles, Table S0201. Suitland, MD, U.S. Census Bureau, 2017. Available at: www.census.gov/acs/www/data/data-tables-and-tools/data-profiles/2017. Accessed August 9, 2020.

U.S. Department of Health and Human Services: Mental Health: Culture, Race, and Ethnicity. A Supplement to Mental Health: A Report of the Surgeon General. Rockville, MD, Substance Abuse and Mental Health Services Administration, 2001. Available at: www.ncbi.nlm.nih.gov/books/NBK44243. Accessed April 12, 2020.

U.S. Department of Housing and Urban Development: The 2018 Annual Homeless Assessment Report (AHAR) to Congress: Part 1: Point-in-Time Estimates of Homelessness. Washington, DC, Office of Community Planning and Development, 2018

CHAPTER 3

A Broad Overview of American Indian, Alaskan Native, and Native Hawaiian/Pacific Islander Cultures

Rebecca Susan Daily, M.D., DFAPA, DFAACAP
Richard Livingston, M.D., DFAACAP
Delores S. Bigfoot, Ph.D.
R. Dakota Carter, M.D., Ed.D.
Stefanie Gillson, M.D.
Joseph T. Bell, M.D.
Joy K.L. Andrade, M.D.
Shaylin P.Y.K. Chock, M.D.

Rebecca Susan Daily, family members: Cherokee, Chickasaw, Kiowa; Richard Livingston, Cherokee; Delores S. Bigfoot, Caddo; Joy K.L. Andrade, Native Hawaiian; Shaylin P.Y.K. Chock, Native Hawaiian; Joseph T. Bell, Lumbee; Stefanie Gillson, Dakota; R. Dakota Carter, Cherokee.

AMERICAN Indian, Alaskan Native, Native Hawaiian, and Pacific Islander (AI/AN/NH/PI) individuals comprise a complex multicultural society with layers within the culture of the United States. Historically, thousands of individual nations in the Americas were decimated, relocated, divided, merged, impoverished, traumatized, and "reeducated" over the past 530 years. The precontact population, estimated between 54 and 100 million, dropped to about 237,000 in North America in 1900, then rose to more than 5.5 million identifying as at least half AI/AN/NH/PI in 2018 (Pumariega and Sharma 2018). There are at least four broad social layers within AI/AN/NH/PI culture: 1) individuals raised on or near tribal/nation lands with strong traditional ties, 2) those who frequently visit tribal/nation lands or participate in tribal traditional activities, 3) those who have rarely participated in activities, and 4) those who have no participation but still strongly identify as AI/AN/NH/PI (Figures 3–1 and 3–2).

Within these layers are youth searching for their identity and belief system as they move through developmental stages while their parents negotiate personal issues involving historical and personal trauma, deciding to stay in, leave, or return to the homeland and whether to keep or leave traditions (Pumariega and Sharma 2018). All of this must be considered and understood by anyone offering care to AI/AN/NH/PI individuals. In this chapter, we offer a basic understanding of the initial approach to AI/AN/NH/PI families and provide guidelines for body language, appropriate queries and interactions, appreciation of differences between tribal identities and belief systems, appreciation for the role of historical trauma in today's Native populations, and approaches to concepts of healing among Native peoples. Because of unique differences between these Native populations, these issues are addressed via sections for each population. Although no chapter could be encompassing of each nuance between subgroups, tribes, and individuals, we hope to explore themes to help develop cultural competency for the psychiatric provider.

Identity Development and Crises: The American Indian

Research and understanding of the developmental processes of the American Indian are limited and poorly understood. Developmentalist Erik Erikson was one of few theorists who studied American Indian children. In 1945, he compared and contrasted children from Lakota and Yurok tribes, noting in both "rapidly disintegrating systems of child training," specifically noting the conflict between the development of Native identity within that of American white culture (Erikson 1945). This kind of cultural fragmentation likely impacts the development of identity that is captured via Joseph Bruchac's illustration of his Abenaki grandfather denying his Native identity: "I got in a fight with a boy who called me Indian" (Bruchac 1993).

Newman (2005) used some of Erikson's principles and an elaborated classification to study identity formation in 96 Lumbee teen-parent dyads. He identified three particularly relevant developmental phases for nonwhite adolescent development: a *self-protective* period, which is marked by awareness of ethnicity without much reflection or exploration; *conformist* status, which reflects an actively positive self-regard as to ethnicity, based on some exploration; and a *cooperative/post-conformist* period, which suggests more agency and social competence and a firmer sense of identity, although not necessarily without distress or conflict. These levels are

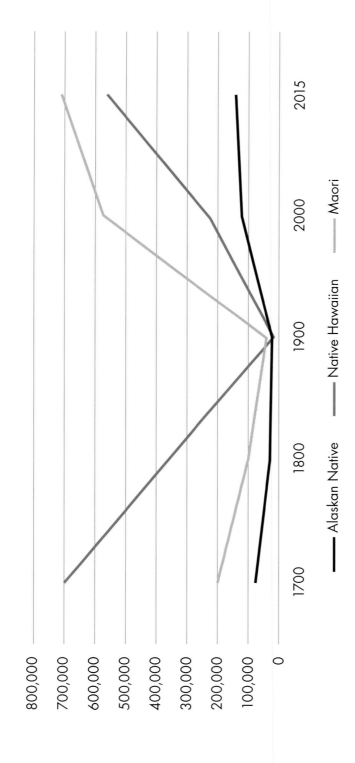

FIGURE 3–1.   Estimated Alaskan Native, Native Hawaiian, and Maori (any blood percentage) population changes, 1700–2015.

Source.   National Congress of American Indians 2020; Thornton 1987; U.S. Census Bureau 2010.

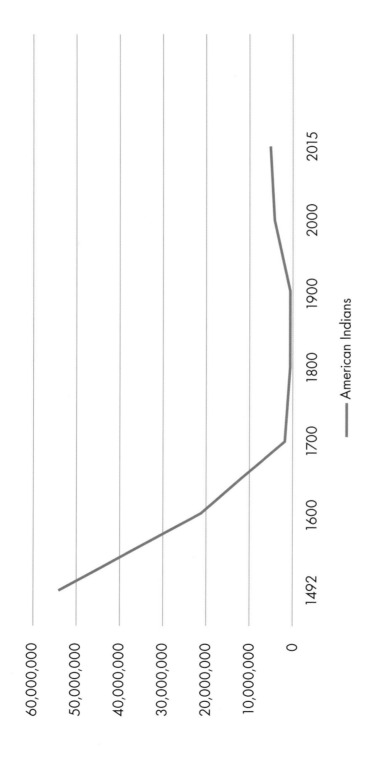

FIGURE 3–2.   **Estimated population of American Indians (any blood percentage), 1492–2015.**

Source.   National Congress of American Indians 2020; Thornton 1987; U.S. Census Bureau 2010.

TABLE 3–1. Erickson levels and Native identity development

Level	Description of identity development
Self-protective (E-3)	Aware of ethnicity but neither very involved nor very reflective about it
Conformist (E-4)	Positive about ethnicity; has harmonious relationships within ethnic group
Post-conformist (E-4)	Has more knowledge, comprehension, and sense of agency as to ethnicity but may experience related distress

Source. Adapted from Newman DL: "Ego development and ethnic identity formation in rural American Indian adolescents." *Child Development* 76(3):734–746, 2005.

presumed to be sequential, and each is labeled with the letter E and a number based on its corresponding Erickson level (Table 3–1). Younger American Indian youth correspond to the E-3 level, self-protective, with many teens emerging into E-4 conformist and cooperative modes as they achieve a degree of pride in their Indian identities, even in youth with mixed white and Native cultural heritage (Newman 2005).

Other researchers have looked more explicitly at the influences on the developmental process when youth have identities in competing cultures. Phinney (1993, 2003) found that youth whose ethnic identity remains unexamined accept the values and mores of the majority (predominantly white) culture. Cultural fragmentation may also involve two minority cultures, as noted among the Garifuna, whose origins are Arawak and Black Caribbean (Guity 2018). Competing cultures can lead some individuals to experience a crisis of identity, often producing rage reactions. A psychiatric provider may need to help American Indian youth navigate cultural fragmentation, or at least recognize its influence on the mental health of this population. Resolution of the crisis phase frequently produces a commitment to the youth's own unique culture.

American Indian and Alaskan Native Youth: Demographic and Mental Health Outcomes

In the summer of 2016, a group of Native youth on Standing Rock Indian Reservation in North Dakota began a movement originating from the desire to protect water and Indigenous rights. As of 2020, this effort is ongoing, and the resulting reactions have produced serious physical and psychological harm. Over many months of encampment by Native opposition to the Dakota Access Pipeline, forceful responses from the state of North Dakota, the federal government, local law enforcement officers, and hired security resulted in many physical confrontations that overwhelmed any attempts at equality, negotiation, and resolution.

Initially started by a small group of American Indians (AIs), this opposition grew to several camps numbering in the tens of thousands that included activists and sympathetic arrivals from around the world to protest the exploitation of Indigenous people and to protect their access to sacred lands and natural resources. This exploitation has been an ongoing method of colonization since European explorers began their initial contact with the so-called New World.

The psychological toil ensuing from these events is illustrated by videos and news accounts describing aggressive encounters and dismissal of the welfare of the Water Protectors (Pember 2016). Narratives like this one illustrate the importance of mental health providers in understanding the impact of traumatic events in the context of historical trauma that lead to common psychiatric findings and current economic and social conditions within AI and Alaskan Native (AN) populations.

Clinical Vignette: Kiowa, Caught-Between

Jay is an intelligent third-grade 8-year-old Kiowa who was referred to the hospital after three fights in one school week, the last one including death threats. His single mom died in a car crash, and he went to stay with his maternal grandparents, but they became too ill to supervise him. He remained, however, in their care. Two acute hospital stays seemingly made no difference, and Jay was admitted for residential care. The fight that preceded admission happened after a white classmate joked about "your mama" to him. Jay fought relentlessly despite being smaller and made several threats while pounding the other boy; two strong men were required to contain him.

Jay demonstrated no interest in completing schoolwork or in interacting with peers. During therapy sessions, he fought back tears often, sometimes after no apparent trigger. Hospital staff repeatedly described him as sad and irritable. After weeks of residential treatment, he began to show a little warmth toward Dr. Raskin, his young white male child psychiatrist, and toward a middle-age Choctaw woman who worked on the unit, calling her "Auntie." He cooperated with fluoxetine treatment. Unfortunately, during month three of treatment, Dr. Raskin killed himself, and Jay's violence bubbled up continuously again for several days. He would not cooperate with medications and usually ate only once a day.

As all this transpired, agencies from two states fought for jurisdiction over Jay's placement. Soon, two county courts, one each in Oklahoma and Arkansas, were attempting to send court orders with conflicting directions. An Arkansas attorney ad litem became involved and invoked the Kiowa nation as possibly having jurisdiction. There were no couples or individuals in any jurisdiction who were attempting to foster or adopt Jay, and as his recurrent aggression became known, hopes for adoption dimmed.

One day, Jay's new psychiatrist explained the situation to him and then ventured a simple interpretation: "You know, I am mad at Dr. Raskin for killing himself." Jay melted into the psychiatrist's arms and cried without letup for a half hour. His behavior improved, and he started taking his medication again. Jay's treatment team arranged a special staffing meeting with his attorney ad litem, representatives from the state social agencies and Kiowa social services, and phone attendance from the two courts. A plan emerged involving tribal jurisdiction to start. The tribe had located one of Jay's great aunts, and after a few visits, a discharge plan to her home was developed. Jay was lost to follow-up but was doing well at last contact.

Numerous reports have indicated the struggles of AI/AN youth. The 2014 U.S. Attorney General's Advisory Committee on AI/AN Children Exposed to Violence report *Ending Violence so Children Can Thrive* (Dorgan et al. 2014) revealed the circumstances that AI/AN youth and their communities are struggling to overcome, which include various health, economic, and social disparities. In another publication, "Tangled Web of Justice" Rolnick and Arya (2008) illustrated a lack of appropriate services and the resulting harm inflicted from inadequate care and jurisdictional quagmires of reservation versus government. AI/AN youth represent the smallest of all ethnic youth populations in the United States (U.S. Department of Health and Human Services

2010), but these youth and their communities are carrying some of the heaviest burdens of health, social, and economic disparities (Dorgan et al. 2014). Disparities AI/AN youth face impact their ability to function within society, leading to overrepresentation of these youth within the child welfare and juvenile justice systems and the potentially homeless population.

AI/AN people continue to die at higher rates than other Americans from many causes, including chronic liver disease and cirrhosis, diabetes mellitus, unintentional injuries, assault or homicide, intentional self-harm or suicide, and chronic lower respiratory diseases. AI/AN/NH/PI children are 2.8 times more likely to have a diagnosis of diabetes than are non-Indian children (Sequist et al. 2011). AI/AN people have long experienced lower health status when compared with other Americans. From 2009 to 2001, diseases of the heart, malignant neoplasm, unintentional injuries, and diabetes were the leading causes of AI/AN deaths. AI/AN children born today have a life expectancy 5.5 years shorter than the all-race U.S. population (73.0 years versus 78.5 years, respectively) (Sequist et al. 2011). Possible causes of this lower life expectancy and disproportionate disease burden include inadequate education, disproportionate poverty, discrimination in delivery of health services, and cultural differences.

AI/AN youth suffer some of the highest rates of mental health disorders and numerous social indicators of poor health. According to the National Center for Children in Poverty, 29% of AI/AN children live in poverty, with approximately 53% living in a single-parent home (Annie E Casey Foundation 2009). Broad quality-of-life issues are rooted in economic adversity and poor social conditions. The Adverse Childhood Experiences (ACEs) Study (Felitti et al. 1998) is the largest and most robust study examining long-term impacts and outcomes of childhood trauma. AI/AN children have higher exposure to all trauma-related areas in the ACEs study (see Chapter 10, "Social Determinants of Child and Adolescent Mental Health"), noting that having any one of these experiences increases risk for poor outcomes. AI/AN youth had higher risk of suicide, PTSD, depression, and polysubstance use (Brockie et al. 2015). For all tribal youth, this status is exacerbated by historical trauma, heightened exposure to violence, discrimination, and extreme poverty.

According to the National Indian Child Welfare Association, AI/AN children have the highest rate of neglect of all populations (Earle and Cross 2001). Child physical abuse, sexual abuse, emotional abuse, or neglect account for AI/AN children being overrepresented in the foster care system, propagated by systemic barriers (socioeconomic, health, and education disparities) that create greater hardship for Native families (Earle and Cross 2001; Hill 2006). Tribal youth have the highest child maltreatment victimization rate among juvenile populations compared with other racial ethnic groups, with one study showing rates of victimization at 15.5 per 1,000 children and another with nearly double the rate of white children at 21.3 versus 11 per 1,000 (U.S. Department of Health and Human Services 2010).

On average, AI individuals experience a violent crime for every 10 residents age 12 years or older—four times the rate of white Americans (Harlow 2003). AI/AN women experience the highest rate of violent assaults and other levels of violence, with a rate 50% higher than that of Black males (Harlow 2003). Additionally, perpetuation of trauma often manifests in the form of gangs, bullying, and human trafficking, especially against those who appear more vulnerable.

Within the context of ACEs and these social conditions, Whitbeck et al. (2004) used the Historical Loss Associated Symptoms Scale to identify frequent emotional responses regarding historical loss among AI/AN populations: sadness, depression, anger, intrusive thoughts, discomfort around non-Natives, and fear and distrust of intentions of non-Natives. This scale highlights the frequency of negative emotions to self-report questions regarding such topics as tribal loss of land, government relocation, broken treaties, family dynamics, language loss, spirituality, and alcoholism. Tribal youth and their families also report negative thoughts related to historical traumas and unresolved grief (Deblinger et al. 2006).

Ongoing intergenerational and historical traumas impact tribal youth and their families in their daily lives. On the community level, effects of chronic trauma and unresolved grief have been directly linked to substance abuse and suicide, which are used to "numb" or "stop" the pain, with serious long-term negative consequences. AI/AN youth have the highest rate of suicide for all groups; these disparities have been documented for Native youth in more than 40 years of research literature. In addition, AI/AN youth lead the nation in death due to injuries and homicides. Understandably, this correlates with high levels of depression, anxiety, and PTSD (Felitti 2009; Newman 2005). Depression rates among AI children are 10%–30%, and suicide among AI males ages 15–24 years accounts for 64% of all AI suicides, a rate 2–3 times higher than that of the general U.S. population (U.S. Department of Health and Human Services 2010). Additionally, incarcerated AI youth suicide rates are almost double that of whites and triple that of other racial/ethnic groups. Rates of depression and suicide are even higher in youth who also identify as members of other minority groups. Historically, lesbian, gay, bisexual, transgender, and queer (LGBTQ) individuals were highly valued in specific tribal cultures as being Two-Spirit. However, because of colonization and intolerance factors, LGBTQ Native youth now have higher rates of victimization, substance abuse, and suicide than do other Native youth.

AI adolescent and transitional-age youth are much more likely than any other ethnic group in the country to be committed to the Federal Bureau of Prisons, representing 70% of all youth committed (Lakota People's Law Project 2015). This statistic generally does not address the number of incarcerated AI/AN juveniles in state and federal custody and those on probation, on parole, or under custody of law enforcement in some fashion. According to Nadia Seeratan of the National Juvenile Defender Center, without question AI/AN youth, along with other racial and ethnic minorities, and youth that are economically disadvantaged, are over-represented in the justice system (Dorgan et al. 2014). Along with higher rates of justice involvement, tribal youth experience higher levels of trauma and related mental health issues, with more restrictive placements and jurisdictional challenges. These issues are compounded by the influence of discrimination, inadequate legal representation, harsher sentencing, the child welfare–juvenile delinquency–prison pipeline, poverty, and limited infrastructure.

The higher incarceration rate of AI/AN youth is in part due to higher rates of disruptive behavior and substance use disorders than in other youth populations (Beals et al. 1997). National statistics reveal that 13% of AI/AN adults are drug dependent, compared with 9% for non-AI/AN adults (Substance Abuse and Mental Health Services Administration 2009). Increased exposure to an alcohol and/or drug abuser in the household is a clear ACE (Felitti 2009). Alcohol-related deaths among AIs ages 15–24 years are 17 times higher than the national average for the same age group (Felitti 2009). A majority of AI/AN incarcerated youth have mental health or substance use disorders (Dorgan et al. 2014).

The Indian Law and Order Commission report *A Roadmap for Making Native America Safer* highlighted the lack of appropriate services; the detrimental social, economic, and health conditions; and the resulting harm inflicted by high rates of violent crime occurring in Indian

TABLE 3–2. **Significant apparel and themes in American Indian/Alaskan Native cultures**

Item	Use or meaning
Clean white scarf, shawl, or wrap	Prayer shawl prayed over by elders and worn by the individual to help with healing
Metal bead necklace	Reduces teething pain
Corn necklace	Maintains health in a child
Strawberry (print, picture, pattern)	Love
Raven	Transformation, trickster, raven mocker (witch)

country. The authors of the report argued that the current criminal justice system resembles antiquated laws and procedures directed at Natives of the nineteenth century (Indian Law and Order Commission 2013). This highlights a unique experience for these youth, especially those incarcerated in states operating under Public Law 280, a federal law that gave jurisdiction over several tribal Nations to state governments. Notably, these jurisdictional concerns highlight an important conflict between reservation and tribal law (autonomy and self-governance) versus state and federal governments that have traditionally violated people's rights, arguably creating the various problems for this population it continues to inadequately address.

Understanding the historical trauma and mental health disparities addressed above are important themes to understand when treating AI/AN youth. Importantly, AI/AN youth may have endured experiences with poverty, juvenile justice, violence and trauma, or experimentation with substance use. When working with AI/AN youth, it is also important to understand cultural beliefs that may have an impact on mental health care. Many AI/AN youth have a preference for natural treatment, and they may have pursued traditional cures, healers, and religious alternatives first, seeking to bring balance back into their life. Native healers are trusted by the community to use traditional healing methods. During sessions with a patient, it can be helpful for the practitioner to be aware of significant clothing or jewelry. Each tribe has its own items of significance, which can range from a very small to a very large part of the individual's wardrobe. These items may relate to beliefs, healing, identity, or stage of life. For examples, see Table 3–2.

Clinical Vignette: Southeastern Tribes

Nan, age 16, presented to the local health clinic with her maternal grandmother and her 14-month-old son, John, reporting feelings of tension, poor sleep, and depression. She had been having thoughts of being better off dead, that her family would be better off without her as a burden and source of shame. She denied a plan for suicide but admitted to having five friends who died from suicide over the past 3 years (overdoses, firearm, and hanging) and four friends who attempted suicide (overdoses and hanging). She has a family history of depression, anxiety, substance abuse, alcoholism, PTSD, and suicide (paternal uncle, paternal grandfather, and maternal aunt). She has no history of prior psychiatric treatment or medication and is anxious about talking with anyone outside the family about her feelings.

Nan gave a history of being raised by her maternal grandparents after age 3 because of her mother's substance abuse and father's alcoholism. Her mother occasionally visited for 2–3 days, then left again for months, whereabouts unknown, leaving Nan and her siblings (one older brother, one older sister, and two younger brothers) at Nan's grandparents' home along with one aunt and three cousins (two younger girls and one older boy). The house has three bedrooms and a den converted into a bedroom for the boys. Nan and John share a room with her aunt and her aunt's infant daughter. She and John sleep on a twin bed, the aunt sleeps in another twin bed, and Nan's cousin sleeps in a crib box. The family raises a garden, but food is often short despite WIC, food stamps, and monthly food bank trips. The family attends the local Baptist church and are active in community gatherings and powwows, where Nan is a jingle dancer.

John's father was an unknown assailant who raped Nan at a party while she was unconscious. Nan reported that after John's birth, she dropped out of school, where she had been a good student. She was unable to find a job and did not feel "normal." She said she gained weight since the delivery. Home most of the time, she did housework, watched YouTube, played video games, and ruminated on ambivalent feelings toward her son, who she fears will grow up to be like his father. During the initial session, the examiner observed Nan's fatigued and sad appearance, with deep circles under her eyes, slumped body posture, and minimal response to John's needs. She did hold him, fixed a bottle, and fed him during session but had minimal eye contact with him and never smiled at him. Her clothing was mildly rumpled except for a white scarf, and she appeared clean with otherwise good grooming. Nan made minimal eye contact with the examiner and kept her head bowed most of the session. There were long pauses before she answered questions. Nan denied homicidal ideation, self-injurious behavior, and hallucinations. She reported intrusive thoughts of dying and her own funeral; feelings of being watched; and guilt, shame, and anger at her situation. She was ministered to by the church with a laying on of hands and an anointing, but the feelings continued. A local healer prayed and smudged her several times, and the home is smudged on a regular basis.

John wore a clean but ill-fitting outfit, socks without shoes, and a metal bead on a string. He actively crawled around the room when not being held. He did not pull up or attempt to walk, sometimes scooted backward, approached the examiner with toys without obvious anxiety, and babbled continuously.

Nan was willing to work with a therapist in individual counseling on issues of abandonment and betrayal related to being the child of an active substance abuser and her experiences of early neglect, rape, single teen parenthood, and poverty. She and her family initially decided to pursue as natural a course as possible with multivitamins and fish oil and building her vitamin D level up to 60 ng/mL along with a nutritional consultation. They worked with a local healer and participated in prayer/healing sessions with the church.

Nan returned to an alternative school setting, where she quickly caught up to her expected level. She progressed over several months but still complained of sadness. Family discussion regarding options for treatment resulted in a prescription for escitalopram 5 mg/day. Further affect brightening and relief of sad feelings resulted within 2 weeks. John was referred for developmental assessment and was found to be slightly delayed. He was enrolled in occupational therapy, resulting in improved motor function. The family reported improved quality of interaction between Nan and John as well.

Native Hawaiian and Pacific Islander Youth

Native Hawaiians (NHs) are the indigenous people of the Hawaiian Islands. As of the 2010 U.S. Census, they are 26% of the 1.4 million people residing in Hawai'i (U.S. Census Bureau 2010). Of the NHs in the United States, approximately 60% live in Hawai'i (Malone and Shoda-Sutherland 2005). Unfortunately, despite being in their own homeland and having strengths and protective factors, such as high family and social support (Carlton et al. 2006), NHs in Hawai'i have overall lower rates of behavioral health well-being (e.g., socioeconomic status, education, mental health) than the general population of Hawaiʻi (Andrade et al. 2019).

Because there are a multitude of factors that should be taken in account when working with NH children and their families, the following guidelines should be considered. These guidelines are based on anecdotal clinical experience and evidence-based cultural competence. Despite the risk factors that may be present and need to be addressed, it is also important to take advantage of the vast strengths, protective factors, and resilience that are built through Native Hawaiian culture.

A NH family is more than just the child and his or her parents and siblings. A family, or *ʻohana*, can include blood relatives, such as grandparents, aunties, uncles, and cousins, as well as nonblood relatives, or *hānai* (informally adopted) nonrelated "aunties," "uncles," "cousins," and close family friends. To the majority of NHs, the family is the center of all relationships. All members of an *ʻohana* are important and influence the child's well-being. Therefore, it is essential to include them when obtaining collateral information or conducting a family meeting. It is important to set aside ample time and enter any family meeting unrushed and without a rigid agenda, allowing everyone to have an opportunity to provide his or her thoughts.

The formal and direct approach used by non-Hawaiian professionals should be avoided when working with a NH family; instead, the professional should start the conversation by "talking story" (Young 1980). *Talking story* is a local term used to describe a conversational style that is freer, less formal, and based on sharing of personal experiences. It can be a way of breaking the ice with an unfamiliar person. Talking story as a method of interviewing creates a relaxed, undirected exchange of information that will often bring forward the problem or chief complaint without the professional's needing to talk about it directly, thus avoiding having the NH family lose face (Young 1980).

Choosing to use Hawaiian Pidgin English (an English-based creole language commonly spoken in Hawaiʻi), speaking Hawaiian, or using a mixture of Hawaiian and other local languages may also help with establishing rapport with the family. However, it may be prudent at first to refrain from speaking Pidgin to a NH child or family, avoiding the assumption that all NHs speak Pidgin, unless they speak to you first using Pidgin. Note that you should speak Hawaiian Pidgin English—a structured language based on a mixture of different vocabularies, languages, and cultures—with patients and families only if you are conversant in it. Likewise, you should speak Hawaiian or use a mixture of Hawaiian words and English only if you are fluent in the Hawaiian language or know the meaning of the words used. Speaking either language when the practitioner is not fluent might offend the family.

The practitioner should not start the interview by directly talking about the problem or chief complaint. Rather, he or she should start the session by doing introductions, letting the family know the purpose of the meeting, and then allowing them to open the interview. The professional may want to avoid asking personal questions at the beginning but may do so later. If the youth's mother or the family matriarch is present, she will usually start the conversation and provide most of the history. However, at some point, the professional should be sure to ask the father or men in the group their thoughts, as well. Avoid assuming that the father's or the men's silence indicates uncaring or being uninvolved with their child. When talking with the men in the group, avoid rushing them or asking too many questions; allow them to speak freely.

The practitioner should also be mindful of his or her body language; the amount of eye contact and space between individuals can be important factors. Engaging in intense direct eye contact may be interpreted as being domineering and hostile. When first meeting a NH family or child, be mindful of their space; avoid getting too close when sitting. Allowing the family to choose where each member sits can give you some insight into the hierarchy of the family. Pointing a finger or singling out someone can be seen as an aggressive gesture and offensive and thus should be avoided.

The family may ask personal questions about the health care professional; this can be the family's way of establishing trust and confidence in the professional. Health care providers should not take offense at these types of personal questions as patients build trust in their traditional culturally based process. Families may ask the practitioner about his or her cultural identity, about family members whom the patient's family may know, and where the professional is from. Regarding the latter, typically, the family is attempting to determine not just which Hawaiian island the professional is from but from what region of the island.

When concluding an interaction, it is common for family members to want to embrace their provider. In the world of mental health boundaries, this may sometimes feel odd or inappropriate; however, culturally, this is a sign that the family finds you trustworthy and is willing to engage in a treatment relationship. Practitioners should be ready for this possibility and not push the family away, which can be seen as offensive and can sever the treatment relationship.

Of course, each child and his or her family must be treated as unique individuals. The large majority of NHs are of mixed ethnicities and cultural identities and therefore cannot be viewed simplistically as a homogeneous group. This blending of culture and ethnicities has created a value system called the Hawaiian way (Young 1980). In addition, the mode of interaction may differ significantly depending on whether the encounter with the NH child and family is in a more laid-back, preventive setting versus one that is more acute and crisis-oriented (e.g., the emergency department). However, the guidelines noted above may help a practitioner establish rapport, complete valid assessments, and provide culturally competent mental health care to NH children and their families.

Clinical Vignette: Native Hawaiian/ Northwestern Tribe

Valerie came to the outpatient clinic with her adoptive grandmother, Helene, reporting ADHD, high levels of anxiety, and trouble socially with being treated as if she were much older than her 11 years. When she took her ADHD medication, her grades were straight As. Valerie's father was Native Hawaiian (NH) and her mother Haida. Her mother, Sandra, had been adopted by a Christian missionary couple along with several other Native children who had all come from abusive situations. Sandra struggled with alcoholism and opioid abuse and was in and out of rehabilitation and jail, which had cost her custody of Valerie several years earlier. She was also in and out of the state and Valerie's life, and Valerie's grandmother believed someday Sandra would stay clean. Valerie struggled between wanting to believe her grandmother's dream and seeing the reality of her mother's presence coinciding with the disappearance of possessions, money stolen, medication missing, and a string of broken promises.

Valerie took her size from her NH ancestors and at 11 years old was 5 feet, 4 inches tall, weighed more than 160 pounds, and was still prepubertal. She identified with both cultural identities but felt a stronger affinity for her NH side, although she had not had much contact with either. She had researched NH and Haida cultures and felt she looked more NH. She was constantly teased at school for her size and was approached by adults as a peer with awkward social interactions. She did have a female friend and a limited social life. She and her grandmother attended a church where there were only a few children, most of whom were in their grandparents' custody for similar reasons. Valerie desperately wanted to connect with people who looked like her. Finding a NH community with similar-age peers was a dream of hers.

As therapy progressed, Valerie expressed a strong desire to protect and not disappoint her grandmother. She felt she had to make amends for her mother's choices and behaviors and wanted to protect her grandmother's fragile health because she feared that, should Helene die, she would have to return to her mother, whom she did not trust to keep her safe. Valerie kept track of her grandmother's medication and hid the medication and valuables whenever her mother showed up.

With family therapy, Valerie and her grandmother were able to communicate their feelings more openly, discussing Helene's health and fear of failing Valerie the way she felt she had failed Sandra. They also discussed where Valerie would go should Helene become unable to care for the two of them. An adoptive aunt (AI Dakota) became actively involved, helping arrange a transition for both Helene and Valerie to her home, where Sandra was not allowed. All visits with Sandra were monitored at a safe location. In addition, an NH community from the same nation as Valerie's father was located near the aunt's home. Valerie was welcomed into the community as a lost child found, with a large celebration at which she, her aunt, and her grandmother were gifted with muʻumu ʻus, ate traditional foods, and learned traditional dances.

Therapeutic Considerations for Native Youth

With 573 federally recognized AI/AN tribes populating the United States, along with more than 100 state-recognized tribes that occupy historical lands within state boundaries, Native people represent a diverse population. Attempts to collectively group AI/AN people have led more toward reinforcing colonization oppression than empowerment and better mental health, highlighting a need for separate cultural considerations for each culturally diverse tribe. The National Survey of Children's Health reports that approximately 60% of AI/AN children have access to mental health services (Child and Adolescent Health Measurement Initiative 2018). However, when these services are available, they often lack cultural appropriateness or specialty health, resulting in challenges related to utilization, outcomes, and sustainability. Comprehensive services necessary to adequately screen, prevent, treat, and support recovery from trauma and mental health–related symptoms are extremely limited in tribal communities. Contemporary or Western approaches focus on deficits of the individual rather than the negative environment, disruption of cultural norms and lifestyles, or harsh social conditions that contribute to poor decision-making, unhealthy coping skills, and problematic social and personal relationships. There is a critical need to focus on addressing the root cause of AI/AN culturally based disparities and improving outcomes for youth related to out-of-home placement, potential involvement in juvenile justice, homelessness, and especially mental health issues.

One such model that incorporates Native identity to treat mental health in this population is Honoring Children—Mending the Circle (HC-MC; BigFoot and Schmidt 2010). HC-MC as a treatment approach has been extensively promoted and implemented in Indian country with the support of the Children's Bureau and the National Child Traumatic Stress Network, which offers a clinical application of trauma-focused cognitive-behavioral therapy (TF-CBT) within an Indigenous framework supporting AI/AN cultural models of well-being (BigFoot and Schmidt 2010; Deblinger et al. 2006). From a complementary perspective, well-being in AI/AN culture is viewed as a healthy balance within and between the spiritual, physical, relational, mental, and emotional aspects of life, both individually and collectively. These aspects work together, and they reflect each other in creating balance and well-being (see the Southeastern Tribes clinical vignette earlier in the chapter).

As trauma creates an imbalance between these aspects of life, addressing the imbalance is important, with the understanding that healing or recovery is required in order to restore the balance (BigFoot and Schmidt 2010). These common principles are incorporated into treatment with core concepts of the TF-CBT Cognitive Triangle model, which contends that there is a direct relationship between thoughts, emotions, and behaviors. This treatment protocol makes extensive use of proven Indigenous teaching approaches and activities (e.g., watching, instruction, modeling, practices) that complement those used in the TF-CBT model (e.g., psychoeducation, relaxation, cognitive coping). Essentially, it seeks to help individuals develop a better understanding of trauma and emotional responses while concomitantly teaching them to acquire the cognitive, emotional, behavioral, and spiritual skills needed to deal effectively with the trauma-related problems or symptoms they are experiencing. This model maintains fidelity to the CBT model while embracing traditional cultural norms (e.g., family, community, language, traditional medicine, spirituality, ceremony, tribal creation stories) to promote healing and well-being for AI/AN youth. The HC-MC adaptation seeks to honor what makes AI/AN youth culturally unique through recognition and respect for beliefs, practices, and traditions within their families, communities, and Tribes that are inherently healing and therapeutic.

With trauma-exposed children, a common symptom is intrusive thoughts that create anxiety and inability to relax. Common physical sensations of rapid heartbeat and breathing result in distress or discomfort. To combat these sensations from a culturally sensitive perspective, the counselor might use traditional instructions used in ceremonial or related activities: "Know that this is a safe place, a place for you. If you have bad or frightening thoughts, you can leave them outside this place. Think about who you are, close your eyes, breathe in, feel how you are sitting, think about who is sitting next to you."

Native youth use digital and social media platforms for sharing cultural teachings, cultivating resiliency, and increasing community connectedness (Pember 2016). This is critically important given the minimal representation and misrepresentation of AIs in mainstream media that consists mostly of mascots (Washington Redskins) or Hollywood film characters from the eighteenth or nineteenth century. Such prominent images are associated with AI youth having lower self-esteem, decreased sense of community worth, and diminished academic future possibilities (Earle and Cross 2001). AI students may progress through their entire academic career without the presence of an American Indian teacher or peer, leading them to question their belonging in a school context (Phinney 2003).

Although research on Native news and digital media is sparse, Native youth are significant users of social media at similar rates to teens in the general population (Rushing and Stephens 2011), despite residing in regions and reservations that do not possess equal access to technology or the Internet (Donnellan 2017). This finding may reflect adaptive development related to historical context. Traditionally, many Native communities used storytelling as the primary instrument to impart lessons generationally as historical record. However, with colonization, Native communities were forced to adapt to the changing environment, including their means of communication—initially by developing written languages and newspapers and now by utilizing digital and social media. These platforms allow AI adults from a variety of backgrounds, cultures, and professions to have increased visibility and to serve as positive role models for AI youth. Further, AI youth often turn to social media as a source of health information.

When working with Native adolescents, it is important to acknowledge the use of digital media as a tool for cultural revitalization as well as a source of health information. Native youth and young adults view health as a priority for their communities and are blending traditional and modern practices when it comes to wellness (Rushing and Stephens 2011). In 2016, out of 675 surveyed Native youth, 78% had regular access to a smartphone, and more than 92% had access to the Internet on a weekly or monthly basis. Further, it was found that 62% of Native youth and young adults obtained their health information online on a weekly or monthly basis, with a large proportion of the information coming from social media sites (Rushing et al. 2018). Native youth also turn to digital media when seeking information on sensitive subjects such as depression, and of those surveyed, 39% felt most comfortable obtaining information online as opposed to in person (Rushing et al. 2018).

Conclusion

AI/AN/NH/PI individuals have a complex, rich heritage intertwined with historical trauma of impressive magnitude. The novel coronavirus SARS-CoV-2 (COVID-19) pandemic of 2020 has only added to this story. The World Health Organization, Doctors Without Borders, and other organizations have identified AI individuals in particular as a high-risk population during this pandemic because of the disparities discussed in this chapter (Conger et al. 2020; Infectious Diseases Society of America 2020). Interestingly, the tribal governments have some of the most consistent recognition of and response to COVID-19 (e.g., quarantine, restricted access and shutdowns, closing tribal borders) anywhere in the United States. Despite being very limited in resources, these governments have utilized every resource available to them efficiently. Still, the costs in human lives and tribal heritage resources has been high.

When working with AI/AN/NH/PI children and families, the most important aspects of psychiatric evaluations and treatment are building trust with the patient and family, understanding historical/generational trauma, and considering the potential exposure to disparities and adverse childhood events that are prevalent in this population. Within Native populations, there is also a wide variation of what is considered the cultural norm related to geography, reservation, tribe, and the individual. Understanding each nation as a separate culture existing within the context of American culture is one of the most frequently missed concepts of health care providers. Overall, time, consistency, and dedication are of the essence in treating these families. The gradual building of trust and understanding is vital to support the mental health needs of vulnerable Native populations.

Clinical Pearls

- Minimal eye contact is a cultural sign of respect and not a sign of depression.
- Healing is about balance in all aspects of life—spiritual, religious, physical, environmental.
- Silence is time for consideration and should be respected. Be patient.

- Long pauses are for all to consider their answers and not necessarily a sign of depression or cognitive slowing. Again, be patient.

- Elders are decision makers in most families. They often have preferential seating, even with regard to height of seating.

- Begin interviews with introductions and connections, not direct questions. Examples of connections include naming the agency or group you work with, naming any ties to or experience with Native or indigenous people, or telling how long you have lived or worked in the area.

- Spirituality may be very important to the family and may be a mixture of traditional and nontraditional beliefs and practices. Ceremony may be very important.

- Trust must be gained through time, keeping your word, and understanding the culture.

- AI/NA/NH/PI children are taught to consider carefully before answering questions or volunteering commentary; thus, there can be long periods of consideration before answering questions.

Self-Assessment Questions

1. Willow is a 12-year-old Apache/Kiowa girl who presents to the outpatient clinic along with her foster mother, Elaine (Kiowas/Pawnee/white). Willow has been in foster care since she was 7 years old; this is her fifth home. She was sexually and physically abused by at least three different men from when she was 2 years old until she was 7 years old. Willow has been treated with trauma-focused cognitive-behavioral therapy and behavior modification to address anger and acting-out behaviors. She is entering puberty and has started having nightmares about the abuse again. Elaine would like to try Honoring Children—Mending the Circle (HC-MC), a therapy she heard about at a recent foster parent meeting. What can you tell her about this therapy?

    A. HC-MC addresses cognitive, emotional, and behavioral skills to help deal with trauma.
    B. HC-MC uses traditional cultural norms for concepts of family, community, language, traditional medicine, spirituality, ceremony, and tribal stories.
    C. HC-MC avoids using ceremonial terms and focuses on calming behavioral techniques.
    D. HC-MC uses nontraditional standards of well-being such as balance between physical, relational, mental, and emotional aspects of life.

2. Phillipa is a 14-year-old American Indian female brought to the clinic by her very angry mother, who is insisting she have a fresh tattoo removed. The tattoo is of a raven. The mother is furious and wants the raven removed immediately, even though the girl has other tattoos (dolphin, flower, cross). A major scene is erupting. What approach would *not* be helpful from a cultural standpoint?

    A. Ask Phillipa and her mother to enter separate spaces where each can calm down.

    B. Ask the mother about the story of the raven and what it represents.

    C. Ask Phillipa about the story of the raven and what it represents.

    D. Ask the mother her reason for allowing Phillipa to keep the rest of her tattoos.

    E. Ask the mother if covering up the tattoo would be adequate and provide a supply of bandages with the hope she will eventually let go of her anger.

3. Contributors to the loss of parenting skills among AI/AN/NH/PI families include all but which of the following?

    A. Removal of children from Native homes for reeducation.

    B. Cultural fragmentation through removal, war, genocide, and disruption of traditional communities.

    C. Loss of connectivity due to living away from traditional lands.

    D. Historical and personal trauma permeating communities and families.

4. AI/AN/NH/PI and other non-white youth pass through three relevant developmental phases. Which of the following is correct?

    A. Self-protective, pre-conformist, conformist.

    B. Pre-conformist, self-protective, conformist.

    C. Self-protective, conformist, post-conformist.

    D. Self-protective, non-conformist, conformist.

    E. Self-protective, pre-conformist, post-conformist.

5. Mark is a 14-year-old Hawaiian/Ute/white male who presents alone to a walk-in adolescent medicine clinic in Reno, Nevada. He has been living on the street for more than a year and has no resources, having supported himself by prostitution and theft. He refuses to give any information about his family of origin except to say they kicked him out when he turned 13 and would never take him back. What should the examiner recommend to child protective services as most appropriate?

    A. Placement in a general foster home with the goal of reuniting with family members.

    B. Placement in a youth shelter with the goal of reuniting with family members.

    C. Placement in a detention center until further information can be gathered.

    D. Placement in a Ute/Hawaiian-approved residential program with counseling services.

    E. Placement in general foster care with counseling services with the goal of emancipation.

Answers

1. B
2. E
3. C
4. C
5. D

References

Andrade NN, Goebert D, Hishinuma E, et al: Task force recommendations for impact (mental and behavioral health and wellness), in E Ola Mau a Mau: The Next Generation of Native Hawaiian Health. Honolulu, HI, Papa Ola Lokahi, 2019

Annie E Casey Foundation: The 2009 KIDS COUNT Data Book. Baltimore, MD, Annie E Casey Foundation, 2009. Available at: www.aecf.org/resources/the-2009-kids-count-data-book. Accessed August 19, 2020.

Beals J, Piasecki J, Nelson S, et al: Psychiatric disorder among American Indian adolescents: prevalence in Northern Plains youth. J Am Acad Child Adolesc Psychiatry 36(9):1252–1259, 1997

BigFoot DS, Schmidt SR: Honoring children, mending the circle: cultural adaptation of trauma-focused cognitive-behavioral therapy for American Indian and Alaska Native children. J Clin Psychol 66(8):847–856, 2010

Brockie TN, Dana-Sacco G, Wallen GR, et al: The relationship of adverse childhood experiences to PTSD, depression, poly-drug use and suicide attempt in reservation-based Native American adolescents and young adults. Am J Community Psychol 55:411–421, 2015

Bruchac J: Notes of a translator's son, in Growing Up Native American. Edited by Riley P. New York, HarperCollins, 1993, p 242

Carlton BS, Goebert DA, Miyamoto RH, et al: Resilience, family adversity and well-being among Hawaiian and non-Hawaiian adolescents. Int J Soc Psychiatry 52(4):291–308, 2006

Center for Native American Youth: 2017 State of Native Youth Report: Our Identities as Civic Power. Washington, DC, Center for Native American Youth at the Aspen Institute, 2017

Child and Adolescent Health Measurement Initiative: National Survey of Children's Health. Rockville, MD, Data Resource Center for Child and Adolescent Health, Maternal and Child Health Bureau, Health Resources and Services Administration, U.S. Department of Health and Human Services, 2018. Available at: www.childhealthdata.org. Accessed August 20, 2020.

Covarrubias R, Fryberg SA: The impact of self-relevant representations on school belonging for Native American students. Cultur Divers Ethnic Minor Psychol, 2014 Epub ahead of print

Conger K, Gebeloff R, Oppel Jr, RA: Native Americans feel devastated by the virus yet overlooked in the data. New York Times, July 30, 2020. Available at: www.nytimes.com/2020/07/30/us/native-americans-coronavirus-data.html. Accessed September 20, 2020.

Deblinger E, Mannarino AP, Cohen JA, et al: A follow-up study of a multisite, randomized, controlled trial for children with sexual abuse–related PTSD symptoms. J Am Acad Child Adolesc Psychiatry 45(12):1474–1484, 2006

Donnellan ES: No connection: the issue of Internet on the Reservation. American Indian Law Journal 5(2):article 2, 2017

Dorgan BL, Shenandoah J, Bigfoot DS, et al; Attorney General's Advisory Committee on American Indian/Alaska Native Children Exposed to Violence: Ending Violence so Children Can Thrive. Washington, DC, U.S. Department of Justice, Office of Juvenile Justice and Delinquency Prevention, Office of Justice Programs, November 2014. Available at: www.justice.gov/sites/default/files/defendingchildhood/pages/attachments/2015/03/23/ending_violence_so_children_can_thrive.pdf. Accessed August 19, 2020.

Earle KA, Cross A: Child Abuse and Neglect Among American Indian/Alaska Native Children: An Analysis of Existing Data. Seattle, WA, Casey Family Programs, 2001

Erikson E: Childhood and tradition in two American Indian Tribes. Psychoanal Study Child 1:319–350, 1945

Felitti VJ: Adverse childhood experiences and adult health. Acad Pediatr 9(3):131–132, 2009

Felitti VJ, Anda RF, Nordenberg D, et al: Relationship of childhood abuse and household dysfunction to many of the leading causes of death in adults: the Adverse Childhood Experiences (ACE) study. Am J Prevent Med 14(4):245–258, 1998

Fryberg SA, Markus HR, Oyserman D, Stone JM: Of warrior chiefs and Indian princesses: the psychological consequences of American Indian mascots. Basic and Applied Social Psychology 30(3):208–218, 2008

Guity NE: Don't get it twisted! in Black Therapists Rock: A Glimpse Through the Eyes of Experts. Edited by Young D. Black Therapists Rock, 2018, pp 105–117

Harlow CW: Educational and correctional populations. Bureau of Justice Statistics: Special Report. Washington, DC, Office of Justice Programs, U.S. Department of Justice, April 15, 2003. Available at: www.bjs.gov/content/pub/pdf/ecp.pdf. Accessed April 13, 2020.

Hill DL: Sense of belonging as connectedness, American Indian worldview, and mental health. Arch Psychiatr Nurs 20(5):210–216, 2006

Indian Law and Order Commission: A Roadmap for Making Native America Safer: Report to the President and Congress of the United States. November 2013. Available at: www.aisc.ucla.edu/iloc/report. Accessed August 19, 2020.

Infectious Diseases Society of America: COVID-19 Policy Brief: Disparities Among Native American Communities in the United States. Arlington, VA, Infectious Diseases Society of America, 2020. Available at: www.hivma.org/globalassets/idsa/public-health/covid-19/covid19-health-disparaties-in-native-american-communities-final.pdf. Accessed September 20, 2020.

Lakota People's Law Project: Native Lives Matter. Bismarck, ND, Lakota People's Law Project, 2015. Available at: https://s3-us-west-1.amazonaws.com/lakota-peoples-law/uploads/Native-Lives-Matter-PDF.pdf. Accessed August 20, 2020.

Malone NJ, Shoda-Sutherland C: Kau Liilii: Characteristics of Native Hawaiians in Hawaiʻi and the Continental United States. Honolulu, HI, Policy Analysis and System Evaluation, Kamehameha Schools, 2005

National Congress of American Indians: Indian Country demographics. Washington, DC, National Congress of American Indians, 2020. Available at: www.ncai.org/about-tribes/demographics. Accessed October 19, 2020.

Newman DL: Ego development and ethnic identity formation in rural American Indian adolescents. Child Dev 76(3):734–746, 2005

Pember MA: DAPL water protectors at risk for PTSD. Indian Country Today, November 14, 2016. Available at: https://newsmaven.io/indiancountrytoday/archive/dapl-water-protectors-at-risk-for-ptsd-_Ek2449xlUCLdUSvl5h-vg. Accessed February 28, 2020.

Phinney JS: A three-stage model of ethnic identity development in adolescents, in Ethnic Identity: Formation and Transmission Among Hispanic and Other Minorities. Edited by Bernal ME, Knight GP. Albany, State University of New York Press, 1993, pp 61–80

Phinney JS: Ethnic identity and acculturation, in Acculturation: Advances in Theory, Measurement, and Applied Research. Edited by Chun KM, Organota PB, Marin G. Washington, DC, American Psychological Association, 2003, pp 63–81

Pumariega AJ, Sharma N (eds): Suicide Among Diverse Youth: A Case-Based Guidebook. Basel, Switzerland, Springer, 2018

Rolnick AC, Arya N: A tangled web of justice: American Indian and Alaska Native youth in federal, state, and tribal justice systems. Las Vegas, NV, William S. Boyd School of Law, UNLV, 2008. Available at: https://scholars.law.unlv.edu/facpub/981. Accessed April 13, 2020.

Rushing SC, Stephens D: Use of media technologies by Native American teens and young adults in the Pacific Northwest: exploring their utility for designing culturally appropriate technology-based health interventions. J Prim Prev 32(3–4):135–145, 2011

Rushing SN, Stephens D, Dog TL Jr: We R Native: harnessing technology to improve health outcomes for American Indian and Alaskan Native youth. J Adolesc Health 62(2):S83–S84, 2018

Sequist TD, Cullen T, Bernard K, et al: Trends in quality of care and barriers to improvement in the Indian Health Service. J Gen Intern Med 26(5):480–486, 2011

Substance Abuse and Mental Health Services Administration: National Survey on Drug Use and Health. Rockville, MD, Substance Abuse and Mental Health Services Administration, 2009. Available at: www.datafiles.samhsa.gov/study/national-survey-drug-use-and-health-nsduh-2009-nid13531. Accessed April 13, 2020.

Thornton R: American Indian Holocaust and Survival: A Population History Since 1492 (Civilization of the American Indian Series, Vol 186). Norman, University of Oklahoma Press, 1987

U.S. Census Bureau: 2010 Census Shows Native Hawaiians and Other Pacific Islanders Surpassed One Million. Suitland, MD, U.S. Census Bureau, 2010. Available at: www.census.gov/newsroom/blogs/random-samplings/2012/06/2010-census-shows-native-hawaiians-and-other-pacific-islanders-surpassed-one-million.html#:~:text=2010%20Census%20Shows%20Native%20Hawaiians%20and%20Other%20Pacific%20Islanders%20Surpassed%20One%20Million,-Tue%20Jun%2005&text=According%20to%20the%202010%20Census,with%20one%20or%20more%20races. Accessed August 19, 2020.

U.S. Department of Health and Human Services: How tobacco smoke causes disease: the biology and behavioral basis for smoking-attributable disease: a report of the Surgeon General. Atlanta, GA, Office on Smoking and Health, National Center for Chronic Disease Prevention and Health Promotion, Centers for Disease Control and Prevention, 2010. Available at: www.cdc.gov/tobacco/data_statistics/sgr/2010/index.htm. Accessed April 13, 2020.

Whitbeck LB, Adams, GW, Hoyt DR, et al: Conceptualizing and measuring historical trauma among American Indian people. Am J Community Psychol 33(3–4):119–130, 2004

Young BBC: The Hawaiians, in People and Cultures of Hawaiʻi: A Psychosocial Profile. Edited by McDermott Jr JF, Tseng W-S, Maretzki TW. Honolulu, HI, University of Hawaiʻi Press, 1980, pp 5–24

CHAPTER 4

Mental Health in Asian American Populations

Annie S. Li, M.D.
Jang E. Cho, M.D.
Janet C. Chen, M.D.

THE need for recognizing and understanding the mental health needs of Asian American and Pacific Islander (AAPI) youth has never been greater. Asian Americans are now the fastest-growing minority group in the United States (Hoeffel et al. 2012). Compounding the population growth is the complexity of *Asian American* as a heterogeneous group comprising multiple sub-ethnic groups, each with its own distinct cultural values, language, religion, and historic relations to America. Misconceptions of Asian American children being the "model minority" with high scholastic achievements, combined with underutilization of mental health services due to stigma, work against AAPI youth, making them vulnerable to the sequelae of untreated mental illness. Such factors result in mental health professionals having to interface with Asian American youths when symptoms are highly acute and being tasked to broker therapeutic relationships that often terminate prematurely.

In this chapter, we draw on current literature and our collective expertise in providing a comprehensive look at the Asian American population, describing cultural factors impacting child and adolescent development and mental health in Asian American youth, and exploring the issue of stigma challenging mental health diagnosing and treatment. We will also highlight application of DSM-5 cultural formulation (American Psychiatric Association 2013) with a clinical vignette. Our hope is to equip mental health providers with culturally informed knowledge to optimize care delivery when working with Asian American youth and families.

TABLE 4–1. Asian American subgroups population

Group	Population
1. Chinese	4.0 million
2. Filipino	3.4 million
3. Indian	3.1 million
4. Vietnamese	1.7 million
5. Korean	1.7 million
6. Japanese	1.3 million
Total Asian American population	17.3 million

Note. Total includes 2.1 million individuals from other subgroups.
Source. Adapted from Hoeffel et al. 2012.

Overview of Asian Americans: Demographics at a Glance

According to the 2010 U.S. Census, Asian Americans make up 5.6% of the total population (17.3 million of 308.7 million) and is the fastest-growing minority group in the United States (Hoeffel et al. 2012). It is projected that Asian Americans ages 17 and younger will make up 7.7% (6 million) of the total youth population in 2050 (Vespa et al. 2018).

Asian Americans trace their roots from countries making up the Far East, Southeast Asia, and the Indian subcontinent. More than 20 subgroups are identified, with at least 83% of Asian Americans falling into one of the 6 large subgroups: Chinese, Filipino, Indian, Vietnamese, Korean, and Japanese (Pew Research Center 2013) (Table 4–1). Additional groups, such as Bangladeshi, Burmese, Cambodian, Hmong, Laotian, Pakistani, and Thai, were aggregated in census data in 2010 to comprise the subcategory "Other Asians" (Pew Research Center 2013). In recent decades, there is a growing population of Asians who identify themselves as Asian combined with another race, referred to as multiple-race Asians.

Asians are concentrated in the bicoastal regions, but one area experiencing a tremendous Asian population growth is the U.S. South (see Table 4–2). Comparison of the 2000 and 2010 U.S. Census shows that the proportion of Asians living in the West has decreased, whereas the proportion in the South has increased (Hoeffel et al. 2012). Among the Asian groups with large concentration in the South are Asian Indians, Koreans, and Vietnamese (Hoeffel et al. 2012).

Socioeconomic Status

The socioeconomic status of Asian Americans spans a spectrum despite generalized trends of higher overall household income, wealth, education attainment, and employment compared with the national average (Pew Research Center 2013). Closer examination of subgroups shows that Hmong (28.3%), Bhutanese (33.3%), and Burmese (35.0%) have higher poverty rates when compared with the national average (15.1%); Filipino, Indian, and Japanese poverty rates range from 7.5% to 8.4% (Pew Research Center 2013).

TABLE 4–2. Top 10 states with the highest Asian population per the 2010 U.S. Census

State	Asian population	Percent of total state population
1. California	5.6 million	14.9
2. New York	1.6 million	8.2
3. Texas	1.1 million	4.4
4. New Jersey	0.8 million	9.0
5. Hawaii	0.8 million	57.4
6. Illinois	0.7 million	5.2
7. Washington	0.6 million	9.0
8. Florida	0.6 million	3.0
9. Virginia	0.5 million	6.5
10. Pennsylvania	0.4 million	3.2

Source. Adapted from Hoeffel et al. 2012.

Religion

Identification of faith and religion varies among Asian subgroups. Christianity is considered the largest religious group in Asian Americans, with Filipinos predominantly identifying as Catholic and a majority of Koreans identifying as Protestant (Pew Research Center 2013). Chinese Americans, who comprise the largest Asian subgroup, are more likely to embrace philosophies of Confucianism, Taoism, ancestry worship, and Buddhism. Hinduism, Islam, and Sikh are principal religions among South Asian Americans. Many Vietnamese, Thai, and Southeast Asian Americans identify themselves as Buddhists (Pew Research Center 2013).

Immigration History

Asians in the United States trace back to the early 1800s and the arrival of Chinese and Japanese immigrants who worked in the agricultural and railway construction industries. Their growing presence was met with heightened xenophobia, resulting in passage of laws such as the Chinese Exclusion Act of 1882, the Gentlemen's Agreement of 1907, and the Immigration Act of 1917, all aimed at restricting entry of Asians into the country. Filipinos were one subgroup spared from such immigration restrictions, in part because of American occupation of their territory from 1898 to the 1940s. Following the Japanese invasion of Pearl Harbor, Executive Order 9066 was signed in 1942, resulting in the internment of more than 100,000 Japanese Americans. Lifting of restrictions for Asian immigration did not occur until 1965, when the Immigration and Nationality Act opened up pathways for Asians to enter the country through family reunification and professional employment visas.

The late 1970s and early 1980s saw an upsurge of immigrants from Vietnam, Cambodia, and Laos who came seeking refugee status as they fled violence, political instability, and the rise of oppressive regimes at home. Today, Asia's rapid economic growth has facilitated a rise in professionals coming to the United States under the H1-B work visa program and in international students coming to the United States to study. There are also an estimated 1.8 million unauthorized Asian immigrants in the United States (Baker 2018).

Child Development and Family Framework

Various constructs influence the process of child development in AAPI youth. From infancy, the child and parents cultivate attachments and relationships informed by Eastern cultural values alongside Western cultures and practices. Growth becomes an experience of navigating intersecting languages, philosophical doctrines, religious faiths, parental expectations, and dietary preferences, culminating in the formation of a *hybrid identity* for Asian American youth (Mistry et al. 2016). The unfolding of such experiences, along with stressors related to immigration, premigration trauma, socioeconomic disparities, and discrimination in the United States, influence Asian youths' mental well-being, development, and identity consolidation (García Coll et al. 1996).

An appreciation of prevailing Eastern principles is fundamental to understanding child development in Asian American youth. Although ethnic subgroup differences abound, as a whole, Asians emphasize collectivism, familial integrity, respect for elders, discipline, promotion of harmony, and avoidance of confrontation as cultural values in everyday life (Ho et al. 2008). Of prominence is the Confucian virtue of *filial piety*, in which an individual imparts respect, reverence, and gratitude to parents, elders, and ancestors. These principles are intended to extend from the home to the greater community and society as the Tao or the Way to promote harmony and peace (Cline 2016).

In general, Asian parents embody a more authoritarian parenting style compared with the nurturing style of their Western European and American counterparts (Ho et al. 2008). In contemporary times, this approach to child rearing is sometimes referred to as *tiger parenting* in association with Amy Chua's (2011) memoir *Battle Hymn of the Tiger Mother*. Emphasis on obedience and adherence to rules become foundations in toddlerhood and preschool years, with children being taught to contain strong affect, wishes, and needs within themselves. Children equate parental strictness and demands with expressions of parental care, love, and involvement. When the child reaches school age, parents cultivate a hard work ethic and discipline in order to attain academic success. Achievement failures may be interpreted as shameful and contribute to the youth's sense of inadequacy. Strict discipline may also manifest in the use of corporal punishment, particularly among Asian American parents of lower socioeconomic status and education attainment, who also may have experienced trauma in their home countries or have a lower degree of acculturation (Tajima and Harachi 2010).

During adolescence, differences in Eastern and Western cultural values can create turmoil for Asian American youth in their pursuit of identity consolidation. Traditions inform parents to focus on academic success, hoping that their children's achievements preserve family honor and prosperity. However, Asian American adolescents may find such expectations restrictive as they strive for independence, autonomy, and peer social belonging. In one study, Huang et al. (2017) observed that parental acculturation directly impacts Asian American adolescents' well-being: the more acculturated their parents are, the more likely adolescents are to be well adjusted and the less likely they are to have mental health issues (Huang et al. 2017).

Immigration experiences and trauma exposure also play a role in self-esteem and identity development in AAPI children and adolescents (García Coll et al. 1996). In low-income Chinese American immigrant families, children born in the United States leave for China in infancy to be cared for by grandparents and then reunite with their parents in the United States years later when they reach school age. Such early disruptive attachments can heighten anxiety related to trust and separation later on in life. In addition, many Asian parents encountered significant trauma in their home countries and endure acculturative stressors on arrival in the United States. It has been documented that unaddressed parental trauma may decrease parental availability to their children and perpetuate intergenerational trauma for these youth (Kiang et al. 2016). Asian American youth who either live without legal status or have parents without legal status in the United States contend with fears of deportation and parental separation and experience legal barriers to achieving higher education and employment.

Asian American youth also experience more peer discrimination and school victimization than other minority groups in the country (Cooc and Gee 2014). Asians have distinct physical attributes delineating their identity at birth, and stereotypes related to physical appearance, accents, and being the model minority may perpetuate negative peer interactions. Discrimination contributes to feelings of inferiority and marginalization, which then dampen a youth's sense of self. Asian American youth identifying as lesbian, gay, bisexual, transgender, or queer are even more vulnerable because they are likely to not have parental embrace of and support for their sexual or gender identity and often experience shame and fear as they conceal their authentic selves from family members.

The cultural characterizations of AAPI youth and their development process are part of a complex and intricate phenomenon requiring full integration of multiple constructs. Clinicians should be mindful of these complexities and try to integrate such constructs when caring for AAPI youth.

Clinical Assessment and the DSM-5 Cultural Formulation Interview

During clinical assessment, mental health professionals need to explore the presenting problem for the Asian American child within a cultural context. The DSM-5 Cultural Formulation Interview (CFI) provides a framework to do this and emphasizes four domains of assessment: cultural definition of the problem; cultural perceptions of cause, context, and support; cultural factors affecting self-coping and past help seeking; and cultural factors affecting current help seeking. In this section, we emphasize each aspect of the CFI in the context of treatment of Asian American families.

Cultural Definition of the Problem

It is important to understand what Asian families may view as the presenting problem. The concept of mind-body connection is prevalent in Asian cultures, and as a result, many patients do not present with actual psychological problems in initial clinical encounters. Somatic complaints may be the chief presenting issue because the parents are not well versed in verbal expression of emotions and their children lack words to describe their psychological distress (Lin 1985). Parents may also bring their children for evaluation only when mental distress manifests in external symptoms or impedes daily functioning. Ignoring the child's internalized turmoil, parents will raise concerns to professionals about their child's aggressive behaviors or declining academic performance and may attribute these symptoms to character pathologies of defiance, disobedience, and laziness (Chung 1997).

Cultural Perceptions of Cause, Context, and Support

Assessment of Asian American children should incorporate psychosocial stressors as well as cultural features of vulnerability and resilience. The tightly knit social structure of Asian American families can be both a support and a source of stress, and obtaining perspectives from both the patient and the parents is important. Identity development, adaptive functioning in varying cultural contexts, and acculturation require adolescents to incorporate aspects of both their original culture and the mainstream culture. The rigid structure and authoritarian hierarchy of most Asian American families preclude many children from positively identifying with mainstream cultural trends, which can lead to conflicts and negative identity formulation (Pumariega et al. 2005). To obtain accurate clinical information and develop a therapeutic alliance with the family, clinicians should assess the parents' cultural and immigration identity, including primary language and communication styles.

Cultural Factors Affecting Self-Coping and Past Help Seeking

In Asian American families, mental illness is often considered to be a family problem, negatively reflecting on their ancestors as well as the family. Many Asians also believe that emotional distress rises not from biological factors but from lack of self-discipline, and such distress is considered a character flaw or personality deficit (Han and Pong 2015). As a result, it is not uncommon for Asian American individuals to delay seeking mental health treatment until symptoms are quite severe. Parents may first try to impose stricter discipline to modify behaviors or may turn to spiritual leaders or an herbalist for help (Han and Pong 2015; Nguyen and Anderson 2005).

Cultural Factors Affecting Current Help Seeking

An important component in the assessment of Asian American youth is examining cross-cultural dynamics such as intergenerational conflicts, degree of acculturation, and marginalization from the family's original or mainstream culture. Level of acculturation strongly influences Asian Americans' attitudes toward seeking mental health treatment: the more acculturated they are, the more positive their attitudes toward mental health and services will be (Tata and Leong 1994; Ying and Miller 1992).

Clinical Vignette

Connor, a 13-year-old Chinese American adolescent male attending eighth grade at an urban private school, presented to the emergency department after calling 911 for suicidal ideations following an argument with his parents at home. He had spent the early evening hours socializing with friends, and when he returned home, his father reprimanded him for not completing extra math exercises. Connor recalled his father berating him for his lack of ambition. accusing him of jeopardizing his prospective college acceptances by not prioritizing his academics. Connor became angry, and said aloud, "Sometimes I wish I was not alive." His mother responded, "Well, if you can't handle this pressure to succeed, then maybe you should go kill yourself." In the emergency department, Connor endorsed feelings of sadness, helplessness, and hopelessness since fourth grade, with intermittent plans of either jumping off his apartment balcony, running into traffic, or taking an overdose.

Connor's parents, both immigrants from China, described him as "a sensitive child, different from us," who they wished would "toughen up." Seeing that their son was "not cut out to be athletic," they determined math as an area in which he could excel. Since fourth grade, Connor's teachers had expressed concern about his mental health and recommended counseling, but his parents never followed through. In the emergency department, Connor's parents insisted on his being discharged and became hostile toward the psychiatry team when extended observation was recommended. His mother accused the psychiatrist of treating them "like slaves and prisoners," and the parents demanded Connor have access to his computer during observation so that he could complete his schoolwork.

The emergency department treatment team collaborated with the dean of Connor's school, who had expressed concern for Connor since grade school, and collectively outlined a treatment contract in which following up with a psychologist was a prerequisite for Connor's return to school. The parents agreed, and Connor was finally able to pursue the treatment he needed and wanted.

Cultural Formulation of Case Vignette

The clinical vignette highlights many of the key challenges in assessing and treating Asian American children. Cultural and intergenerational differences between the immigrant Chinese parents and the patient, Connor, an American-born child, are played out. The parents strongly emphasize education and success, perceiving their son's struggles as a character flaw that should be remediated through tough love and self-discipline. Meanwhile, Connor, feeling hopeless and helpless, senses that he may have depressive symptoms and desperately seeks out emergent professional help on his own, an intervention atypical for youth his age. The deep-rooted stigma regarding mental health felt by the parents can be appreciated in their dismissal of the school's recommendation for therapy, hostility to the psychiatrist in the emergency department, and resistance to engaging with the treatment team.

In cases such as this one, the physician's primary focus is to broker with the parents a commitment to ensure that the patient will undergo treatment. Leveraging with external support systems, particularly schools, can be instrumental. The school administration can intervene, advocate for the youth's well-being, and encourage parents to seek treatment for their child. Parents may be more inclined to listen to the school rather than jeopardize their child's school standing. In Connor's case, the emergency department treatment team worked with the dean of the school to help him obtain needed treatment.

Opportunities for psychoeducation and exploration of parent-child dynamics through cultural variables can occur when the patient is involved in mental health treatment. Clinicians need to be gradual and patient in their approach because the paradigm of mental health treatment may be a novel and foreign experience for Asian families. Any small steps toward change (e.g., parents listening to their children, consistent attendance at sessions, youth reaching out to the therapist or psychiatrist when in crisis) should be recognized and lauded.

Mental Health Conditions in Asian American Youth

Common mental health conditions may manifest differently for Asian American children and adolescents, and Asian American youth may present differently from other children. There are Asian culture-bound syndromes to consider, but given how infrequently they are seen in children, adolescents, and young adults, they will not be included here. For a review of common child and adolescent psychiatric diagnoses, their documented lifetime prevalence, and clinical presentations, see Table 4–3.

Treatment and Management of Mental Health Disorders in Asian American Children, Adolescents, and Young Adults

Challenges and Barriers to Mental Health Treatment

There are unique challenges when engaging and implementing treatment in Asian American youth. Stigma is by far the largest barrier and impacts every stage of treatment, from widely documented low rates of mental health utilization to high rates of medication nonadherence and treatment attrition (Abe-Kim et al. 2007; Akutsu et al. 2004; Alegria et al. 2004; Le Meyer et al. 2009). The National Latino and Asian American Study (NLAAS) reported that only 8.6% of Asian Americans sought out mental health treatment compared with 17.9% of the general population (Alegria et al. 2004).

Mental illness is deeply associated with shame, fear, and embarrassment in Asian countries, and these sentiments persist when immigrants come to the United States. Denial of the illness

TABLE 4–3.   Psychiatric diagnoses in AAPI youth and clinical presentation

Pediatric psychiatric condition or diagnosis	Incidence and prevalence in AAPI youth	Clinical presentation in cultural context
Depression	Most cross-cultural studies of depression indicate that Asian American adolescents report lower rates of depression than do youth of other ethnic groups. One study quoted a prevalence of 2.9% in Asian American adolescents compared with 12% for Mexican American adolescents (Choi 2002). Another study noted that 17% of Asian American youth reported depressive symptoms, compared with 18% of white, 22% of Hispanic, 29% of American Indian, and 15% of African American youth (Saluja et al. 2004).	Asian experience of depression integrates body and mind, which can lead to presentation with somatic symptoms in place of affective symptoms. Instead of a chief complaint of sadness, the patients and families may come to the doctor complaining about headaches, backaches, stomachaches, insomnia, and fatigue (Kalibatseva and Leong 2011). Asian adolescents may have a hard time expressing their feelings and may try to conceal their emotional struggles. The first signs of depression may be that the patient is starting to fall behind academically, is falling asleep in class, is tardy for school, or lacks focus and has become more withdrawn and introverted (Choi 2002).
Suicide	Among females ages 15–24 years, AAPI have the highest rate of suicide deaths (14.1%) compared with other racial/ethnic groups (white 9.3%, Black 3.3%, and Hispanic 7.4%) (Lee et al. 2009). AAPI males in the same age range have the second-highest rate of suicide deaths (12.7%) compared with other racial/ethnic groups (white 17.5%, Black 6.7%, and Hispanic 10%) (Lee et al. 2009).	Asian American teenagers, particularly first-generation immigrants arriving in the United States at an older age, with lower acculturation status and experiences of parent-child conflict are at increased risk of suicide (Balis and Postolache 2008).
Anxiety	In a national study of more than 35,000 U.S. children, 9% of Asian American children met criteria for adjustment disorder—1.7 times more than non–Asian Americans (Nguyen et al. 2014). Asian American adolescents report elevated levels of social anxiety and score in the clinical range more frequently than do adolescents from other ethnic groups (Brice et al. 2015).	Asian American children are more likely than non-Asian American children to receive a diagnosis of anxiety disorder or adjustment disorder. Discrimination from peers, which has been found to be more frequent among Asian Americans than other ethnic minorities, may increase risk for social anxiety (Brice et al. 2015).

TABLE 4–3.   Psychiatric diagnoses in AAPI youth and clinical presentation (continued)

Pediatric psychiatric condition or diagnosis	Incidence and prevalence in AAPI youth	Clinical presentation in cultural context
Substance abuse	Lifetime illegal drug use rate of Asian American adolescents (12–17 years) has been reported at 17.9%, lower than the rate for whites (30.3%), Hispanics (29.8%), and African Americans (28.1%) (Wu et al. 2011). Asian American adolescents reported a marijuana use rate of 8.2% compared with 21.4% of whites, 19.6% of Hispanics, and 17.1% of African Americans (Wu et al. 2011). The rate of ecstasy use in Asian Americans adolescents (3.7%) was comparable to that of whites (3.8%) and higher than that of Hispanics (2.8%) and African Americans (0.9%) (Wu et al. 2011).	Rates of illicit drug use are generally lower among Asian American youth compared with the other three major racial/ethnic groups. Substance use is perceived as taboo, and there is strong parental disapproval of substance use in Asian American adolescents and young adults. The worry of bringing shame to the family may be a protective factor against substance use. This buffer may be reduced for Asian American adolescents living in high-density metropolitan areas, where they are more likely to initiate and experiment with drug use (Wu et al. 2011).
Eating disorder	Studies including high school and college-age students suggest that whereas Asian American and white women share similar levels of body dissatisfaction, Asian Americans have lower rates of bulimia nervosa and other eating disorders (Cummings and Lehman 2007; Nicdao et al. 2007). In a large-scale epidemiological study, Project Eating Among Teens (EAT), Asian American and African American boys were found to be at greater risk for potentially harmful weight-related concerns and behaviors than white boys (George and Franko 2010; Neumark-Sztainer et al. 2002).	Studies regarding diagnosis of eating disorders in AAPIs are limited. There is concern that the low prevalence rates may be misleading because current diagnostic criteria are informed by Western values and lack sensitivity to subtle cultural behaviors. Definitions of beauty and attractiveness vary not only between Asian and non-Asian populations but also within Asian subgroups. Eating behaviors such as binge eating may be perceived in Asian cultures as an acceptable mechanism for exercising emotional restraint when coping with stress. Exploring these constructs is important when assessing for eating disorders in Asian American patients (Cheng 2014).

TABLE 4-3. **Psychiatric diagnoses in AAPI youth and clinical presentation** *(continued)*

Pediatric psychiatric condition or diagnosis	Incidence and prevalence in AAPI youth	Clinical presentation in cultural context
Autism spectrum disorder (ASD)	The 1998–2009 National Health Survey reported a 0.32% ASD prevalence rate in the AAPI population (Mehta et al. 2013). In more recent studies, the crude rates of ASD diagnosis in AAPI children varied. Reported prevalence ranged from 30 to 210 cases per 10,000 AAPI children (Becerra et al. 2014). In studying adjusted risks, diagnosis of ASD was 43% higher in foreign-born Vietnamese children and 25% higher in foreign-born Filipino children. However, children with mothers born in China and Japan had ~30% lower risk of ASD compared with white U.S.-born children (Becerra et al. 2014).	Asian American parents may perceive diagnosis of ASD and other intellectual disabilities as a disruption of harmony, an interference of supernatural forces, or an ancestral punishment for misdeeds in current or past lives (Ennis-Cole et al. 2013). In South Korea, autism is viewed as a punishment for the family's sins (Hwang and Charnley 2010). Speech or language delays and social skills deficits may go undetected because parents feel the child will eventually catch up, which delays diagnosis and initiation of early intervention services. Degree of parental acculturation may determine when AAPI children with ASD interface with mental health professionals. Immigrant parents of children with ASD from lower socioeconomic status and limited English proficiency may not interface with psychiatrists until the school system makes a referral because of the child's poor academic and milestone achievements during early school years. Asian Americans may be less receptive to professional support and educational services, perceiving such interventions as intrusive, and may depend on family involvement instead. Families seeking those services might encounter difficulties due to scarce availability of bilingual, culturally informed trained professionals.

TABLE 4-3. **Psychiatric diagnoses in AAPI youth and clinical presentation** *(continued)*

Pediatric psychiatric condition or diagnosis	Incidence and prevalence in AAPI youth	Clinical presentation in cultural context
ADHD	Prevalence by race (ages 3–17) is Asian 0.8%, white 8.7%, Black 9.8%, and Hispanic 5.1% per the CDC in 2009 (Bloom et al. 2009). Research suggests that ADHD is less prevalent among Asian Americans than other ethnic minority groups (Nguyen et al. 2014). Although rates for ADHD among whites, Blacks, and Hispanics have been increasing, rates of ADHD among AAPI have remained unchanged over time (Getahun et al. 2013).	Asian American parents are less likely to report externalizing behavioral problems, primarily because of stigma associated with reporting behavioral or emotional problems. Thus, AAPI youth tend to score lower on externalizing scales and are less frequently diagnosed with conduct problems. Asian children who are struggling academically may not come to the attention of teachers or clinicians as quickly as children from other groups because of biases suggesting Asians are the "model minority" who generally perform well academically.
Trauma-related disorders	Asian Americans report lower rates of PTSD compared with other minority groups: 1.9% of Asians ages 18 and older report a lifetime prevalence of PTSD, compared with 7.8% of African Americans, 6.9% of non-Latino whites, 6.3% of Afro-Caribbeans, and 4.6% of Latinos (Alegría et al. 2013).	Trauma-related disorder rates are higher in Southeast Asians compared with other Asian subgroups. This is largely related to family experiences of fleeing war-torn home countries, being displaced as refugees, and facing acculturative stressors. Unresolved trauma in parents may reduce their availability to nurture children's development. The sequelae of intergenerational trauma include externalized behaviors in youth, with increases in violence and delinquency. AAPI youth who experienced or witnessed violence related to discrimination also self-report PTSD symptoms. In one study, college-age AAPI students reported depressed mood, dissociation, and hypervigilance as the most common phenotypes of PTSD (Gómez 2017).

Note. AAPI=Asian American and Pacific Islander; CDC=Centers for Disease Control and Prevention.

results in treatment avoidance and perpetuates isolation, hopelessness, and helplessness among patients and families. Anxiety and depression may be viewed not as medical conditions but as character flaws or weaknesses requiring self-discipline and training to overcome. Chronic conditions such as autism spectrum disorder or schizophrenia are often concealed within the family. Families seeking help are at risk of losing face and experiencing significant discrimination within their community (Webster and Fretz 1978). Therefore, Asian Americans may first seek guidance from family members, close friends, or religious community members before accessing professional help.

Asian Americans who have acculturated to American culture are more likely to access mental health treatment (Alegria et al. 2004). Second- and third-generation immigrants are more likely to seek help than first-generation immigrants, and the further they depart from household Asian cultural values, the more likely they are to seek treatment (Gloria et al. 2008; Ting and Hwang 2009). AAPI youth with less supportive parents are less likely to express distress in order to avoid disappointing their families (Meneses et al. 2006).

Poor mental health literacy is another challenge. It is not uncommon for Asian patients to present with somatic symptoms of physical pain and after a series of medical evaluations be diagnosed with a psychiatric illness. Mental health care is perceived as indicated only for the seriously ill, making the threshold to access care very high. Parents may seek psychiatric care only when the child exhibits significant decline in functioning such as poor academic performance (Kearney et al. 2005). This delay translates into higher acuity and urgency in the child's illness, with families seeking care during crisis and through emergency services.

Scarcity of resources is another factor to consider when treating Asian American youth. There is a shortage of bilingual and bicultural child and adolescent mental health professionals, so by default, primary care providers are often the first-line treatment provider during clinical encounters. Wraparound services for patients with autism spectrum disorder or intellectual disabilities may be unavailable because of the limited availability of bilingual trained professionals.

Strategies to Promote Mental Health Treatment in Asian American Youth

Treating Asian American youth requires a holistic and integrated approach. Focusing on family strengths and their good intentions is important in order to lessen guilt and shame. When parents feel that the clinician is working with them, receptiveness to treatment increases. Parents and children should be encouraged to work on direct, open communication to express emotions.

Reluctance to engage in treatment and high attrition rates make the initial evaluation crucial. All family members should be invited to the initial evaluation. Clinicians are encouraged to impart authority and expertise because Asian families are more likely to respond positively to recommendations from a respected professional figure. The initial appointment should also function as a treatment session in case the family does not return. Treatment plans should be created and may include complementary and alternative remedies. Short-term, problem-focused approaches with results-oriented solutions such as cognitive-behavioral therapy may align with Asian cultural expectations better than play therapy or long-term psychodynamic therapy (Chung 2002).

Once the dyadic relationship is established, it is vital for the clinician to create a scaffold to reinforce the relationship. Strengthening the collaboration with the primary care physician or pediatrician is one way to promote treatment adherence (Yeung et al. 2006). Other formal service systems and community resources such as schools, support groups within Asian American organizations, faith-based spiritual leaders, and local government-sponsored psychoeducation workshops can also be immensely helpful.

Approaching and involving the school in treatment may create mixed sentiments for Asian American families. Asian American parents are reluctant to have the clinician communicate with the school for fear this may negatively impact the child's academic reputation. At the same time, building collaboration with the school can often serve as a protective factor for treatment adherence given how strongly parents emphasize academic achievements. In fact, when school-based mental health services are available, they can be used as an asset because youth can access treatment without disrupting their academic obligations. Unfortunately, Asian American youth are less likely than Hispanic students to be referred to school-based mental health care services (Guo et al. 2014).

Asian Americans and Psychopharmacology

Psychotropic medication response involves a complex interplay between culture and genetics. There are special considerations to bear in mind when prescribing psychotropics to Asian Americans. The activity of cytochrome P450 enzymes involved in drug metabolism has been shown to be slower in Asians when compared with whites (Wong and Pi 2012), which may account for Asian individuals' increased sensitivity to medication side effects. Prescribers should be aware that Asian patients respond to lower doses of medications (neuroleptics, antidepressants, mood stabilizers, and benzodiazepines) than those taken by white patients (Wong and Pi 2012). Therefore, when prescribing for Asian patients, it is important to start medications at lower doses and to monitor closely.

When treating Asian American youth, it is always important to ask about herbal remedies, traditional Chinese medicine, and foreign imported pharmaceutical products because they can increase the side effects of medication or even potentially increase efficacy through pharmacodynamic synergism (Sarris et al. 2010). It is also important to recognize that adherence to psychopharmacological treatment is lower in the Asian population (Wong and Pi 2012). This may be attributed to cultural expectations and beliefs about medication. Many Asian patients believe that Western medications are more potent than traditional Eastern treatments and have reservations about medication overpowering the body's balance. Providing culturally informed psychoeducation can help with medication adherence.

Conclusion

As the Asian American population increases, mental health providers will continue to be tasked with addressing the mental health needs and unique challenges of Asian American children, adolescents, and young adults. Clinicians must appreciate cultural factors and intergenerational differences present in Asian American communities; with each successive generation comes a more acculturated cohort, and the movement to reduce stigma within the Asian community is growing stronger, particularly with the proliferation of technology and social media. Meeting the mental health needs of the AAPI community will require expansion of the mental health workforce to include more culturally sensitive, bilingual practitioners.

Clinical Pearls

- Asian Americans are the fastest-growing minority group in the United States.

- Stigma, suboptimal mental health literacy, and scarcity of resources are factors impacting mental health treatment in Asian American youth. Their reluctance to seek care unfortunately often leads to higher acuity of illness on presentation in clinical settings.

- When working with Asian American families, clinicians can use the Cultural Formulation Interview to map intergenerational and cultural differences between members of the family.

- Clinicians working with Asian American youth can strengthen treatment relationships through active collaboration with primary care providers and school systems, as well as emphasizing the family's strengths and promoting open communication between parents and their child.

Self-Assessment Questions

1. Which of the following statements accurately describes child development in Asian American youth?

    A. The degree of parental acculturation has no impact on Asian American child development.
    B. Parent-child conflicts emerge in adolescence for Asian Americans because Confucian values of collectivism and filial piety are at odds with pursuits of individual autonomy.
    C. Parental discipline and focus on academic achievements is fundamental to a positive identity formation for Asian American young adults.
    D. Discrimination is a rare phenomenon for Asian American youth and does not impact identity development.

2. When it comes to treatment of mental health in the Asian American youth population, which of the following statements is *not* correct?

    A. Asian patients respond to higher doses of psychotropic medications than white patients do. Therefore, it is important to start medications at higher doses when prescribing for Asian patients.

    B. Stigma against mental health is often the largest barrier to Asian American youth receiving mental health treatment.

    C. Asian Americans will often present to the doctor with complaints of somatic symptoms of physical pain instead of the typical symptoms of a psychiatric disorder.

    D. Asian American youth are less likely than their Hispanic counterparts to be referred to school-based mental health care services.

3. Which of the following is *not* a helpful strategy for providers when engaging with the Asian American youth population and their families?

    A. Incorporate treatment as part of the session in case the family does not return after the first appointment.

    B. Establish a strong collaboration with the primary care physician for better treatment adherence.

    C. Downplay the authority and expertise of the provider in order to overcome treatment noncompliance and the family's reluctance to trust the provider.

    D. Cytochrome P450 enzyme activity should be considered in pharmacological intervention for Asian American patients.

Answers

1. B
2. A
3. C

References

Abe-Kim J, Takeuchi D, Hong S, et al: Use of mental health-related services among immigrant and US-born Asian Americans: results from the National Latino and Asian American Study. Am J Public Health 97(1):91–98, 2007

Akutsu PD, Tsuru GK, Chu JP: Predictors of non-attendance of intake appointments among five Asian American client groups. J Consult Clin Psychol 72(5):891–896, 2004

Alegria M, Takeuchi D, Canino G, et al: Considering context, place, and culture: the National Latino and Asian American Study. Int J Methods Psychiatr Res 13(4):208–220, 2004

Alegría M, Fortuna LR, Lin JY, et al: Prevalence, risk, and correlates of posttraumatic stress disorder across ethnic and racial minority groups in the United States. Med Care 51(12):1114–1123, 2013

American Psychiatric Association: Diagnostic and Statistical Manual of Mental Disorders, 5th Edition. Arlington, VA, American Psychiatric Association, 2013

Baker B: Population estimates: illegal alien population residing in the United States: January 2015. Washington, DC, Office of Immigration Statistics, U.S. Department of Homeland Security, 2018. Available at: www.dhs.gov/sites/default/files/publications/18_1214_PLCY_pops-est-report.pdf. Accessed April 14, 2020.

Balis T, Postolache TT: Ethnic differences in adolescent suicide in the United States. Int J Child Health Hum Dev 1(3): 281–296, 2008

Becerra TA, von Ehrenstein OS, Heck JE, et al: Autism spectrum disorders and race, ethnicity, and nativity: a population-based study. Pediatrics 134(1):e63–e71, 2014

Bloom B, Cohen RA, Freeman G: Summary health statistics for U.S. children: National Health Interview Survey, 2009. Vital Health Stat 10(247):1–82, 2010

Brice C, Warner CM, Okazaki S, et al: Social anxiety and mental health service use among Asian American high school students. Child Psychiatry Hum Dev 46(5):693–701, 2015

Cheng H-L: Disordered eating among Asian/Asian American women: racial and cultural factors as correlates. Couns Psychol 42(6):821–851, 2014

Choi H: Understanding adolescent depression in ethnocultural context. ANS Adv Nurs Sci 25(2):71–85, 2002

Chua A: Battle Hymn of the Tiger Mother. New York, Penguin, 2011

Chung H: The challenges of providing behavioral treatment to Asian Americans. West J Med 176(4):222–223, 2002

Chung W: Asian American children, in Working With Asian Americans: A Guide for Clinicians. Edited by Lee E. New York, Guilford, 1997, pp 165–174

Cline EM: Families of Virtue: Confucian and Western Views on Childhood Development. New York, Columbia University Press, 2016

Cooc N, Gee KA: National trends in school victimization among Asian American adolescents. J Adolesc 37(6):839–849, 2014

Cummings L, Lehman J: Eating disorders and body image concerns in Asian American women: assessment and treatment from a multicultural and feminist perspective. Eat Disord 15(3):217–230, 2007

Ennis-Cole D, Durodoye BA, Harris HL: The impact of culture on autism diagnosis and treatment: considerations for counselors and other professionals. Family Journal 21(3):279–287, 2013

García Coll C, Lamberty G, Jenkins R, et al: An integrative model for the study of developmental competencies in minority children. Child Dev 67(5):1891–1914, 1996

George JB, Franko DL: Cultural issues in eating pathology and body image among children and adolescents. J Pediatr Psychol 35(3):231–242, 2010

Getahun D, Jacobsen SJ, Fassett MJ, et al: Recent trends in childhood attention-deficit/hyperactivity disorder. JAMA Pediatr 167(3):282–288, 2013

Gloria AM, Castellanos J, Park YS, et al: Adherence to Asian cultural values and cultural fit in Korean American undergraduates' help-seeking attitudes. J Counsel Dev 86:419–428, 2008

Gómez JM: Does ethno-cultural betrayal in trauma affect Asian American/Pacific Islander college students' mental health outcomes? An exploratory study. J Am College Health 65(6):432–436, 2017

Guo S, Kataoka S, Bear L, et al: Differences in school-based referrals for mental health care: understanding racial/ethnic disparities between Asian American and Latino youth. School Mental Health 6:27–39, 2014

Han M, Pong H: Mental health help seeking behaviors among Asian American community college students: the effect of stigma, cultural barriers, and acculturation. Journal of College Student Development 56(1):1–14, 2015

Ho C, Bluestein DN, Jenkins JM: Cultural differences in the relationship between parenting and children's behavior. Dev Psychol 44(2):507–522, 2008

Hoeffel E, Rastogi S, Kim MO, et al: The Asian population: 2010. 2010 census briefs C2010BR-11. Suitland, MD, U.S. Census Bureau, March 2012. Available at: www.census.gov/prod/cen2010/briefs/c2010br-11.pdf. Accessed April 14, 2020.

Huang K-Y, Calzada E, Cheng S, et al: Cultural adaptation, parenting and child mental health among English speaking Asian American immigrant families. Child Psychiatry Hum Dev 48(4):572–583, 2017

Hwang S, Charnley H: Making the familiar strange and making the strange familiar: understanding Korean children's experiences of living with an autistic sibling. Disability and Society 25(5):579–592, 2010

Kalibatseva Z, Leong FTL: Depression among Asian Americans: review and recommendations. Depress Res Treat 2011:320902, 2011

Kearney LK, Draper M, Baron A: Counseling utilization by ethnic minority college students. Cultur Divers Ethnic Minor Psychol 11:272–285, 2005

Kiang L, Tseng V, Yip T: Placing Asian American child development within historical context. Child Dev 87(4):995–1013, 2016

Lee S, Juon H-S, Martinez G, et al: Model minority at risk: expressed needs of mental health by Asian American young adults. J Community Health 34(2):144–152, 2009

Le Meyer O, Zane N, Cho Y, et al: Use of specialty mental health services by Asian Americans with psychiatric disorders. J Consult Clin Psychol 77(5):1000–1005, 2009

Lin TY: Mental disorders and psychiatry in Chinese culture: characteristic features and major issues, in Chinese Culture and Mental Health: An Overview. Edited by Tseng WW, Wu YH. Orlando, FL, Academic, 1985, pp 369–394

Mehta NK, Lee H, Ylitalo KR: Child health in the United States: recent trends in racial/ethnic disparities. Soc Sci Med 95:6–15, 2013

Meneses LM, Orrell-Valente JK, Guendelman SR, et al: Racial/ethnic differences in mother-daughter communication about sex. J Adolesc Health 39(1):128–131, 2006

Mistry J, Li J, Yoshikawa H, et al: An integrated conceptual framework for the development of Asian American children and youth. Child Dev 87(4):1014–1032, 2016

Neumark-Sztainer D, Croll J, Story M, et al: Ethnic/racial differences in weight-related concerns and behaviors among adolescent girls and boys: findings from Project EAT. J Psychosom Res 53(5):963–974, 2002

Nguyen L, Arganza GF, Huang LN, et al: Psychiatric diagnoses and clinical characteristics of Asian American youth in children's services. J Child Fam Stud 13(4):483–495, 2014

Nguyen QC, Anderson LP: Vietnamese Americans' attitudes toward seeking mental health services: relation to cultural variables. J Community Psychol 33:213–231, 2005

Nicdao EG, Hong S, Takeuchi DT: Prevalence and correlates of eating disorders among Asian Americans: results from the National Latino and Asian American Study. Int J Eat Disord 40(suppl):S22–S26, 2007

Pew Research Center: The rise of Asian Americans. Washington, DC, Pew Research Center, updated April 4, 2013. Available at: www.pewsocialtrends.org/2012/06/19/the-rise-of-asian-americans. Accessed April 14, 2020.

Pumariega AJ, Rogers K, Rothe E: Culturally competent systems of care of children's mental health: advances and challenges. Community Ment Health J 41(5):539–555, 2005

Saluja G, Iachan R, Scheidt PC, et al: Prevalence of and risk factors for depressive symptoms among young adolescents. Arch Pediatr Adolesc Med 158(8):760–765, 2004

Sarris J, Kavanagh DJ, Byrne G: Adjuvant use of nutritional and herbal medicines with antidepressants, mood stabilizers, and benzodiazepines. J Psychiatr Res 44:32–41, 2010

Tajima EA, Harachi TW: Parenting beliefs and physical discipline practices among Southeast Asian immigrants: parenting in the context of cultural adaptation to the United States. J Cross-Cultural Psychol 41(2):212–235, 2010

Tata SP, Leong F: Individualism-collectivism, social-network orientation, and acculturation as predictors of attitudes toward seeking professional psychological help among Chinese-Americans. Couns Psychol 41(3):280–287, 1994

Ting JY, Hwang WC: Cultural influence on help-seeking attitudes in Asian American students. Am J Orthopsychiatry 79(1):125–132, 2009

Vespa J, Armstrong D, Medina L: Demographic turning points for the United States: population projections for 2020–2060. Current Populations Rep P25-1144. Suitland, MD, U.S. Census Bureau, 2018. Available at: www.census.gov/content/dam/Census/library/publications/2020/demo/p25-1144.pdf. Accessed April 14, 2020.

Webster DW, Fretz BR: Asian-American, black and white college students' preference for helping services. J Couns Psychol 25(2):124–130, 1978

Wong FK, Pi EH: Ethnopsychopharmacology considerations for Asians and Asian Americans. Asian J Psychiatr 5(1):18–23, 2012

Wu P, Liu X, Kim J, et al: Ecstasy use and associated risk factors among Asian-American youth: findings from a national survey. J Ethn Subst Abuse 10(2):112–125, 2011

Yeung A, Yu S-C, Fung F, et al: Recognizing and engaging depressed Chinese Americans in treatment in a primary care setting. Int J Geriatr Psychiatry 21:819–823, 2006

Ying YW, Miller LS: Help-seeking behavior and attitude of Chinese Americans regarding psychological problems. Am J Community Psychol 20(4):549–556, 1992

CHAPTER 5

Bridging the Gap in Psychiatric Care of Latinx Youth and Families

Maria Jose Lisotto, M.D.

Andrés Martin, M.D., M.P.H.

Lisa R. Fortuna, M.D., M.P.H.

Demographics and Latino Heterogeneity

Latinos/Hispanics are the largest ethnic minority in the United States. In 2014, Hispanics comprised 17.4% of the U.S. population (55.4 million), and projections estimate that by 2060, 29% (119 million) of the U.S. population will be of Hispanic origin (Colby and Ortman 2015). More than 27 million (23%) Latinos will be younger than age 18 by 2060, making them the nation's largest and youngest racial and ethnic group.

In this chapter, we use Latino/Latina and Hispanic interchangeably; however, there are distinctions between these terms that are important when it comes to understanding and providing care to the Latinx community. The term *Hispanic* refers to a common language and describes those whose ancestry derives from Spain or Spanish-speaking countries. The term Latino/Latina, most recently replaced by the gender-neutral alternative Latinx (Merriam-Webster 2020), refers to geography and indicates Latin America origin. Because most of the federal data and academic research continue to use the term Latino/Latina, we will use Latino/Latina at times in this chapter, with the understanding that the most appropriate and sensitive adjective is, in fact, Latinx.

The U.S. Latino population is quite heterogeneous and includes non-U.S.-born individuals originally from South America, Central America, the Caribbean, and North America. In 2015, Hispanics of Mexican origin accounted for 63.3% (36 million) of the nation's Hispanic population; Puerto Ricans were the second-largest group, representing 9.5% of U.S. Hispanics (Flores 2017). According to the 2010 Census, Hispanic/Latino refers to "a person of Cuban, Mexican, Puerto Rican, South or Central American, or other Spanish culture or origin regardless of race" (Ennis et al. 2011). The federal government recognizes just one ethnic group in its classification system, which unfortunately can lead to simplifications and overgeneralizations by collective labeling of various self-sustained ethnicities into one all-encompassing "Latino/Hispanic group." In a 2011 national bilingual survey of 1,220 Latino adults, most Latinos preferred to use their family's country of origin (e.g., Puerto Rican, Cuban, Mexican) over pan-ethnic terms when describing their identity (Taylor et al. 2012). As we demonstrate throughout this chapter, homogenization of Latinos can lead to misconceptions and stereotyping that not only promote discrimination but also fail to recognize the diversity and utility of a Latino subgroup-specific model of care, especially when treating children, adolescents, and families.

The Latino population in the United States reached nearly 58 million in 2016 and has been the principal driver of U.S. demographic growth, accounting for half of national population growth since 2000 (Flores 2017). However, since the year 2000, there has been a shift in terms of the primary source of Latino population growth, moving from immigration to U.S. births (Krogstad and Lopez 2014). In the year 2000, foreign-born Latinos comprised 40% of the total Latino population in the United States, whereas in 2015, the share of foreign-born Latinos declined to 34.4%. The share of U.S.-born Latinos, or second-generation Latinos (children born in the United States to at least one foreign-born parent) increased from 59.9% in 2000 to 65.6% in 2015 (Flores 2017).

The prevalence and symptom presentation of mental health illness vary among Latino subgroups. Latinos are a highly diverse group, so it is not surprising that there is so much variation in terms of lived experiences and circumstances around migration of patients and their families, as well as prevalence and clinical presentation of mental illness. A more nuanced understanding of the specific challenges that Latinos face as a highly heterogeneous yet often stereotyped group is necessary in order to promote respectful interactions with patients and families.

Minority Status Impacting Psychiatric Illness and Access to Care

Latinx individuals in the United States face inequities in terms of education, socioeconomic status, and access to care; unfortunately, such inequities are often exacerbated by language barriers as well as undocumented immigration status. The Institute of Medicine seminal report *Unequal Treatment* notes that racial and ethnic minorities tend to receive lower quality of health care than do nonminorities, even after controlling for access-related factors (Smedley et al. 2003), and Hispanic Americans "face greater barriers than any other racial and ethnic groups in the U.S." (Smedley et al. 2003).

There are many risk factors that place Latinos in the United States at higher risk for mental illness. Poverty and mental illness interact in a negative cycle: people who live in poverty are at increased risk of mental illness, and, in turn, there is an increased likelihood that those living with mental illness will drift into or remain in poverty (Lund et al. 2011). Almost 20% of Latinos live below the poverty line (compared with less than 9% of non-Hispanic whites), which correlates with poverty rates among Latinx children and adolescents (26% vs. 11%, respectively) when compared with non-Hispanic whites (Annie E Casey Foundation 2017). Food insecurity, a social determinant of mental health, is associated with a heightened risk of past-year mood, anxiety, and substance use disorders in Latino children (McLaughlin et al. 2012).

When it comes to educational outcomes, data show that each year from 2000 to 2016, Latinx students' high school dropout rates were higher than rates in white and black youth (McFarland et al. 2018). Although there has been significant improvement (Latinx high school dropout rates were almost 28% in 2000, compared with 8.6% in 2016), Latinx students continue to lag behind their same-age white, Asian American, and African American peers in terms of high school completion, high-technology education, and college admission rates (McFarland et al. 2018). Latinx children as a group are then more likely to become or remain poor (Adelman 2007), which, as stated above, further deepens the socioeconomic divide for Latinx future generations. Educational and socioeconomic status are linked to both physical and mental health (Adelman 2007). Therefore, it is difficult to understand how Latinos, despite being the largest ethnic minority group in the United States, still struggle with accessing health care services and are more likely to receive less and inferior mental health services as compared with non-Latino whites (Alegría et al. 2010b).

There are a multitude of barriers interfering with timely access to psychiatric services for Latino families, including financial need (high cost of mental health services and low wages among Latino parents), location of services and availability of transportation, lack of adequate insurance, poorly understood bureaucratic procedures, scarce community-based psychoeducation, cultural stigma associated with mental health, and lack of linguistic support (Pumariega et al. 2013). Rates of mental health care access are lower among Latino youth than among non-Latino youth (Jiménez et al. 2019), and even when minority children and families receive services, the services are often interrupted prematurely by these barriers.

Data from the National Comorbidity Survey Replication Adolescent Supplement showed that Latinx youth were less likely than non-Hispanic white youth to receive services for severe ADHD (Merikangas et al. 2011), and despite having higher rates of mood and anxiety disorders, Latinx adolescents were less likely than white adolescents to receive treatment (Merikangas et al. 2011). Although Latinx youth continue to have a higher rate of suicide attempts compared with non-Latino white students (8.2% vs. 6.1%) (Kann et al. 2018, p. 26), they are less likely to receive assistance when they endorse suicidal ideation (Freedenthal 2007). Knowledge and counseling about medications are associated with willingness among adolescents to seek active treatment (Fortuna et al. 2015). Because Latinx youth report lower average scores on knowledge of antidepressants and counseling compared with white teenagers (Chandra et al. 2009), it is not surprising that Latinx adolescents have lower rates of mental health service use (Alegría et al. 2002).

Evidently, there is an urgent need for mental health interventions specifically directed toward Latinx youth. An intersectional approach that considers the complex interaction between social determinants of health and Latinx group heterogeneity would allow for better understanding and more effective recognition of the elevated risk for poor health outcomes among Latinx communities.

Diversity, Cultural Humility, and Microaggressions

It is vital to remember the level of socioeconomic, political, and ethnic diversity within Latino/Hispanic subgroups when it comes to caring for Latinx communities. The understanding of both medical and psychiatric illness also varies greatly depending on the Latinx subgroups' place of origin, history, and religious beliefs, as well as patterns and effects of immigration. Providers should not only understand these variables but also strive to provide comprehensive care that builds on concepts of cultural competence and cultural humility.

Culturally competent psychiatric care is meant to improve the psychiatric treatment of immigrant and minority individuals, often identified by the cultural mainstream as "others" (Qureshi et al. 2008). This model focuses on eliminating cultural barriers to quality care and values the patient's culture and perception of illness. On the other hand, the cultural humility model promotes self-reflection into the provider's ethnic background and how the provider's cultural experiences can inform and affect patient care, focusing on the aspects of cultural identity that are "most important to the [patient]" (Hook et al. 2013, p. 2).

Racial bias and discrimination can be subtle and imperceptible and may be present even when there is no intention to discriminate. Comments or actions, often unconscious or unintentional, that express prejudice toward a minority group, known as *microaggressions*, have detrimental and pervasive effects that create anxiety and crises of belonging within culturally diverse individuals. For many people, given the huge diversity within Latinx subgroups, being labeled as "Latino/Latina" or "Hispanic" might symbolize a loss of identity and could be interpreted as a form of microaggression. Common microaggressions described by Latinx individuals include the assumption that all Latinx/Hispanics have similar customs and backgrounds (e.g., food preferences, weather in their native countries), political beliefs, values, phenotypes, and idioms of expression. Comments such as "You don't look Latina/Latino," "You don't look as dark," or "You look European" or statements about a person's accent, especially within academic environments (e.g., "You speak really good English" or "You don't even sound Latina/Latino") constitute other examples of microaggressions. The recipients of such comments are often left wondering whether the comments were meant as a compliment, as a reminder that they do not belong, or a statement that people from Latinx backgrounds are "less than" the majority culture. If the recipient were to inquire about the intention of such a statement, they would run the risk of being labeled as "too sensitive," "overreacting," or "dramatic" ("Maybe you just watched too many *telenovelas*"). Judgmental comments such as these only further accentuate the stereotyping of, discrimination against, and prejudice toward Latinx groups.

Both direct and indirect perceived discrimination can hinder an individual's self-worth, increasing vulnerability for depressive symptoms (Lisotto et al. 2018). Latinx youth commonly report episodes of perceived discrimination, which have been associated with lower self-esteem and more depressive symptoms (Umaña-Taylor and Updegraff 2007). Given that evidence suggests that minorities with higher levels of ethnic identity exploration and resolution have higher levels of self-esteem (Umaña-Taylor and Updegraff 2007), clinicians and educators should focus on enhancing youths' positive self-concept, as well as promoting their ethnic pride, in order to help mitigate some of the negative effects of perceived discrimination among Latinx youth.

Clinical Vignette 1

Michael is a 16-year-old high school student from Puerto Rico who moved to New York City with his family 2 years ago. Michael wanted to stay in Puerto Rico, but because of significant economic problems on the island after Hurricanes Irma and Maria, his family decided to move to the mainland. Michael is homesick, misses his grandparents and cousins back in Puerto Rico, and feels guilty about leaving home. He is adjusting well to New York but often feels like an "outsider." He has experienced several instances of discrimination, such as when a school peer recently posted hateful comments about minorities on social media. He has been feeling increasingly sad, has trouble focusing in school, and says he worries a lot. At home, he has been irritable to the point of seeming explosive toward his parents.

When Michael went to his pediatrician for a well visit, he was screened for depression, scoring in the moderate depression range. The integrated behavioral health specialist at the clinic evaluated Michael and started to work with him using cognitive-behavioral therapy. The pediatrician discussed starting an antidepressant as an option, but the family decided to start with therapy first. Michael responded well to therapy, and his depression symptoms improved. He felt motivated to join his school's baseball team, and he began making new friends.

Cross-cultural skills among practitioners play a significant role when it comes to providing psychiatric care for children, adolescents, and families, especially when it comes to recognizing *cultural syndromes*, complex expressions of psychological or emotional distress that are unique to a given culture. For example, a common cultural syndrome among Latinos of Caribbean origin, *ataque de nervios*, a reaction combining anxiety, agitation, and dissociation, can be confused with a psychotic reaction (Pumariega et al. 2013). Conversely, clinicians could mistakenly categorize similar symptoms in a Latino patient as *ataque de nervios*, just on the basis of the patient's cultural background, dismissing other potential diagnoses such as panic attacks, psychosis, substance-induced illness, or even organic illness.

Providers must examine their own cognitive and affective processes during medical decision-making because implicit social attitudes and stereotypes may be retrieved from memory, unintentionally influencing medical care (Smedley et al. 2003). Clinicians practicing from a model of cultural humility will be better equipped to understand their own countertransferential reactions and the effects that implicit biases can have in the care of culturally diverse populations. In turn, continuous self-assessment, clinical curiosity, and approaching Latinx patients and families with a nonjudgmental stance will lead to stronger therapeutic alliances and better treatment outcomes.

Language

There are more than 577 million Spanish speakers in the world, representing 7.6% of the global population (Instituto Cervantes 2018). More than 42 million people in the United States speak Spanish at a native or equivalent level, with more than 16 million of those Spanish speakers having only "limited competence" (Instituto Cervantes 2018). Given that one in four children in the

United States is Latinx, with 61% coming from immigrant families living in Spanish-speaking homes (Garcia and Jensen 2009), understanding language acquisition, skills, and use in Latinx youth is of paramount importance.

Dual-language development is dependent, among other factors, on the type and amount of exposure and the age at which children begin acquiring their second language (Toppelberg and Collins 2010). *Sequential bilinguals* acquire their first language during the period of rapid language acquisition before age 3 years and a second language later; *simultaneous bilinguals* acquire both languages as first languages (Toppelberg and Collins 2010). Most Latinx children in the United States are sequential bilinguals (Toppelberg and Collins 2010). The term *dual-language* children has become favored over *bilingual* because it does not presuppose full proficiency in both languages, recognizing individual differences in bilingual development and wide variability between first and second languages (Genesee et al. 2004; Gutiérrez et al. 2010). Sequential bilinguals have varying degrees of skills in each language, especially around domains highly dependent on language exposure (Oller et al. 2007). For example, Spanish-English dual-language children tend to have stronger English-based school-related vocabulary, whereas Spanish is stronger around home-related vocabulary.

Because of assimilative forces propelling immigrant children to learn English quickly, a language shift or loss can occur when children begin school. This leads to *subtractive bilingualism*, a process in which a second language is acquired at the expense of the first language (Toppelberg et al. 2006, p. 161). Societal and school pressures to assimilate and the subsequent loss of the home/primary language can have detrimental developmental and socioeconomic consequences for Latinx children. Maintaining the first language guarantees access to family and community support, which can lead to stronger identification and internalization of Latinx cultural values. There has been a poorly substantiated but widespread practice of recommending parents to "discontinue exposure to one of the languages (typically the home language) when a child is facing cognitive, language, or learning delays" (Toppelberg and Collins 2010, p. 707), with little consideration of the impact this might have on the family and attachment system. This practice has little or no empirical support (Toppelberg et al. 2006), with research suggesting instead that even children with language impairment can learn two languages (Genesee et al. 2004). The linguistic ability of the parents, as well as the potential for family distancing in the case of Spanish-speaking only caregivers, should be carefully considered before making recommendations to discontinue exposure to the Spanish language.

Between 2000 and 2015, the proportion of Latino students enrolled in public elementary and secondary schools increased from 16% to 26% and is projected to reach 29% by 2027 (National Center for Educational Statistics 2017). Schools have had to adjust their curriculum and teaching practices in order to effectively teach English to children who are still developing language skills in Spanish (Collins 2014). Typical language demands of schooling can be overwhelming for many dual-language Latinx children, with ensuing implications for educational attainment, self-esteem, and socioeconomic status.

Because English language proficiencies are often the only ones being assessed during school language assessments (Toppelberg et al. 2006, p. 161), difficulties in at least one language frequently go undetected in dual-language children of Latinx background. One cannot infer competence in one language based on competence in another language (Toppelberg et al. 2006, p. 161). Language assessment services that can recognize normal and delayed dual-language development

TABLE 5–1. **Psychotherapy considerations in dual-language youth and their families**

Psychotherapy should be delivered in the language of greatest mastery for each patient.

Reduced language competence in dual-language children limits their ability to communicate with family members and compromises their ability to participate in verbally mediated psychotherapies.

Once a relationship is established, psychotherapy can serve as a vehicle to provide additional exposure to linguistic experiences by slowly challenging and expanding the child's cognitive linguistic capacity (Toppelberg et al. 2006, p. 162).

Child and family–based psychotherapies can help promote adaptive outcomes through the development of emotion-based vocabulary that can allow for better identification, expression, and interpretation of difficult emotions. In turn, this can increase emotional regulation and encourage more harmonious family relationships.

of English-language learners is of paramount importance. Educators and providers should also be able to recognize "the wide range of language competences young children of immigrants have in their first and second language" (Toppelberg and Collins 2010, p. 707). Dual-language competence is critically associated with the emotional well-being and school functioning of Latino children of immigrants (Collins et al. 2011), making dual-language assessments absolutely necessary.

Language deficits are also present in many psychiatrically referred dual-language children (Toppelberg et al. 2006, p. 156), with multiple studies showing an association between deficits in linguistic competence and psychopathology in children (Toppelberg and Shapiro 2000; Toppelberg et al. 2002). Language deficits predict increased prevalence and greater severity of ADHD and externalizing disorders, language-based learning disorders (e.g., dyslexia), and depressive and anxiety disorders (Beitchman et al. 1996a, 1996b). Effective language ability assessment in both languages as well as treatment of language difficulties is crucial when designing targeted therapeutic and remedial strategies for dual-language children. Furthermore, assessment of parents' ability to understand English instructions is also of vital importance when caring for Latinx youth. Efforts should be made to communicate diagnostic and treatment recommendations to the child or adolescent as well as to caregivers, using the language in which each feels most comfortable or proficient. It is important that providers never assume a patient's language competency and should ask for translation services as needed. Providers should use language as a tool to immerse themselves in the patient's own culture while delivering effective, conscientious, and culturally humble care. Table 5–1 includes important considerations when providing psychotherapy for dual-language youth and their families.

Immigration, Acculturation, and Consequences of Border Separation

Migratory movements from Latin American countries into the United States continue to be a highly controversial topic despite the fact that massive migrations have shaped the United States throughout its history. Clinicians caring for Latinx youth need to understand culturally mediated factors relevant to the patient and family's experience, including discrete patterns of migration

(Figure 5–1), acculturation, and adaptation narratives, as well as premigration experiences. As a reflection of Latinx heterogeneity, the reasons for migration as well as the process and rates of migration vary significantly depending on the country of origin. As portrayed in Table 5–2, there are noticeable differences between U.S. Latinx subgroups. Mexicans are the most ubiquitous Latinx subgroup, with almost 36 million Mexicans living in the United States, of whom 32% are foreign born. By comparison, 57% of 274,000 Argentinians living in the United States are foreign born.

The unique values and sociopolitical characteristics of the different Latinx subgroups, coupled with different premigration circumstances, make the experiences of migration and acculturation different among Latinos (see Glossary for definition of acculturation). Many migrants dream of the "land of opportunities" but are often dismayed to find themselves socially and economically isolated on arrival. Negative public perceptions increase feelings of failure and shame, which in turn increase acculturative stress and lead to further separation between parents and U.S.-born children. Acculturation directly affects the developmental task of identity. Culturally diverse youth face significant pressures to assimilate into mainstream society, while also experiencing pressure from the family to retain their parents' cultural heritage. Development of bicultural identity, in which the child or adolescent is able to remain connected with their culture of origin while acquiring the necessary knowledge and interpersonal skills to navigate mainstream culture, leads to the best adaptational outcomes (Rothe et al. 2010).

Acculturation stress describes the experience of internal conflict that results from "the adaptation to a new host culture, including internal cultural value conflicts and external pressures to assimilate, and facing the host society's hostility in the form of racism and discrimination" (Pumariega et al. 2013, p. 1107). Acculturation stressors such as discrimination, parental acculturative stress, and peer victimization have been identified as potential contributors to Latinx children's psychosocial maladjustment (Alegría et al. 2010a) and may increase the risk of psychopathology (Duarte et al. 2008). Parental stress and family separations can adversely affect acculturative stress, leading to family discord and less effective parenting practices, and positive family relationships can mitigate such stress (Rothe et al. 2010). Orientation to mainstream American culture coupled with internalization of the family's native heritage and cultural practices is associated with lower rates of conduct disorders and substance abuse among Latinx youth (Pumariega et al. 2013).

Clinical Vignette 2

Andrea is a 12-year-old girl born in New York City whose family is from El Salvador. She has an 8-year-old brother, Elmer, who was also born in New York and was diagnosed with autism spectrum disorder. Her 15-year-old sister, Rita, was born in El Salvador and is a Dreamer, an immigrant who entered the United States as a minor. Andrea's parents are both undocumented immigrants. Andrea's family is like many "mixed-status" families, with children and parents of different immigration status living together in the United States. The family lives in a government-subsidized apartment on a relatively safe block. Andrea loves school and wants to become a doctor when she grows up. Both of her parents work 10-hour shifts at minimum wage jobs, 6 days a week. Andrea looks forward to Sunday mornings, when the entire family attends a nearby Catholic church, calls her grandmother back in El Salvador, walks in the park, and makes a huge family lunch.

Andrea has become increasingly anxious because of immigration raids in nearby communities and the media's negative messages about immigrants. She is worried about what will happen to her and her siblings if her parents are deported. Andrea begins having trouble sleeping and eating,

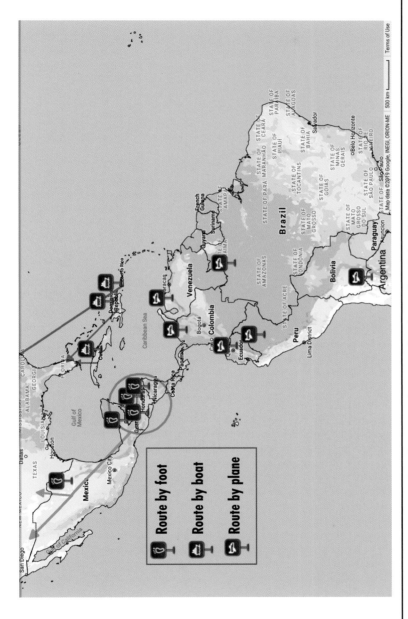

FIGURE 5–1. **Process of migration from Latin America into the United States.**

The most common means of migration into the United States is by foot (which includes other terrestrial means of transportation, i.e., vehicles). Migrants from islands (Cuba, Dominican Republic, or Puerto Rico) enter by boat. Individuals from South American countries mostly enter the United States by plane. Nowadays, migrants entering by foot or by boat can also enter the United States by plane.

TABLE 5-2. **Characteristics of U.S. Latinx subgroups**

Population rank[a]	Latinx subgroups[b]	Median age (years)	Foreign born[c]
1	Mexicans	26	32%
2	Puerto Ricans	29	2%
3	Salvadorans	30	59%
4	Cubans	40	56%
5	Dominicans	30	54%
6	Guatemalans	28	61%
7	Colombians	36	61%
8	Hondurans	29	63%
9	Spaniards	34	15%
10	Ecuadorians	33	59%
11	Peruvians	37	63%
12	Nicaraguans	35	58%
13	Venezuelans	35	71%
14	Argentineans	37	57%
	All Latinos/Hispanics (surveyed in this study)	28	34%

[a]Reference population rank in count: rank 1=35,758,000 individuals; rank 14=274,000 individuals. All Hispanics=56,477,000 individuals.
[b]No data available for the remaining Latino/Hispanic countries.
[c]Individuals born outside the United States or its territories whose parents are not U.S. citizens.
Source. Adapted from Flores 2017 and based on data from the Pew Research Center tabulations of the 2015 American Community Survey (1% IPUMS). The American Community Survey is the largest household survey in the United States with a sample of >3 million addresses. The specific data sources for this table are the 1% samples of the 2015 American Community Survey, IPUMS=Integrated Public Use Microdata Series.

and although her parents worry about her, they feel uncomfortable communicating with school staff because they worry about the prospect of being separated from their children because of their immigration status. Andrea's teacher recommended that she meet with the school therapist because she has appeared sad and distracted during classes and her grades have started to decline.

The school therapist knew that culturally appropriate care and treatment in Spanish was critical for Andrea and her family. The therapist began to use narrative therapy with Andrea and later included conjoint sessions with her family. Narrative therapy focuses on helping people to therapeutically express and define their own story. In a family setting, narrative therapy allows the technique of externalizing problems, identifying how the problem has challenged the core strength of the bond and helping parents with coping and supporting their children's and their own well-being. The therapist then obtained permission from the family to involve a family navigator, who helped them address essential needs, connecting the family to social services, health care, and legal resources for addressing immigration issues. Andrea felt supported, her anxiety symptoms improved, and she was much more focused in school.

Tragically, despite evidence showing the detrimental effects of family separation and its negative long-lasting effects on development and mental health, the federal government approved the "zero tolerance" immigration policy in 2018. Under this policy, the Department of

Justice prosecuted all adult aliens apprehended while crossing the border illegally, with no exception for asylum seekers or those with minor children (Congressional Research Service 2019). Any children accompanying these "adult aliens" were put into shelters or foster care. Most of the separated families were parents with young children fleeing violence and poverty in Central America, trying to provide a better life for their children. The actual number of children separated by immigration authorities is unknown because thousands may have been separated from their families before accounting by the court began.

Developmental studies have shown the importance of consistent and attuned care that meets children's needs; this is certainly not the type of care immigrant children receive on arrival at the U.S. border. There is significant evidence demonstrating the devastating effects of child separation from caregivers. Migrant children have often been exposed to *premigration trauma* after fleeing violence and even war in their home countries. Their parents also likely endured traumatic experiences, and given growing evidence showing transmission of detrimental effects of childhood trauma across generations (Buss et al. 2017), it is not hard to see how Latinx migrant children would be more susceptible to further traumatization on separation and placement in detention centers. Childhood adversity is a risk factor for later psychiatric illness and worse financial and educational outcomes, as well as diabetes, stroke, and premature mortality (Anda et al. 2006). Parents' vulnerability to deportation affects their emotional adjustment and ability to financially and emotionally support their children, as well as the children's emotional well-being and school performance (Brabeck and Xu 2010).

Both the American Psychiatric Association and the American Academy of Child and Adolescent Psychiatry have issued position statements vehemently opposing any policy that separates immigrant children from their families. In their statements, they underscore the importance of parental support, especially when it comes to "protecting children and helping children recover from the negative impacts of stress and trauma" (American Academy of Child and Adolescent Psychiatry 2018). Both statements focus on the mental health sequelae of forced separation, which "can cause lifelong trauma, as well as an increased risk of other mental illnesses, such as depression, anxiety, and posttraumatic stress disorder (PTSD). The evidence is clear that this level of trauma also results in serious medical and health consequences for these children and their caregivers" (American Psychiatric Association 2018). Expert opinion is clear: children should remain with their families as they seek asylum, and any policy that forces separation of children from caregivers places already vulnerable children at increased risk for adverse mental and medical outcomes.

Clinicians working with undocumented families have the opportunity to not only provide clinical care but also to act as advocates for Latinx youth and families. Caring for diverse and/or undocumented immigrants is complex. Clinicians should seek supervision, focus on self-care, and attend to their own transferential reactions in order to avoid burnout and vicarious traumatization.

Media and Latinx Youth

Although the Latinx population grew more than 43% from 2000 to 2010, the rate of Latinx depictions in the media stayed stagnant or grew only slightly, at times proportionally declining

(Ennis et al. 2011). The paucity of Latinx media representation, coupled with the often homogeneous and stereotypical depiction of Latinx communities in the rare opportunities when they are in fact portrayed in the media, unfortunately plays a significant role in shaping children's and adolescents' view of Latinx culture.

Mass media shape knowledge and beliefs of the majority about minority groups and, in turn, influence minority responses to the majority (Faber et al. 1987). Because children and adolescents use media (television and films, literature, music, and social media) to understand and develop higher-order thinking skills and make sense of the world (Lisotto et al. 2018), it is not surprising that media would play such an important role in shaping their concepts of minority groups. The media are thought to promote development by providing new information or stimulating children's learning. However, according to *cultivation theory*, media content can also affect viewers' beliefs about the world and, consequently, alter their behavior (Gerbner et al. 2002). In recent years, we have unfortunately seen an uprise in xenophobic, anti-immigration, and divisive social media posts, as well as an increase in access to videos depicting violent content and aggression toward minority groups in different media outlets. False ideas about a group can be validated by the media, and stereotypes may serve to develop norms of treatment of certain groups which, in turn, may create an unequal power structure (Berg 1990). "Viewed as a tool of the dominant ideology, the creation and perpetuation of stereotypes in the media function to maintain the status quo by representing dominant groups as 'naturally' empowered and marginal groups as disenfranchised" (Berg 1990, p. 282). The portrayal of Hispanics as illegal aliens coming to "steal American jobs" inherently exacerbates the power differential and divisiveness between groups.Given that youth in the iGen (youth born in the mid-1990s and later) and millennial (youth born in the 1980s through the mid-1990s) generations spend a significant amount of their time connected through different media platforms, one wonders about the effects that anti-immigration rhetoric conveyed through the media will have on future generations' understanding and tolerance of cultural minorities.

A 2010 study from the Kaiser Family Foundation including 2,000 youngsters showed that 8- to 18-year-olds "spend more time with media than in any other activity besides (maybe) sleeping—an average of more than 7½ hours a day, seven days a week" (Rideout et al. 2010, p. 1). The report underscored the massive role that mobile devices play in fueling media use: 20% of media consumption occurs on mobile devices. Tweens and early teenagers (11- to 14-year-olds) seem to be higher than any other age group in terms of media consumption (Rideout et al. 2010). Differences in media use in relation to race and ethnicity are more pronounced, even after controlling for age, parental education, and number of parents in the household. Hispanic youth, similar to Black youth, average 13 hours of media exposure a day, significantly higher than usage by white youth, who average 8.5 hours a day. This report also showed that the likelihood of parents imposing rules on children's time spent on media was very similar regardless of race, although parents of white children were more likely to attempt to impose controls on media content.

Communication and media allow immigrants to become acculturated to their new social environment. As part of the complex process of acculturation, or cultural identity formation, Latinx youth, more so than older immigrant groups, turn to different media outlets to become acquainted with the new host culture. There is a strong relationship between acculturation and achievement of developmental milestones in Latinx youth, with media playing a crucial role in facilitating their connection. Developmental domains such as individual identity formation, as well as social interactions—within and between cultural groups—are likely to be influenced by how the media portrays Latinos (Lisotto et al. 2018). Media can serve as a vehicle to promote positive Latinx role models to developing youth. Unfortunately, mass media can also further perpetuate stigmatization and Latinx homogenization by portraying Latinx males as either criminals, drug lords, or seductive but uneducated individuals and relegating Latinx females to portraying roles of sensual brunettes with voluptuous bodies or maids with minimal ability to speak English. The portrayal in media of successful, strong, intelligent Latinx individuals who embrace their cultural heritage while simultaneously adapting to and incorporating American culture can reinforce positive development and inspire Latinx youth. Prime-time television has tried to promote positive Latinx role models by depicting characters such as Betty Suarez from *Ugly Betty*, Dr. Callie Torres from *Grey's Anatomy*, Detective Nina Moreno-Torres from *New York Undercover*, Jane Villanueva from *Jane the Virgin*, and Aaron Shore from *Designated Survivor*. This, in turn, will mitigate the effects of negative Latinx stereotypes portrayed in different media sources, hopefully discouraging negative cognitive associations often perpetuated by limited exposure to diverse and successful Latinx characters.

Providers are also greatly influenced by media representation of minorities, leading in some cases to stereotyping, unconscious bias, racial prejudice, and even discrimination (Smedley et al. 2003). Providers educated in a model of cultural humility can use media to inform and enrich their clinical care because doing so stimulates them to reflect on their own cultural background and promotes self-analysis of the care provided to minority youth (Lisotto et al. 2018). Clinicians must remain cognizant of the influence that media can have on the creation and perpetuation of racial stereotypes and of media's effect on children's development.

Culturally Tailored Treatment Approaches for Latinx Youth and Families

When caring for Latinx youth and families, it is important to differentiate the ethnic identity of Latinx subgroups, minimize generalization and ethnic stereotyping, and avoid pathologizing normal processes. However, it is worth remembering that Latinx groups also share certain commonalities that can inform therapeutic interventions.

The Latinx cultural value of *familismo* (see "Clinical Pearls" for definition and significance in treatment), a collectivistic perspective that places greater value on needs of the family over needs of individuals, is shared by most Latinx subgroups. Maintaining family ties and connections appears to be protective against psychiatric disorders in Latino adolescents (Alegría et al. 2007). In our collective experience, treatment of Latinx children and adolescents without including the child or adolescent's primary caregivers is likely doomed to fail. Evidence suggests that Latinos are often more responsive to treatment approaches that incorporate family members, collectivistic perspectives, and values (Cardemil and Sarmiento 2009). When considering whom to include in the identified patient's treatment, providers should carefully consider which family members are most important to the child because extended family members (grandparents, aunts and uncles, cousins), play a central role in most Latinx youths' lives.

Stigma can be a powerful barrier to timely access to psychiatric care. In many cultures, mental illness has major negative connotations, leading to the fear of *double discrimination* (as a result of being culturally different and perceived as "crazy"), which prevents minority families from accessing services (Pumariega et al. 2013). In addition, culturally diverse families are more vulnerable to perceived or actual power differentials with respect to health care professionals. They may mistrust mental health services, given the history of discrimination and disregard for cultural needs. Some Latinx patients might reject the physician's advice out of fear of being "tricked" or "overmedicated." Other Latinx patients might be reticent to trust providers who practice medicine by promoting autonomy instead of paternalism. In fact, many patients and families might even request a medication or believe that unless they leave the office with a prescription, the visit was a waste of time. Clinicians should therefore be attentive to the different perceptions around medications as well as address the realities and perceptions of power differentials that may interfere with therapeutic relationships (Alegría et al. 2010b).

It has been posited that differences in perceived need may contribute to underutilization of mental health services among minorities (Ruiz 1993). There is considerable difference between Hispanic adults and non-Hispanic whites when it comes to the presence of an underlying psychiatric disorder and the perception that one needs help (Jang et al. 2014). Latinos, especially those with low incomes, often interpret symptoms as normal responses to stressful life situations and tend to report somatic symptoms in the face of psychiatric disorders (Cabassa et al. 2008). This can lead to delays in appropriate and/or specialized care as well as mischaracterization of illness.

Providers should remember that individuals from Latinx subgroups will experience medical and psychiatric symptoms differently depending on each subgroup's history of origin, particular values, and even effects of immigration. The symptom profile and/or ability to seek care for Latinx youth might vary greatly depending on which subgroup the patient and family identify with. Recognizing and adopting intersectional approaches to understanding perceived need within Latinx communities might help uncover social processes that lead to disparities in mental health care. Exploring the patient's and family's migration history and acculturation experiences will provide important information about premigration socioeconomic and political circumstances, which, in turn, will inform the clinical formulation and help create individualized treatments. Treatment considerations when caring for Latinx youth are presented in Table 5–3.

Conclusion

Latinx culture can serve as a buffer by promoting values within the family and through the community that can serve as sources of resilience and potentially even protect Latinx youth against physical and mental illness. Latinx children are extremely resilient despite risk and adversity and usually have the advantage of linguistic competence in both Spanish and English. In treatment of adolescents, family-based interventions with exploration of intergenerational and intercultural conflicts are effective, underscoring the importance of open dialogue and communication (Sullivan et al. 2007). Development of educational and health care strength-based models integrating and promoting Latinx culture-based and individual attributes will positively impact behavioral, emotional, and academic well-being of future generations of Latinx youth.

TABLE 5–3. Treatment considerations with Latinx patients

Narrative therapy

Therapy focuses on stories or narratives created by the individual to make sense of their world (White 2007)

Narratives are self "constructed" through culturally mediated social interactions and can convey how people perceive themselves (White and Epston 1990)

Construction of their own narrative can lead to problematic behavior and distress if patients believe that "the problems of their lives are a reflection of certain truths about their nature and their character" (White 2007, p. 9)

Goals of treatment:

1. Help the patient separate from problematic narratives by questioning pervasive cultural assumptions and by challenging internalized stories of discrimination

2. Empower the patient to create a more constructive narrative of their life

Importance for Latinx youth and families:

- Latinx families benefit most from treatments like narrative therapy because of the attention to contextual and environmental factors (Taylor et al. 2006)

- Narrative therapy can provide Latinx adolescents space to explore and help them externalize themes of discrimination, acculturative stress, and mental health issues

- Narrative therapy empowers Latinx youth to identify new and alternative narratives, exerting new meanings of their Latinx heritage

Ethnic matching

Matching between patients and therapists is based on ethnicity

Studies in adults have yielded mixed results, and there is scarce research for treatment of children and adolescents, but it has been linked to achieving culturally sensitive treatments (Flicker et al. 2008)

A study of almost 2,000 children and adolescents in community mental health centers found no difference among ethnicities, age groups, or ethnic match on Global Assessment of Functioning dependent measure (Gamst et al. 2004)

Meta-analysis (Cabral and Smith 2011) found that patients tend to perceive therapists of their own race/ ethnicity somewhat more positively than other therapists, likely because of patients' belief that the therapist shares their same worldview. Ethnic matching did not affect patient's evaluation of the therapist or clinical outcomes.

Given the diversity within Latinx communities and shortage of Latinx mental health clinicians, ethnic matching can be cumbersome or unrealistic. Rather than ethnic matching, it might be more effective to provide culturally adapted treatments, taking language into consideration and having the therapist align with youngsters' and caregivers' worldview.

Providers' understanding of patients' sociocultural background as well as their ability to empathize with the child and/or families' lived experiences—likely including experiences of discrimination—will have important effects on treatment adherence and likelihood of seeking future care. Targeting efforts toward increasing clinicians' self-awareness of implicit attitudes, decreasing provider stigmatization and Latinx homogenization, and promoting care stemming from a model of cultural humility should be key components of medical education.

The Latinx community is on track to become nearly one-third of the United States population by the mid twenty-first century. In several states and cities across the country today, Latinx individuals are not the majority minority; they are majority, period. The remarkable Latinx growth upends and challenges traditional notions of what it is to be a linguistic or cultural minority in this country. With these demographic realities in mind, it behooves mental health professionals to become familiar with this heterogeneous population because cultural competence has, in essence, become clinical competence. Clinicians are not expected (although they are welcome!) to learn Spanish, but they are encouraged to approach this community and other immigrant communities with respect, humility, and legitimate curiosity and interest. We have much to learn and to give back to a community that has been in the United States for a very long time (the first Western settlers in the United States came from Spain, not England) and that is today one of the newest and neediest groups, as can be gleaned from those fighting for their lives at our southern border.

COVID-19, the Syndemic, and Latinx Communities

The novel coronavirus SARS-CoV-2 (COVID-19) has had disproportionate impacts on Latinx communities and among the poor in the United States, with higher contagion and fatality rates (Fortuna et al. 2020). Latinx children have been impacted more severely by coronavirus, with higher pediatric case rates, hospitalizations, and virus-related complications as compared with the non-Latinx white population (Aguilera 2020). These findings mirror similar reports across the nation of adults in minority communities being hit harder by COVID-19 (Webb Hooper et al. 2020). Furthermore, toxic stress resulting from racial and social inequities have been magnified during the pandemic, with implications for poor physical and mental health and socioeconomic outcomes for children and their families.

Inequities in the social determinants of health, such as poverty and poor health care access, affecting many Latinx groups are interrelated and influence a wide range of health and quality-of-life outcomes and risk during the COVID-19 pandemic (Belmonte 2020). Latinx communities are disproportionately represented in essential work settings such as health care facilities, farms, factories, grocery stores, and public transportation (U.S. Bureau of Labor Statistics 2019). Individuals who work in these settings have more chances to be exposed to the virus that causes COVID-19 because of several factors, such as close contact with the public or other workers, not being able to work from home, and not having paid sick days. Because of housing costs in urban settings, many Latinx and immigrant families frequently live in high congregate situations, further increasing the risk and degree of exposure. Children and families in immigration detention settings (Kerwin 2020) or experiencing homelessness and living in shelters (Fortuna et al. 2020) have similarly endured disproportionate risk of exposure.

Preexisting inequities in health care access, education, and mental health services have contributed to poor outcomes and increased morbidity. Disproportionate death rates among Latinx, as high as eight times the death rate of non-Latinx whites according to recent data (Webb Hooper et al. 2020), have had profound mental health and economic impacts on children. Poor access to reliable or sustainable teletechnology has worsened health care access and exacerbated gaps in educational attainment. Health care barriers, including lack of insurance and immigration fears, have contributed to worsening of preexisting health conditions (e.g. asthma, diabetes) and delay in COVID-19 treatment during acute illness and for aftercare (Adams et al. 2020). The COVID-19 pandemic, combined with racial-ethnic disparities, otherwise known as the syndemic, has highlighted the need to address the underlying disparities faced by Latinx communities. We must do a better job as mental health professionals and as a country in addressing existing socioeconomic and health care inequities, working within our profession, with health care policy, and with communities in addressing the social determinants and structural inequities and bias that place so many of our children and families at risk of poor outcomes.

Clinical Pearls

- Language switches: Be attentive to switches from English to Spanish or vice versa because they can provide important information regarding a patient's emotional states, psychological defenses, and ability to or difficulties with discussing certain topics in their native tongue versus second language.

- Assumption of linguistic intimacy trap: Spanish-speaking clinicians should not assume that because they speak the patient's language, they already know or will be able to immediately connect with Latinx patients. Just because you speak the same language as your patient does not mean you understand their worldview. Avoid falling for this common feel-good "trap." The corollary is to remain humble in all clinical encounters.

- *Familismo* (family first): Latinos' cultural value of *familismo,* which encompasses connectedness, interdependency, and strong attachment to one's family of origin, can be misunderstood and pathologized as codependency, leading to more confusion and stress among youth already struggling to balance individuation with family and cultural (ethnic) belongingness. Treatment of Latinx youth is enriched and more effective when family members are involved.

- Double discrimination and trauma: Latinx patients can often feel doubly discriminated against: not only as mentally ill but as a cultural minority as well. And it is not only their feelings that may be hurt: the rate of trauma among Latinx individuals is higher than among other groups and is likely to worsen given recent misguided and aggressive federal immigration policies, including the unconscionable forced separation of children from their parents.

Self-Assessment Questions

1. Mental health risk factors for Latinx youth differ from those of their non-Latinx counterparts in which of the following ways?

    A. They are less likely than African American youth to drop out of school.
    B. They are more likely to receive mental health services for severe ADHD as compared with white youth.
    C. They have a higher rate of suicide attempts compared with non-Latinx white youth.
    D. They demonstrate less mental health knowledge compared with white youth.

2. In regard to language development in Latinx children, all of the following are true *except*:

    A. Sequential bilinguals acquire their first language during the period of rapid language acquisition before 3 years of age.
    B. Simultaneous bilinguals acquire both languages as first languages.
    C. Most Latinx children in the United States are sequential bilinguals.
    D. There is substantial empirical support for recommending that parents discontinue exposure to Spanish at home when a child is facing learning delays in English at school.

3. Treatment considerations that could improve care with Latinx children and their families include which of the following?

    A. Assisting the patient and family with internalized stories of discrimination.
    B. Providing culturally adapted treatments taking language into consideration.
    C. Aligning with the child's and caregivers' worldview and practicing cultural humility.
    D. All of the above

4. What specific questions will you add to your usual base of interview questions to include content from this chapter?

5. How might you adjust your current rubric for patient conceptualization to include these concepts?

6. As you reflect, how does the information in this chapter inform your future practice?

Answers

1. C
2. D
3. D

References

Adams ML, Katz DL, Grandpre J: Population-based estimates of chronic conditions affecting risk for complications from coronavirus disease, United States. Emerg Infect Dis 26(8):1831–1833, 2020

Adelman L: Unnatural causes: is inequality making us sick? Prev Chronic Dis 4(4):A116, 2007

Aguilera E: The virus and the vulnerable: Latino children suffer higher rates of COVID-19. Sacramento, CA, CalMatters, July 7, 2020. Available at: https://calmatters.org/children-and-youth/2020/07/the-virus-and-the-vulnerable-latino-children-suffer-higher-rates-of-covid-19. Accessed August 12, 2020.

Alegría M, Canino G, Ríos R, et al: Mental health care for Latinos: inequalities in use of specialty mental health services among Latinos, African Americans, and non-Latino whites. Psychiatr Serv 53(12):1547–1555, 2002

Alegría M, Shrout PE, Woo M, et al: Understanding differences in past year psychiatric disorders for Latinos living in the U.S. Soc Sci Med 65(2):214–230, 2007

Alegría M, Mulvaney-Day N, Carson N, et al: A sociocultural framework for understanding the mechanisms behind behavioral health and educational service disparities in immigrant Hispanic children, in Growing Up Hispanic: Health and Development of Children of Immigrants. Edited by Landale NS, McHale S, Booth A. Washington, DC, Urban Institute Press, 2010a, pp 275–303

Alegría M, Vallas M, Pumariega AJ: Racial and ethnic disparities in pediatric mental health. Child Adolesc Psychiatr Clin N Am 19(4):759–774, 2010b

American Academy of Child and Adolescent Psychiatry: Policy statement: separating immigrant children from their families. Washington, DC, American Academy of Child and Adolescent Psychiatry, June 2018. Available at: www.aacap.org/AACAP/Policy_Statements/2018/Separating_Immigrant_Children_From_Their_Families.aspx. Accessed April 15, 2020.

American Psychiatric Association: APA statement opposing separation of children from parents at the border. Washington, DC, American Psychiatric Association, May 30, 2018. Available at: www.psychiatry.org/newsroom/news-releases/apa-statement-opposing-separation-of-children-from-parents-at-the-border. Accessed April 15, 2020.

Anda RF, Felitti VJ, Bremner JD, et al: The enduring effects of abuse and related adverse experiences in childhood: a convergence of evidence from neurobiology and epidemiology. Eur Arch Psychiatry Clin Neurosci 256(3):174–186, 2006

Annie E Casey Foundation: Children in poverty by race and ethnicity in the United States. Baltimore, MD, Kids Count Data Center 2017. Available at: https://datacenter.kidscount.org/data/tables/44-children-in-poverty-by-race-and-ethnicity?loc=1andloct=1#detailed/1/any/false/871,870,573/12,1,13/any. Accessed April 15, 2020.

Beitchman JH, Wilson B, Brownlie EB, et al: Long-term consistency in speech/language profiles, I: developmental and academic outcomes. J Am Acad Child Adolesc Psychiatry 35(6):804–814, 1996a

Beitchman JH, Wilson B, Brownlie EB, et al: Long-term consistency in speech/language profiles, II: behavioral, emotional, and social outcomes. J Am Acad Child Adolesc Psychiatry 35(6):815–825, 1996b

Belmonte A: "Structural inequalities": These areas of America are particularly vulnerable to coronavirus. Yahoo Finance, April 27, 2020. Available at: https://finance.yahoo.com/news/coronavirus-vulnerable-cdc-145303772.html. Accessed August 12, 2020.

Berg CR: Stereotyping in films in general and of the Hispanic in particular. Howard J Commun 2(3):286–300, 1990

Brabeck K, Xu Q: The impact of detention and deportation on Latino immigrant children and families: a quantitative exploration. Hisp J Behav Sci 32(3):341–361, 2010

Buss C, Entringer S, Moog NK, et al: Intergenerational transmission of maternal childhood maltreatment exposure: implications for fetal brain development. J Am Acad Child Adolesc Psychiatry 56(5):373–382, 2017

Cabassa LJ, Hansen MC, Palinkas LA, et al: Azúcar y nervios: explanatory models and treatment experiences of Hispanics with diabetes and depression. Social Sci Med 66(12):2413–2424, 2008

Cabral RR, Smith TB: Racial/ethnic matching of clients and therapists in mental health services: a meta-analytic review of preferences, perceptions, and outcomes. J Couns Psychol 58(4):537–554, 2011

Cardemil EV, Sarmiento IA: Clinical approaches to working with Latino adults, in Handbook of U.S. Latino Psychology: Developmental and Community-Based Perspectives. Edited by Villarruel FA, Carlo G, Grau JM, et al: Los Angeles, CA, Sage, 2009, pp 329–345

Chandra A, Scott MM, Jaycox LH, et al: Racial/ethnic differences in teen and parent perspectives toward depression treatment. J Adolesc Health 44(6):546–553, 2009

Colby SL, Ortman JM: Projections of the size and composition of the U.S. population: 2014 to 2060. Population estimates and projections. Current Population Rep P25-1143. Suitland, MD, U.S. Census Bureau, March 2015. Available at: www.census.gov/content/dam/Census/library/publications/2015/demo/p25-1143.pdf. Accessed April 15, 2020.

Collins BA: Dual language development of Latino children: effect of instructional program type and the home and school language environment. Early Child Res Q 29(3):389–397, 2014

Collins BA, Toppelberg CO, Suárez-Orozco C, et al: Cross-sectional associations of Spanish and English competence and well-being in Latino children of immigrants in kindergarten. Int J Soc Lang 2011(208):5–23, 2011

Congressional Research Service: The Trump Administration's "Zero Tolerance" Immigration Enforcement Policy. Washington, DC, Congressional Research Service, updated February 26, 2019. Available at: https://fas.org/sgp/crs/homesec/R45266.pdf. Accessed July 31, 2020.

Duarte CS, Bird HR, Shrout PE, et al: Culture and psychiatric symptoms in Puerto Rican children: longitudinal results from one ethnic group in two contexts. J Child Psychol Psychiatry 49(5):563–572, 2008

Ennis SR, Rios-Vargas M, Albert NG: The Hispanic population: 2010. 2010 Census Brief C2010BR-04. Suitland, MD, U.S. Census Bureau, May 2011. Available at: www.census.gov/prod/cen2010/briefs/c2010br-04.pdf. Accessed April 15, 2020.

Faber RJ, O'Guinn TC, Meyer TP: Televised portrayals of Hispanics: a comparison of ethnic perceptions. Int J Intercult Relat 11(2):155–169, 1987

Flicker SM, Waldron HB, Turner CW, et al: Ethnic matching and treatment outcome with Hispanic and Anglo substance-abusing adolescents in family therapy. J Fam Psychol 22(3):439–447, 2008

Flores A: How the U.S. Hispanic population is changing. Washington, DC, Pew Research Center, September 18, 2017. Available at: www.pewresearch.org/fact-tank/2017/09/18/how-the-u-s-hispanic-population-is-changing. Accessed September 1, 2018.

Fortuna LR, Jimenez A, Porche MV: Understanding and responding to the mental health needs of Latino youth in a cultural framework, in Cultural Sensitivity in Child and Adolescent Mental Health. Edited by Parekh R, Gorrindo T, Rubin DH. Boston, MA, MGH Psychiatry Academy, 2015, pp 155–178

Fortuna LR, Tolou-Shams M, Robles-Ramamurthy B, Porche MV: Inequity and the disproportionate impact of COVID-19 on communities of color in the United States: the need for a trauma-informed social justice response. Psychol Trauma 12(5):443–445, 2020

Freedenthal S: Racial disparities in mental health service use by adolescents who thought about or attempted suicide. Suicide Life Threat Behavior 37(1):22–34, 2007

Gamst G, Dana RH, Der-Karabetian A, et al: Ethnic match and treatment outcomes for child and adolescent mental health center clients. J Couns Dev 82(4):457–465, 2004

Garcia E, Jensen B: Early educational opportunities for children of Hispanic origins. Social Policy Report, Vol XXIII, No II. Ann Arbor, MI, Society for Research in Child Development, 2009. Available at: https://files.eric.ed.gov/fulltext/ED509217.pdf. Accessed April 15, 2020.

Genesee F, Paradis J, Crago MB (eds): Dual Language Development and Disorders: A Handbook on Bilingualism and Second Language Learning. Baltimore, MD, Paul H Brookes, 2004

Gerbner G, Gross L, Morgan M, et al: Growing up with television: cultivation processes, in Media Effects, 2nd Edition. Edited by Bryant J, Zillmann D, Oliver MB. New York, Routledge, 2002, pp 53–78

Gutiérrez KD, Zepeda M, Castro DC: Advancing early literacy learning for all children: implications of the NELP report for dual-language learners. Educational Researcher 39(4):334–339, 2010

Hook JN, Davis DE, Owen J, et al: Cultural humility: measuring openness to culturally diverse clients. J Couns Psychol 60(3):353–366, 2013

Instituto Cervantes: El español: una lengua viva. Informe 2018. Madrid, Instituto Cervantes, 2018. Available at: https://cvc.cervantes.es/lengua/espanol_lengua_viva/pdf/espanol_lengua_viva_2018.pdf. Accessed April 15, 2020.

Jang Y, Park NS, Kang SY, et al: Racial/ethnic differences in the association between symptoms of depression and self-rated mental health among older adults. Community Ment Health J 50(3):325–330, 2014

Jiménez AL, Alegría M, Camino-Gaztambide RF, et al: Cultural sensitivity: what should we understand about Latinos? in The Massachusetts General Hospital Textbook on Diversity and Cultural Sensitivity in Mental Health. Edited by Parekh R, Trinh NHT. Totowa, NJ, Humana Springer, 2019, pp 201–228

Kann L, McManus T, Harris WA, et al: Youth Risk Behavior Surveillance—United States, 2017. MMWR Surveill Summ 67(8):1–114, 2018

Kerwin D: Immigrant Detention and COVID-19: How a Pandemic Exploited and Spread through the US Immigrant Detention System. New York, Center for Migration Studies of New York, 2020. Available at: https://cmsny.org/publications/immigrant-detention-covid. Accessed August 12, 2020.

Krogstad JM, Lopez MH: Hispanic nativity shift: U.S. births drive population growth as immigration stalls. Washington, DC, Pew Research Center, April 29, 2014. Available at: www.pewhispanic.org/2014/04/29/hispanic-nativity-shift. Accessed April 15, 2020.

Lisotto MJ, Fortuna L, Powell P, et al: Media's role in mitigating culturally competent understanding of Latino youth, in Child and Adolescent Psychiatry and the Media. Edited by Beresin EV, Olson CK. Philadelphia, PA, Elsevier Health Sciences, 2018, pp 153–164

Lund C, De Silva M, Plagerson S, et al: Poverty and mental disorders: breaking the cycle in low-income and middle-income countries. Lancet 378(9801):1502–1514, 2011

Merriam-Webster: Latinx. Springfield, MA, Merriam-Webster, 2020. Available at: www.merriam-webster.com/dictionary/Latinx#h1. Accessed April 15, 2020.

McFarland J, Hussar B, Wang X, et al: Status dropout rates, in The Condition of Education 2018. NCES 2018-144. Washington, DC, National Center for Education Statistics, U.S. Department of Education, 2018, pp 136–139. Available at: https://files.eric.ed.gov/fulltext/ED583502.pdf. Accessed April 15, 2020.

McLaughlin KA, Greif JG, Alegría M, et al: Food insecurity and mental disorders in a national sample of U.S. adolescents. J Am Acad Child Adolescent Psychiatry 51(12):1293–1303, 2012

Merikangas KR, He J, Burstein ME, et al: Service utilization for lifetime mental disorders in U.S. adolescents: results of the National Comorbidity Survey Adolescent Supplement (NCS-A). J Am Acad Child Adolescent Psychiatry 50(1):32–45, 2011

National Center for Educational Statistics: Indicator 6: elementary and secondary enrollment, in Status and Trends in the Education of Racial and Ethnic Groups. Washington, DC, National Center for Education Statistics, 2017. Available at: https://nces.ed.gov/programs/raceindicators/indicator_rbb.asp. Accessed April 15, 2020.

Oller DK, Pearson BZ, Cobo-Lewis AB: Profile effects in early bilingual language and literacy. Appl Psycholinguist 28(2):191–230, 2007

Pumariega AJ, Rothe E, Mian A, et al: Practice parameter for cultural competence in child and adolescent psychiatric practice. J Am Acad Child Adolescent Psychiatry 52(10):1101–1115, 2013

Qureshi A, Collazos F, Ramos M, et al: Cultural competency training in psychiatry. Eur Psychiatry 23(suppl 1):49–58, 2008

Rideout VJ, Foehr UG, Roberts DF: Generation M2: Media in the Lives of 8-to 18-Year-Olds. Menlo Park, CA, Henry J. Kaiser Family Foundation, January 2010. Available at: https://files.eric.ed.gov/fulltext/ED527859.pdf. Accessed April 15, 2020.

Rothe EM, Tzuang D, Pumariega AJ: Acculturation, development, and adaptation. Child Adolesc Psychiatr Clin N Am 19(4):681–696, 2010

Ruiz P: Access to health care for uninsured Hispanics: policy recommendations. Hosp Community Psychiatry 44(10):958–962, 1993

Smedley BD, Stith AY, Nelson AR (eds): Unequal Treatment: Confronting Racial and Ethnic Disparities in Health Care. Institute of Medicine, Committee on Understanding and Eliminating Racial and Ethnic Disparities in Health Care. Washington, DC, National Academies Press, 2003

Sullivan S, Schwartz SJ, Prado G, et al: A bidimensional model of acculturation for examining differences in family functioning and behavior problems in Hispanic immigrant adolescents. J Early Adolesc 27(4):405–430, 2007

Taylor BA, Gambourg MB, Rivera M, et al: Constructing cultural competence: perspectives of family therapists working with Latino families. Am J Family Ther 34(5):429–445, 2006

Taylor P, Lopez MH, Martinez J, et al: When labels don't fit: Hispanics and their views of identity. Washington, DC, Pew Research Center, April 4, 2012. Available at: www.pewhispanic.org/2012/04/04/when-labels-dont-fit-hispanics-and-their-views-of-identity. Accessed April 15, 2020.

Toppelberg CO, Collins BA: Language, culture, and adaptation in immigrant children. Child Adolesc Psychiatr Clin N Am 19(4):697–717, 2010

Toppelberg CO, Shapiro T: Language disorders: a 10-year research update review. J Am Acad Child Adolesc Psychiatry 39(2):143–152, 2000

Toppelberg CO, Medrano L, Morgens LP, et al: Bilingual children referred for psychiatric services: associations of language disorders, language skills, and psychopathology. J Am Acad Child Adolescent Psychiatry 41(6):712–722, 2002

Toppelberg CO, Munir K, Nieto-Castañon A: Spanish-English bilingual children with psychopathology: language deficits and academic language proficiency. Child Adolesc Mental Health 11(3):156–163, 2006

Umaña-Taylor AJ, Updegraff KA: Latino adolescents' mental health: exploring the interrelations among discrimination, ethnic identity, cultural orientation, self-esteem, and depressive symptoms. J Adolesc 30(4):549–567, 2007

U.S. Bureau of Labor Statistics: Labor force characteristics by race and ethnicity, 2018. Washington, DC, U.S. Bureau of Labor Statistics, October 2019. Available at: www.bls.gov/opub/reports/race-and-ethnicity/2018/home.htm. Accessed August 13, 2020.

Webb Hooper M, Nápoles AM, Pérez-Stable EJ: COVID-19 and racial/ethnic disparities. JAMA 323(24):2466–2467, 2020

White MK: Externalizing conversations, in Maps of Narrative Practice. New York, WW Norton, 2007, pp 9–60

White M, Epston D: Story, knowledge, and power, in Narrative Means to Therapeutic Ends. New York, WW Norton, 1990, pp 1–37

CHAPTER 6

The Role of Culture, Stigma, and Bias on the Mental Health of Arab American Youth

Balkozar Adam, M.D.

Omar M. Mahmood, Ph.D.

ARAB Americans are residents of the United States who trace their heritage and ethnic origin to one of 22 countries in an area most commonly described as the Middle East and North Africa, as well as the African countries of Somalia, Djibouti, and Eritrea. Representing various countries, religions, and races, Arab Americans are one of the most diverse ethnic groups in the United States (Abuelezam et al. 2018; Amer and Hovey 2007). Their skin color can vary from fair to dark, and they may identify as white, black, or brown. The term *Arab* is broad and encompasses wide cultural variations, but unifying factors include language, cultural identity, geography, and historic experiences (Abuelezam et al. 2018; Amer and Hovey 2007).

Arab Americans are considered relatively recent immigrants to the United States, arriving before the turn of the nineteenth century (Amer and Hovey 2007; Semaan 2013; Suleiman 2010). They migrated primarily in three waves, with the first group arriving more than a century ago between the late 1800s and World War I. This wave came primarily from Greater Syria. The majority were Christian, and many were farmers or merchants. The second wave, comprising many professionals and students, arrived around the time of World War II in the early to mid-1940s. The passage of the Immigration and Nationality Act of 1965 paved the way for the third wave. Many Arabs, along with other non-Europeans, immigrated to the United States during this time. Some came to escape political instability or join family already in the country, whereas others came to study or had specialized skills they hoped would offer them a stable economic future. It is worth noting that a more recent fourth wave began arriving in 2010 after the so-called Arab Spring, with many arriving as refugees.

The Arab region is the birthplace of the three major world religions, and, as such, Arab Americans include Muslims, Christians, and Jews. Islam is the predominant religion in the Arab world, with the exception of Lebanon. The Pew Research Center reported that 93% of the Arab population is made up of Muslims, and Christians make up 4% of the population of the Middle East and Africa (Wormald 2016). Given the first migration wave, however, the majority of Arab Americans are Christian (Naff 1980). The Arab identity is closely associated with Islam, in part because Arabic is the language of the Qur'an, Islam's holy book. Arab Americans of all religions often struggle with teaching their children Arabic in a country where it is not the dominant language. Some parents struggle to find the time or resources to teach their children a second language; others opt for weekend or full-time schools to help preserve the language and culture. The assimilation process also plays a role. Some parents decide against teaching their children Arabic in hopes of their children fitting in better, and some children clash with their parents over speaking a foreign language.

There are an estimated 3.6 million Arab Americans living in the United States (Arab American Institute Foundation 2018). However, the exact number of Arab Americans is not known because they may be reluctant to identify themselves as being of Arab descent out of concern for possible negative social repercussions. Another complicating factor is that the U.S. Census Bureau classifies Arab Americans as white, which affects their consideration as a minority group (Beydoun 2016). There has been a push in recent years to add a Middle East or North Africa category to the census, but officials announced it would not occur in time for the 2020 census.

Traditional Arab Culture

Family, respect, spirituality, generosity, honor, and education are some common Arab American values. Family is at the center of Arab American culture, and the father is often considered the head of the family. Although traditional Arab culture is both patriarchal and hierarchical, the mother also has an esteemed place in the family. Elders in general, ranging from parents to grandparents or great-grandparents, are to be respected. It is not unusual to see multiple generations of Arab Americans living together in the same house, especially in metropolitan areas with large Arab American populations such as New York, Detroit, Los Angeles, and Chicago. The culture is a collectivist one that values family and community over the individual. Communities often form around country of origin, making it easier for community members to bond over their shared traditions, dialects, and food.

In Arab American families, the mother's role has traditionally been one of caretaker. Raising and teaching the children are seen as primarily her responsibility, although some Arab American families have seen a shift away from the traditional roles in recent years. An increasing number of women are pursuing careers outside the home, and familial duties now often are split between husband and wife. The mother has an elevated status in Islam, which often is reflected in the respect and attention she is given in the family. Children are viewed as a gift from God to be treasured, nurtured, and protected. Boys, especially firstborn, are expected to care for their parents when they grow old and help them financially if needed. The sons carry the family name, and some parents are known by their eldest son's name (e.g., "Father of Omar," "Mother of Khalid"). In many Arab American families, boys are given fewer responsibilities inside the home and more freedom to stay out late. They are seen as the protectors of their sisters, who were traditionally expected to live at home until they got married. However, this trend also is changing.

Education is highly valued in Arab American communities in part because of the emphasis on seeking knowledge and in part because of the financial stability it can provide for the family. Statistically, Arab Americans far exceed Western Americans in obtaining postgraduate education (Wingfield 2006). More than 40% of Arab Americans are college educated, which is significantly higher than the roughly 25% of Americans who earned their college degrees (Wingfield 2006). A similar pattern is seen in graduate education, with 17% of Arab Americans obtaining an advanced degree compared with 9% for their American counterparts (Wingfield 2006).

Many Arab Americans work to balance their traditional values with American values, but it can be a challenge, especially when it comes to religion. Arab Americans, whether Christian, Muslim, or Jewish, tend to value spirituality and the moral guidance it can provide. Putting those teachings into practice may create dissonance as individuals toggle between American and Arab cultures. Arab Americans who also are Muslim are asked to dress and act modestly, which can present and be interpreted in many vastly different ways. Some women choose to wear hijab, a headscarf that covers their hair. Some may cover their hair with a turban or hat. Some women wear an abaya, a long dress, while others wear hijab with jeans. Some do not cover their hair at all. This personal choice is informed by spirituality, culture, identity, and often family.

In Muslim Arab American communities, modesty is expected from both genders (Odeh Yosef 2008). This has encouraged some individuals to focus on developing a deeper, more authentic self. However, it also has hindered some female youth from accessing family planning or obtaining information about safe sex (Munro-Kramer et al. 2016). The focus on modesty and chastity also may influence the decision by teenagers and young adults to abstain from sex before marriage, decreasing the risk for sexually transmitted infections and unplanned pregnancies. From a religious perspective, Islam prohibits premarital sex. From a cultural lens, premarital sex is considered disreputable, especially for women. As with other Arab American cultural norms, the double standard between men and women is pronounced when it comes to premarital sex. This can lead to some families turning a blind eye when their son engages in sexual relations outside marriage, but traditional Arab American families do not tolerate the same from their daughters.

Connection with extended family and a feeling of responsibility to one's family have been shown to protect against sexual and other risk behaviors in other cultures (Barry and Murray 2006). For example, research has shown that modesty and duty to family promote abstinence before marriage among adolescent girls and young women in Latino communities (Barry and Murray 2006). Many Arab Americans tend to feel a heightened loyalty to their families, and in Arab American youth, spirituality and sexual activities are significantly related, such that those who reported high spirituality were less likely to participate in sexual activities (Munro-Kramer et al. 2016). Those who engage in minimal health risk behaviors are more likely to be abstinent, have experienced positive life events, and have supportive systems in their lives.

Given their cultural expectations and values, Arab American youth may not want to discuss their sexual activities or disclose high-risk behaviors. Male youth are more likely than female youth to be sexually active. In addition, Arab American youth, especially males, have slightly higher rates of smoking than their non-Arab peers. Unfortunately, the stigma surrounding mental illness in the Arab American community persists. As noted, honor is an important concept in Arab American families. If a youth feels his or her action might embarrass the family, he or she may not want to share that action with the treating clinician. Therefore, it is important to emphasize confidentiality and to be open and nonjudgmental. Practicing cultural humility will help promote a candid and honest dialogue.

Immigration and Acculturation

Like other marginalized groups, Arab Americans have faced a history of prejudice and discrimination. Long before the September 11 attacks, Arab Americans were the victims of hate crimes, housing discrimination, media bias, and workplace prejudice. From movies to cartoons, they were portrayed as terrorists or oppressed daughters and wives. The men were characterized as violent and uncivilized, and the women ostensibly lived to serve them and had no agency over their lives. These negative depictions go back decades and have a dehumanizing effect (Shaheen 2015).

Discrimination and hate crimes against Arab Americans increased post–September 11 (Ibish and Stewart 2003). Racial and ethnic profiling produced the term "flying while Arab," a modification of "driving while Black" (Baker 2002). Children and adults alike have internalized these harmful images, acts, words, and experiences. This causes a ripple effect that negatively impacts cultural identity development, a phenomenon that is consistent with the experiences of other marginalized groups throughout U.S. history (Ogbuagu 2013). Finding the strength to dismiss the stereotypes and fight against discrimination so deeply entrenched in the society at large has been challenging. One study, which found that Arab Americans look to community for support, highlighted the connection between increased sense of ethnic identity, elevated self-esteem, and decreased depression (Fakih 2013).

Arab American youth in particular face an increased risk of the damaging effects of Islamophobia. Anti-Arab sentiment has been linked to negative mental health outcomes, including psychological distress and decreased happiness (Samari 2016). Arab American children experience bullying, depression, and anxiety. Girls have had their hijabs pulled off. Some youth have questioned their identity, abused substances, and had suicidal thoughts. However, research shows that Arab American youth are less likely to seek the psychological help they need (Jaber et al. 2015). Given the sociopolitical climate, more recent Arab immigrants to the United States who take part in cross-border media consumption (watching media from home) may experience increased mental health problems compared with more established Arab Americans (Samari 2016).

Immigration can compound the effects of Islamophobia. Arab American immigrants may have experienced trauma and stress before, during, and after migration. They struggle with the loss of their homeland, family, and friends they left behind and feeling unwelcome in their new land. Interestingly, a study by Amer and Hovey (2007) found that Christian patterns of acculturation and mental health were consistent with acculturation theory, but Muslim integration was not associated with better mental health. Religiosity was predictive of better family functioning and less depression. Experience with social injustice may bias them against a mental health professional who is not Arab American or familiar with Arab culture. They also may feel the provider is capable but is unable to understand their specific culture-related issues or provide them with the support they need. This creates an additional barrier for Arab Americans seeking care (Amer and Hovey 2007).

If they are able to get past that obstacle, Arab American youth want a clinician who can provide culturally sensitive care. Some Arab American patients are reluctant to express their emotional issues out of fear that doing so will reflect poorly on them or their culture. They also do not want to feel that they are validating prejudices or reinforcing stereotypes. It may take longer for them to trust their clinicians. In addition, some Arab Americans may feel more comfortable with a provider who is the same gender as them.

Some new immigrants may genuinely feel that they do not need treatment. They survived war and persecution and may minimize their symptoms in comparison. They may feel that many of their friends and family experienced similar trauma but did not seek treatment, so why should they? However, research shows that their experience with war and trauma places them at greater risk for mental health disorders. It is well documented that immigrants who have experienced such trauma are at increased risk for depression, anxiety, and PTSD (Abuelezam et al. 2018). However, political instability in their region of origin may prevent some immigrants from sharing their thoughts out of fear that the information may somehow reach their country of origin and negatively affect the family members who remain there.

Acculturation stress and language barriers add to Arab Americans' vulnerability to mental illness. However, the overall prevalence of depression and other adverse mental health outcomes in Arab Americans is still relatively unknown. A study of Arab American adolescents living in Dearborn, Michigan, estimated that 14% of the respondents endorsed clinically significant symptoms of depression (Jaber et al. 2015). Additional research has noted the preference of Arab Americans to receive emotional support from their families and hesitancy to get that support from outside their families (Martin 2014).

Adolescence

Arab American youth have many protective factors to help them navigate their daily life. Arab American youth rely on their families and communities for social support (Fakih 2013). The extended family may provides stability, emotional support, guidance, and financial assistance. In a collectivist culture, the extended family is an important source of support to youth. In addition, religious values, among other important factors, contribute to the psychological well-being of Arab Americans.

Those factors are often at odds with the many risk factors facing Arab American youth. Arab American youth are often the subject of discrimination, marginalization, microaggressions, and bullying because of their ethnicity. Although the current political climate has led to heightened concerns, stigmatization and discrimination of Arab Americans have been on the rise for two decades (Abuelezam et al. 2018). Discrimination based on religious affiliation or ethnicity may lead some Arab American Muslim youth to attempt to conceal their identity (Amer and Hovey 2007). One common practice is the use of a nickname that does not sound like an Arab name, such as Mohammad being shortened to Mo. Women who wear hijab may instead use a hat or turban to cover their hair.

Although adolescents and parents may face the acculturation process together, adolescents are typically able to master the acculturation process before their parents do. This may reflect the adolescents' cognitive abilities and emotional flexibility. Role reversal may occur when the parents count on their children to communicate with others. This may be seen in small or large interactions, ranging from ordering food at a restaurant to translating court documents.

Smoking in general is a concern among Arab American youth. Water pipe smoking, known as hookah, is a cultural practice that has endured. A pilot study of American Muslim college students of predominantly Arab and South Asian backgrounds found that lifetime hookah smoking was reported by almost half the participants (Arfken et al. 2015). One study found that high schoolers were more likely to smoke hookah, which contains tobacco, if someone in the family did (Weglicki et al. 2008). Although hookah smoking used to be more common in young men, their female counterparts are closing that gap. Religiosity, and the Islamic teaching strongly discouraging smoking, is not a deterrent (Arfken et al. 2015). Acculturation studies of Arab American adults linked the connection with Arab culture to increased smoking (Jadalla and Lee 2012). Smoking is prevalent in the Middle East, which normalized it for many youth who grew up around it. Historically, cigarettes have been relatively easy to access in much of the Arab world. They are used as a way to cope with stress and trauma and are viewed as the lesser evil compared with drugs and alcohol.

Some Arab American youth, however, have moved beyond tobacco. The extent to which this is happening is virtually unknown because of the dearth of research on his issue. One study by the Family and Youth Institute (Abu-Ras et al. 2010) found that nearly 50% of American Muslim college students who participated in the study reported consuming alcohol in the past 12 months. Despite religious teachings or cultural expectations, Arab American youth are at risk for substance abuse. As such, providers need to develop proper interventions and continue research on this subject.

Such interventions should cover the role of the family. Many parents are unaware of the adolescent's substance use issue until there is outside involvement with the school, police, or other officials. The use of alcohol and drugs is considered shameful in many Arab American families, especially for Muslim Arab Americans because of the religious prohibition against the substances. The parents' feeling of disappointment and shame may exacerbate the youth's negative feelings. In addition, the stigma surrounding substance abuse and mental health treatment often means families typically do not seek professional help until the issue has reached a critical point.

Arab American parents may be uncomfortable discussing issues around intimate relationships. Dating is a taboo in some Arab American families. As a result, teenagers may resort to secret online relationships. If they meet someone at school or around town, they often will try to keep that relationship hidden. The secrecy and shame can lead to the youth staying in an abusive relationship. Youth may also struggle with depression and suicidal ideation if they are going through a breakup alone. Still, in order to avoid negative repercussions, they may prefer to suffer in silence rather than sharing the relationship with their family. If family members discover the youth's depression, they may prefer to deal with it as a family unit.

Stigma

Perhaps the greatest obstacle to seeking treatment is stigma. This comes as no surprise given the broader stigma around mental health care. That stigma is heightened by some Arab Americans' perception that seeking therapeutic interventions could bring shame to the family or that it is somehow an affront to God's will. Unfortunately, these perceptions may persist across Arab American communities despite immigration status or religious affiliation. Many new immigrants bring with them a tainted and distorted understanding of mental illness from their home country. They often view mental disorders as a personal shortfall or disgrace. Usually, they do not think of a spectrum of disorders but instead perceive any level of emotional struggle as a severe psychiatric illness that may require hospitalization. The premigration and postmigration traumas experienced by Arab American immigrants are intertwined with higher psychological stress observed post–September 11. This may vary depending on country of origin. For example, Iraqi refugees report higher incidence of PTSD. Unfortunately, Iraqi refugees also report a number of barriers to seeking care for their children, including lack of insurance, provider availability, and language barriers (Vermette et al. 2014).

Other Arab Americans may link mental illness to supernatural forces. For example, some Muslims may see mental illness as a punishment from God for their bad deeds or a test that they need to be patient with until He wills it to be resolved. The concept of the "evil eye" is prevalent in some Arab American communities. They refer to it as *hasad* and may wear khamsa jewelry (referring to the five fingers of a hand) to block someone's envy. Some also believe in black magic, jinn, and demonic possession, which are all used to explain someone's behavior or mental status rather than accepting a mental health diagnosis.

If symptoms continue, individuals may seek help from the community, whether through a healer, a religious leader, or a revered elder or family member. They may prefer natural interventions such as black seed or honey or other dietary modifications. They want to avoid the embarrassment of having other people, including family members and friends, discover that they went to a clinician for what they perceive is a nonmedical problem. They also may fear the finality of a mental health diagnosis. This is concerning because, as noted earlier, Arab Americans—and especially youth—are at high risk for mental illness and substance use disorders. One study found that half of the respondents met depression criteria (Amer and Hovey 2012).

Arab American parents may have difficulty accepting a psychiatric diagnosis, especially if they are new immigrants or refugees. Relying on mental health services may be perceived as an inability to cope with "weakness" or resolve emotional issues within the confines of the family; therefore, there is pervasive reluctance to seek mental health support outside the family structure (Martin 2014). Arabs may view help-seeking behavior as a threat to the group or as disloyalty to the family. They may try to normalize certain behaviors, such as a child's ADHD, by pointing out other family members who have similar behaviors. The parents may get offended by a doctor's recommendation of medication, even on a trial basis, so these discussions must be handled with sensitivity and care. Parents may prefer talk therapy before any psychopharmacological intervention.

Psychosis has a negative connotation in Arab American communities. Historically, in traditional Arab communities, a person suffering from mental illnesses was considered "crazy," and the family tried to protect youth from that negative perception. Therefore, instead of seeking medical treatment, the family might ask a Muslim religious healer to make Ruqyah, reading certain prayers and verses of the Qur'an to help rid the person of the Jinn or the evil spirit. The religious healer can help the youth and parents minimize the pathology and decrease the stigma involved. Depending on the specific circumstances, it may be worth asking the family if there is a religious healer involved in conjunction with psychiatric services.

Involving the family is also a consideration. Of course, this may be pursued only if the patient is completely in agreement, separate of any familial pressure. In a collectivist culture, one of the roles of the family is to provide a neutral form of social support to its members. When an Arab patient sees a mental health provider, he or she typically will be accompanied by a family member. The family member will then often play a vital role in determining the course of treatment. While respecting this dynamic, it is imperative to ensure that the extent of family involvement does not compromise patient confidentiality. The Arab American youth may be uncomfortable working with a clinician who has social ties to the patient's family or community.

Help-Seeking and Therapeutic Considerations

In addition to the role the family plays in the care of Arab American youth, the sense of fatalism that Arab Americans have toward illness (including mental illness) plays a role in help-seeking behavior. This reflects the common conception among traditional Arab communities throughout the world that emotional and mental illness emanates from supernatural forces or God's will. This belief leads to toleration of symptomatology as a type of acquiescence to divine will (Hamdan 2008). Boulos (2011) studied the role of acculturation, ethnic identity, and religious fatalism in attitudes toward seeking psychological help among Coptic (Egyptian Christian) Arab Americans. She reported that ethnic identity and acculturation are strong predictors of fatalistic religious beliefs. Individuals who identify as having greater Arab ethnic identity and less assimilation to the dominant culture have stronger religious fatalistic beliefs than do those who identify more with Western culture and an American ethnic identity. Results showed a significant negative relationship between stigma and attitudes toward counseling (Boulos 2011). Smith (2011), who sampled first- and second-generation Muslim Arab Americans, found that stigma and negative feelings regarding counseling prevent involvement in therapy. These include the beliefs that mental health workers may not honor confidentiality, that they may be biased, and that they may lack specific culture competency training (Smith 2011). Boulos (2011) reported that Christian Arab Americans tend to be skeptical of the formal mental health system and prefer to seek emotional support and help from their family and religious leaders.

Significant negative self-stigma and negative attitudes toward counseling are found in the Arab American population. Avoidance of counseling may be a result of wanting to save face for the family and protecting the family's image. Therefore, psychoeducation and empowering Arab American patients is recommended (Soheilian and Inman 2009). Public education forums about the importance of psychological health are also recommended.

The journey to mental health treatment for many Arab Americans begins with their primary care physician. Many Arab Americans may be more accepting of discussing depression and anxiety with their primary care physician, who also may recognize the somatic presentation of the mental illness (Eldeeb 2017). Arab Americans have a tendency to display emotional pain through physical complaints (Erickson and al-Timimi 2001). If the symptoms are so severe that they are able to overcome the stigma and go to a mental health provider, they may prefer a therapist who adopts more of an expert role rather than a patient-centered approach (Erickson and al-Timimi 2001). Some may expect detailed advice and explicit directions.

One significant complication is that many mental health practitioners report feeling less competent working with Arab Americans compared with other ethnic groups (Sabbah et al. 2009). There remains a lack of knowledge and research-based expertise when it comes to Arab American culture and practices. The use of a cultural broker has been recommended for people of minority cultures (Singh et al. 1999) and may help with Arab patients; al-Krenawi and Graham (2001) advocated for the use of a cultural mediator to broker contact between the formal mental health system and Arab patients who have traditional perspectives on mental health. A person who is intimately familiar with the patient's culture or who is a member of that culture could help to make the available mental health treatment more culturally relevant (al-Krenawi and Graham 2001).

Working with Arab American patients demands a high level of cultural competency and sensitivity (al-Krenawi and Graham 2000; Graham et al. 2010). The DSM-5 Outline for Cultural Formulation and Cultural Formulation Interview (American Psychiatric Association 2013) are particularly helpful in incorporating ethnographic techniques into the clinical encounter. The "Practice Parameter for Cultural Competency in Child and Adolescent Psychiatry Practice" (Pumariega et al. 2013) consists of principles that include bias, language, use of interpreters, immigration, traditional extended families, and cultural strengths; these principles are listed in Table 1–4 in Chapter 1, "Introduction to Cultural Psychiatry." Each of these tools is of value in the assessment of Arab American youth.

Case Examples

One of the best ways to increase cultural humility and proficiency is by becoming more familiar with Arab Americans and their distinct experiences. This is a heterogeneous population, and no two cases are exactly alike. Three individual cases are included that illustrate various aspects of Arab American mental health care.

Clinical Vignette 1

Layla is a 16-year-old female. She is a refugee from Iraq who left the country with her parents and two younger siblings when she was 14. The family had been living in a village that was completely destroyed by ISIS. Layla was referred to a male primary care physician by the Christian social service agency that sponsored the family's resettlement in the United States. Her mother, Mrs. Sadiq, denied a history of abuse of Layla or any history of mental illness in the family.

Mrs. Sadiq asked the primary care physician for vitamins because Layla had been failing her classes in the past year, which was unusual considering how well she did in school in Iraq. Mrs. Sadiq refused to allow the physician to see Layla alone because she had always been with her daughter during all previous doctor visits. Layla grew upset at her mother and lashed out, telling her to stop taking her to "weird places." It was later learned she was referring to a folk healer.

With her mother present, Layla described how she withdrew from her family and school. She isolated herself and was easily agitated, sometimes even abusive, to her younger siblings. The primary care physician found no physical reasons for the symptoms. He noted an odd affect and observed that Layla wore a bracelet with blue beads and a necklace with a hand charm with foreign writing.

Mrs. Sadiq later reported that she was concerned about her daughter's behavior. Layla talked to herself when nobody was around and sometimes smiled for no apparent reason. Her parents believed somebody who remained in Iraq was jealous of Layla and her family for being fortunate enough to come to America. They started reading verses from the Qur'an and made special supplications, then blew on Layla's face, all in hopes of ridding her of the "evil eye." Layla, however, thought that her parents were trying to harm her with these rituals. She continued to show signs of depression. She lost weight and missed school. When the support provided by the religious healer was insufficient, Mrs. Sadiq agreed to a trial of a low dose of antidepressant medication. The family noted some improvement in Layla's moods and allowed the physician to further adjust her medication. Layla was successfully treated for major depression with psychotic features.

Clinical Vignette 2

Mona is a 17-year-old Arab American female whose mother found her cutting in her bathroom one evening. She was brought to the emergency department by her parents and was observed overnight before she and her family agreed to a safety plan. During the initial evaluation, several psychosocial stressors were identified. Mona reported she argued constantly with her father about several of her life choices, including what career she hopes to pursue, whom she socializes with, and how she dresses. Mona endorsed significant depressive symptoms and frequent thoughts about death.

Mona's family identifies as religiously conservative Muslims. Mona does not consider herself to be "practicing," but she still holds on to many of the beliefs and teachings of Islam. She stated that her belief that suicide results in being sent to hell was the one thing that prevented her from attempting suicide. Her parents were understandably shocked by just how much emotional turmoil Mona was reporting because the topic of psychological distress had never been discussed in the family. When asked about family history, Mona's father stated that he has two sisters who may have depression but were never treated by any mental health professional.

Mona's symptoms were so severe that the emergency department psychiatrist decided to recommend psychopharmacological and psychotherapy treatments. Mona was agreeable to this, but her parents were reluctant and preferred to seek help from traditional healers in their religious community.

Moving forward, a considerable amount of psychoeducation is needed to provide both Mona and her parents with an understanding of what therapy entails and to clear up many misconceptions they may have about mental illness. The treatment team will have to be flexible, perhaps starting with talk therapy alone, building trust and a therapeutic alliance and being open to allowing the family to simultaneously seek traditional treatments from religious scholars in the community. The therapy also will have to address Mona's bicultural struggles as a child of Arab immigrants who was brought up in a conservative household but goes to public schools and has adopted many of the mainstream views of her peers in the greater society. Family work will also be beneficial in helping the parents communicate better with their daughter, learn how to identify depressive symptoms and warning signs, and accept that psychiatric illness is a real phenomenon that has diagnostic criteria and empirically established treatments.

Clinical Vignette 3

Nashaat is a 15-year-old Arab American male who lives with his parents and two younger sisters. He was born on the East Coast 6 months after his father arrived in the United States to pursue a higher education degree. The family moved to the Midwest a few years ago for the father's job. They did not have any extended family in the United States but kept in touch with their family back home through visits and phone calls. While the family assimilated, they kept close ties with local Arab families. Nashaat is a good student without behavioral problems.

Over the course of several months, Nashaat's teachers noticed deterioration in his interest in academics. He also seemed to no longer care about his passion for running. He began to argue frequently with his friends, resulting in the loss of multiple friendships. At home, Nashaat refused to join the family at dinner and spent increasing amounts of time alone in his room either sleeping or on his phone or computer. He kept his blinds shut because he was worried someone might be watching him. He repeatedly shouted at his parents and sisters and felt that his parents favored his siblings. He claimed they falsely blamed him for things for which he wasn't responsible.

The family first sought support from elders and other respected Arab members of the community. The elders and community members talked to Nashaat, but his behaviors persisted. He continued to struggle with both his personal and academic life. The school administrators recommended seeing a doctor for an evaluation. With much hesitancy, Nashaat went to see a psychiatrist. After the psychiatrist reassured Nashaat that what he said would be confidential, Nashaat told him that he was possessed by demons. He said he had betrayed his parents' trust by watching pornography, and that was why the demons took over his soul. He was sure that he deserved the punishment because everything leading up to it was his own doing.

The psychiatrist used the DSM-5 Cultural Formulation Interview (CFI; American Psychiatric Association 2013) to understand the impact of cultural beliefs on Nashaat's presentation. The use of the core version and the Informant Version of the CFI helped the psychiatrist realize that Nashaat was presenting with depression, not schizophrenia.

Nashaat's case reflects a number of common themes related to mental health treatment in Arab American communities: Nashaat linked his mental condition to supernatural forces, he considered his symptoms as punishment for his deeds, and his family initially went to nonmedical providers for assistance. In fact, another member of his community reported a similar experience. Understanding the sociocultural context of patients can help clarify key points, such as that Nashaat's symptoms were consistent with depression, not schizophrenia. It helps guard against misdiagnosis and lead to appropriate treatment.

Conclusion

Arab Americans are a relatively recent immigrant group to the United States. They are a heterogeneous group who are predominantly Christian and Muslim and trace their origin to 22 different countries in the Middle East and North Africa. Some Arab Americans were forced to flee war and persecution in recent years. Others are the descendants of immigrants who arrived in the United States more than a century ago. Some came to pursue work opportunities or advanced education. All of these individuals came to this country in search of a better life for themselves and their families. The stressors they face, in addition to the acculturation process, may leave youth struggling with depression, anxiety, PTSD, substance abuse, and bicultural identity, among other issues. In addition, many Arab Americans have faced discrimination and marginalization.

Although Arab American youth have specific stressors and risks for mental illness, they also have a number of protective factors, including ethnic identity, religiosity, and being part of a collectivist culture. Traditional Arab culture emphasizes the role of the family, which is both a protective and a risk factor. Stigma, limited awareness of mental illness, a sense of fatalism, and an emphasis on not bringing shame or embarrassment to the family may keep Arab American youth from seeking mental health treatment. To better serve this population clinically, more research is needed on the prevalence of various psychiatric disorders and risk-taking behaviors. There has been some recent growth in research on the mental health of American Muslim adolescents; however, most study samples include a mixture of races and ethnicities (e.g., South Asian, Arab, Black), which makes it difficult to draw conclusions that are unique to Arab American youth. In order to increase the chances for successful treatment, the clinician should understand the nuances of Arab culture and be trained in providing culturally competent care. Sample interview questions and cultural expectations to consider are listed in Tables 6–1 and 6–2, respectively.

TABLE 6–1. Possible interview questions

How do you identify ethnically? Religiously? Culturally?

What role does culture play in your life?

What are your expectations regarding treatment?

Is there anything you want me to know before we move forward?

Do you think your culture or religion could affect your treatment process? If so, how?

Have you faced harassment or experienced discrimination based on your culture, ethnicity, or religion?

Do you feel that you struggle to fit in? If so, how?

Do you feel accepted in America? Why or why not?

What causes you stress in your life?

How would you describe your relationship with your family and extended family?

TABLE 6–2. Phrases and cultural expectations to consider

When you have a Muslim Arab American patient

- Some Muslim patients may prefer a clinician who is the same gender.
- Some patients may not feel comfortable shaking hands with someone of the opposite gender. It is recommended to wait and see if the patient or family members extend their hands first.
- Some patients may be reluctant to have the session in a closed-door setting. It is important to ask what physical setting would be most comfortable for the patient (i.e., to be seen separately or to have a family member present).
- Confidentiality remains critical, and permission from the patient to obtain and share information with the parents is necessary to ensure that confidentiality is not jeopardized.
- It is important not to make assumptions based on dress, such as whether a woman wears hijab. Spirituality, experiences, and values will vary widely.

For Arab Americans in general

- Remember how powerful and persistent stigma can be. It is one of the primary reasons that Arab Americans are hesitant to seek mental health treatment.
- The family's reputation and honor are a primary concern. Therefore, it is critical for the provider to stress confidentiality.
- Work on building rapport before asking questions about sexual behavior, substance use, or other issues that may be considered invasive or that can trigger feelings of shame.
- A lack of familiarity with Western approaches may make the patient and family wary of treatment. It may be helpful to explain the interview process to the patient and family at the initial meeting and describe what to expect in order to help establish an environment of trust and comfort.
- The family may want to be heavily involved in the treatment. Assess the benefits and drawbacks of their involvement on a case-by-case basis, but always ensure that confidentiality is never compromised.
- Evaluate the need for an interpreter or translator.
- There may be a lack of confidence in a provider who does not share the same cultural or ethnic background. It is helpful to be open and respectful while also cognizant of your own personal feelings, biases, and prejudices.
- Keep in mind that the experience of Arab Americans differs greatly depending on whether they are immigrants, refugees, or American-born.

Clinical Pearls

PRIOR TO TREATMENT

- The effects of discrimination and bias on the mental health of most Arab American teenagers are similar to those of other ethnic minority youth. General awareness of how racism impacts psychological functioning will be helpful when conceptualizing new cases.

- Clinicians must keep in mind that not all Arab American youth will present the same way. Both the role of culture and the role of individual differences in a particular patient's presentation must be considered and explored. It may be that a teenager does not agree with the views of his or her family.

DURING TREATMENT

- Stigma can have an outsize effect on a family's engagement in the treatment process. Therefore, clinicians must take advantage of the first time a patient presents because this may be the only opportunity to provide psychoeducation and guidance to the patient and family before the patient discontinues treatment prematurely.

- Accurately assessing how much acculturative stress an Arab American youth is experiencing in relation to mainstream society is critical in the clinical formulation of the case because it informs the clinician which psychosocial interventions may be needed, if any.

AFTER TREATMENT

- Connecting the patient to sources of social support and further psychoeducation in the community is helpful for monitoring at-risk patients and limiting relapse. The same external factors that may have exacerbated the mental health struggles of the youth in the first place likely will continue to exist in the community as a chronic stressor.

INTERGENERATIONAL FAMILY CONFLICT

- Arab American youth are better able to acquire a new language and can assimilate to American culture before their parents do. As a result, they may assume a parentified role, which can lead to a role reversal.

- Arab American youth often fight with their parents about clothes, relationships, education, and careers. Clinicians should be aware of any intergenerational family conflict and help the youth and the family work on resolving disagreements and improving their relationship.

Self-Assessment Questions

1. What mental health advantages do Arab American youth have from belonging to their cultural network?

2. What are some acculturative stressors faced by Arab American youth?

3. How does the culture of Arab American youth affect their clinical care?

4. What are some ways clinicians can help Arab American youth deal with discrimination?

5. How does the stigma of mental illness complicate the assessment and treatment of Arab American youth?

6. What specific questions will you add to your usual base of interview questions to include content from this chapter?

7. How might you adjust your current rubric for patient conceptualization to include these concepts?

8. As you reflect, how does the information in this chapter inform your future practice?

Answers

1. Arab American youth can gain support, confidence, and a sense of belonging from being a part of their cultural network. Being part of the cultural network also can help them develop a healthy bicultural identity. In addition, such a network can reinforce the protective factors of their culture.

2. Arab American youth struggle with a wide range of stressors depending on their personal experiences. Arab American refugees and immigrants may face challenges specific to premigration and postmigration, including PTSD, learning a different language, and understanding new cultural norms. Others who were born in the United States or who arrived at a young age may struggle with identity, self-esteem, and dissonance surrounding their family's values and those of the dominant culture. Regardless of immigration status, they may confront anti-Arab discrimination or Islamophobia. As such, they may struggle with related trauma, depression, or anxiety.

3. Arab American youth need clinicians who are culturally aware and sensitive. Arab American culture may lead youth to shy away from seeking care out of a fear that they may embarrass the family or disclose information that will reflect poorly on them, their families, or their culture. Family can be a support or barrier to care. Families often prefer to handle issues within the family unit or with help from community elders or religious leaders.

4. One step is to help youth develop positive coping strategies. For many Arab American youth, discrimination is not limited to the playground. They experience it from their teach-

ers, at the grocery store, and even from their friends. Helping them understand the effects of discrimination and how to cope can go a long way. Teachers and school staff can be partners if they are made aware of the issues.

5. Stigma is a major obstacle to marginalized groups seeking care, and Arab American youth are no different. Their reluctance to seek care in hopes of protecting the family's honor and reputation may mean they do not come in until their symptoms are severe. Once they are in care, patients and their families may not be immediately forthcoming. They may be distrustful of the clinician, afraid that he or she harbors bias against them, or concerned that the clinician is not capable of understanding the nuances of their culture.

References

Abuelezam NN, El-Sayed AM, Galea S: The health of Arab Americans in the United States: an updated comprehensive literature review. Front Public Health 6:262, 2018

Abu-Ras W, Ahmed S, Arfken CL: Alcohol use among U.S. Muslim college students: risk and protective factors. J Ethn Subst Abuse 9(3):206–220, 2010

al-Krenawi A, Graham JR: Culturally sensitive social work practice with Arab clients in mental health settings. Health Soc Work 25(1):9–22, 2000

al-Krenawi A, Graham JR: The cultural mediator: bridging the gap between a non-western community and professional social work practice. Br J Social Work 31(5):665–685, 2001

Amer MM, Hovey JD: Socio-demographic differences in acculturation and mental health for a sample of 2nd generation/early immigrant Arab Americans. J Immigr Minor Health 9(4):335–347, 2007

Amer MM, Hovey JD: Anxiety and depression in a post-September 11 sample of Arabs in the USA. Soc Psychiatry Psychiatr Epidemiol 47(3):409–418, 2012

American Psychiatric Association: Cultural formulation, in Diagnostic and Statistical Manual of Mental Disorders, 5th Edition. Arlington, VA, American Psychiatric Association, 2013, pp 749–759

Arab American Institute Foundation: Demographics. Washington, DC, Arab American Institute, 2018. Available at: https://censuscounts.org/wp-content/uploads/2019/03/National_Demographics_SubAncestries-2018.pdf. Accessed September 4, 2020.

Arfken CL, Abu-Ras W, Ahmed S: Pilot study of waterpipe tobacco smoking among US Muslim college students. J Relig Health 54(5):1543–1554, 2015

Baker E: Flying while Arab-Racial profiling and air travel security. Journal of Air Law and Commerce 67(4):1375–1405, 2002

Barry MG, Murray A: Protective processes of Latina adolescents. Hisp Health Care Int 4(2):111–124, 2006

Beydoun KA: Boxed in: reclassification of Arab Americans on the U.S. census as progress or peril. Loyola University Chicago Law Journal 47(3):693–760, 2016

Boulos SA: The role of acculturation, ethnic identity, and religious fatalism on attitudes towards seeking psychological help among Coptic Americans. Doctoral dissertation, Texas A&M University, College Station, 2011. Available at: https://core.ac.uk/download/pdf/9069277.pdf. Accessed January 25, 2020.

Eldeeb SY: Understanding and addressing Arab-American mental health disparities. Scholarly Undergraduate Research Journal at Clark vol 3, article 1, April 2017

Erickson CD, al-Timimi NR: Providing mental health services to Arab Americans: recommendations and considerations. Cultur Divers Ethnic Minor Psychol 7(4):308–327, 2001

Fakih RR: Ethnic identity among Arab Americans: an examination of contextual influences and psychological well-being. Doctoral dissertation, Wayne State University, Detroit, MI, 2013. Available at: https://digitalcommons.wayne.edu/oa_dissertations/881. Accessed January 25, 2020.

Graham JR, Bradshaw C, Trew JL: Cultural considerations for social service agencies working with Muslim clients. Social Work 55(4):337–346, 2010

Hamdan A: Cognitive restructuring: an Islamic perspective. J Muslim Ment Health 3(1):99–116, 2008

Ibish H, Stewart A: Report on hate crimes and discrimination against Arab Americans: the post-September 11 backlash, September 11, 2001–October 11, 2002. Washington, DC, American-Arab Anti-Discrimination Committee, 2003. Available at: www.mbda.gov/sites/mbda.gov/files/migrated/files-attachments/September_11_Backlash.pdf. Accessed January 29, 2020.

Jaber RM, Farroukh M, Ismail M, et al: Measuring depression and stigma towards depression and mental health treatment among adolescents in an Arab-American community. Int J Cult Ment Health 8(3):247–254, 2015

Jadalla A, Lee J: The relationship between acculturation and general health of Arab Americans. J Transcult Nurs 23(2):159–165, 2012

Martin U: Psychotherapy with Arab Americans: an exploration of therapy-seeking and termination behaviors. Int J Cult Ment Health 7(2):162–167, 2014

Munro-Kramer ML, Fava NM, Saftner MA, et al: What are we missing? Risk behaviors among Arab-American adolescents and emerging adults. J Am Assoc Nurse Pract 28(9):493–502, 2016

Naff A: Arabs, in Harvard Encyclopedia of American Ethnic Groups. Edited by Thernstrom S. Cambridge, MA, Belknap, 1980, pp 128–136

Odeh Yosef AR: Health beliefs, practice, and priorities for health care of Arab Muslims in the United States: implications for nursing care. J Transcult Nurs 19(3):284–291, 2008

Ogbuagu BC: Constructing America's 'new blacks': post 9/11 social policies and their impacts on and implications for the lived experiences of Muslims, Arabs, and others. Mediterr J Soc Sci 4(1):469–480, 2013

Pumariega AJ, Rothe E, Mian A, et al: Practice parameter for cultural competence in child and adolescent psychiatric practice. J Am Acad Child Adolesc Psychiatry 52(10):1101–1115, 2013

Sabbah MF, Dinsmore JA, Hof DD: A comparative study of the competence of counselors in the United States in counseling Arab Americans and other racial/ethnic groups. Int J Psychol 4(1):29–45, 2009

Samari G: Cross-border ties and Arab American mental health. Soc Sci Med 155:93–101, 2016

Semaan G: Arabs in America: an historical perspective. Presentation at the 2013 Hawaii University International Conferences Arts Humanities and Social Sciences, Honolulu, HI, January 6–8, 2013. Available at: www.huichawaii.org/assets/semaan_gaby_ahs_2013.pdf. Accessed January 25, 2020.

Shaheen JG: Reel Bad Arabs: How Hollywood Vilifies a People. Northampton, MA, Olive Branch, 2015

Singh NN, McKay JD, Singh AN: The need for cultural brokers in mental health services. J Child Fam Stud 8(1):1–10, 1999

Smith J: Removing barriers to therapy with Muslim-Arab-American clients. Doctoral dissertation, Antioch University, Yellow Springs, OH, 2011

Soheilian SS, Inman AG: Middle Eastern Americans: the effects of stigma on attitudes toward counseling. J Muslim Ment Health 4(2):139–158, 2009

Suleiman M (ed): Arabs in America: Building a New Future. Philadelphia, PA, Temple University Press, 2010

Vermette D, Shetgiri R, Al Zuheiri H, et al: Healthcare access for Iraqi refugee children in Texas: persistent barriers, potential solutions, and policy implications. J Immigr Minor Health 17(5):1526–1536, 2014

Weglicki LS, Templin TN, Rice VH, et al: Comparison of cigarette and water-pipe smoking by Arab and non-Arab-American youth. Am J Prev Med 35(4):334–339, 2008

Wingfield M: Arab Americans: into the multicultural mainstream. Equity Excell Educ 39(3):253–266, 2006

Wormald B: Projected religious population changes in the Middle East and North Africa, in The Future of World Religions: Population Growth Projections, 2010–2050. Washington, DC, Pew Research Center, May 10, 2016. Available at: www.pewforum.org/2015/04/02/middle-east-north-africa. Accessed January 25, 2020.

PART II
Cultural Concepts

CHAPTER 7

Gender and Sexuality in the Twenty-First Century

Cultural Psychiatry for Children, Adolescents, and Families

R. Dakota Carter, M.D., Ed.D.
Aron Janssen, M.D.

THE twenty-first century has seen tremendous advancements toward structural, legal, and cultural advancement for lesbian, gay, bisexual, transgender, and queer/questioning (LGBTQ+) youth. However, LGBTQ+ youth continue to face tremendous stigma, bias, and bullying both at home and in their communities that lead to alarmingly high rates of anxiety, depression, and suicide attempts that are orders of magnitude more than rates of their cisgender, heterosexual peers. These effects are mitigated by supportive parents, communities, and legal protections— all things over which youth have no control. LGBTQ+ youth are in many ways a hidden minority because in most cases they do not share a core element of their identity with their parents and as a result often are forced to hide their identity across facets of their lives.

In this chapter, we hope to elucidate the universal development of gender identity and sexual orientation. We also describe how families and communities can best support and celebrate the different developmental trajectories of LGBTQ+ youth and describe common psychiatric needs of LGBTQ+ youth, including risk of depression, anxiety, suicidal ideation and attempts, disordered eating, and substance use disorders. We explore mental health, medical, and structural interventions to reduce the disparities faced by LGBTQ+ youth; discuss intersectionality and influence on outcomes in this population; and review best treatment practices, including the most recent guidelines for transgender youth wishing to transition.

Identity Formation: LGBTQ+ Youth

Developmentally, childhood and adolescence are marked with pivotal physical, emotional, cognitive, and social milestones, progressing a youth toward adulthood; these developmental achievements include sexual maturation and the determination of an individual's gender and sexual identity. During this time, youth also begin the development of self and understanding of their place in the world. This idea of *self-concept* recognizes both a personal identity and a group identity that highlight the natural and created connections with family, friends, community, and other demographic-related memberships (e.g., race, ethnicity, religion, sexuality, gender). This natural phenomenon can be challenging for youth who identify as nonheterosexual or gender nonconforming as they progress through identity formation and then integration. The formation and integration of identity can be greatly influenced by individual experience in addition to intersectionality of identity that can impact health. These processes are variable, nonlinear, and individual; although variability is normal, challenges in identity formation and integration, especially for LGBTQ+ youth, can lead to negative mental health outcomes. Clinicians must recognize the psychosocial stressors faced by these youth specifically and understand the nuanced dynamics between sexual and gender identity, race/ethnicity, geographic location, religion, immigrant status, socioeconomic level, and other aspects at play between development and culture.

As practitioners who treat children, adolescents, and transitional-age youth, child mental health providers are aware of the mental health needs of this large population. Statistically, LGBTQ+ youth make up 5%–10% of the population; it is important to note that this percentage does not capture questioning or closeted youth. LGBTQ+ youth carry higher rates of depression, anxiety, substance use, and disordered eating than do their heterosexual, gender-conforming peers (Marshal et al. 2011). Fifty-four percent of lesbian, gay, and bisexual youth have been diagnosed with an eating disorder, and 21% believe they have an undiagnosed eating disorder; a vast majority of these youth (85% or more) report serious thoughts of suicide in addition to disordered eating (Ackard et al. 2008; The Trevor Project et al. 2018). Although research is limited, substance use disorders can be seen in 20%–30% of this population, compared with 9% in the general population (Marshal et al. 2008; Medley et al. 2016). Other research indicates that LGBQ+ youth may have a 190% higher risk of substance use disorders than do their heterosexual, gender-conforming peers, with even higher numbers in bisexual youth and lesbians (Marshal et al. 2008; Medley et al. 2016).

According to the Centers for Disease Control and Prevention, suicide is the third leading cause of mortality in children ages 10–14 years and second in those ages 15–24 years (Kann et al. 2018). Data and studies indicate a higher rate of suicidal ideation for lesbian, gay, and bisexual adolescents, ranging from two to three times higher than rates for their heterosexual peers and a suicide attempt rate four times or higher (Kann et al. 2011; Mustanski et al. 2010). Those youth coming from families who reject their identity are 8.4 times more likely to attempt suicide than are the heterosexual cohort. Forty percent of transgender individuals report attempting suicide, with more than 90% attempting before age 25 (Mustanski et al. 2010).

Research has shown that LGBTQ+ youth are more likely than their heterosexual counterparts to fight, experience dating violence, or experience forced sexual intercourse. These youth are also more likely than their peers to experience in-person victimization or online cyberbullying. Rejection and isolation from family can lead to homelessness and increased *survival crimes*, such as sex work with risky sexual behavior, drug use, and theft. It is estimated that 20%–40% of the ~2.8 million homeless youth population identify as a member of this cohort, with an alarming number of LGBTQ+ youth facing homelessness within the next year (Choi et al. 2015; Mustanski et al. 2010). Of this population, gender-nonconforming and transgender youth have a higher likelihood of homelessness at an earlier age than the lesbian, gay, and bisexual cohort (Choi et al. 2015; Mustanski et al. 2010).

Although many LGBTQ+ youth have high levels of resiliency, they are predisposed to negative health outcomes because of the social stigmatization they experience, not because of inherent factors related to their identity. These negative health outcomes have been shown to be directly related to stress caused by belonging to an often-stigmatized population facing discrimination, prejudice, intolerance, and bullying. Each incident of discrimination, prejudice, rejection, or victimization, including harassment or abuse, can increase self-harming behavior by 2.5 times on average (Mustanski et al. 2010). Importantly, researchers and policy makers have identified this rampant stress as a significant public health crisis with clear solutions, noting that sexual and gender minority youth who feel supported in socially, emotionally, and physically safe environments can build resiliency and have outcomes similar to those of their peers, becoming healthy adults.

Clinical Vignette

Brooke, age 10, and her parents visit a psychiatrist for an initial evaluation. Brooke is the oldest of two siblings and lives at home with her mother and father. Brooke was assigned female at birth and has no formal past psychiatric history. During her current fifth grade year, she started experiencing conflict within her social circle and began to withdraw from friendships. Although Brooke has been a high-achieving student, her grades began to slip over the course of this year. Her parents note that she has been more irritable and has stopped wanting to participate in the usual family weekend outings, which typically involve a church-based service and social function. They brought her in because of concern about these changes and fear that she is depressed.

During the initial evaluation with Brooke, the psychiatrist notes clear depressive symptoms, along with a recent conflict over attraction to a girl in her class who was her best friend. They were sexually active once, and afterward her friend rejected her and has been systematically isolating her from their shared friends. Brooke self-identifies as a lesbian, but she has internalized conflict around her burgeoning sense of self and fears that her parents and her community will reject her on the basis of their religious beliefs if she reveals her sexual orientation.

Over the course of a few months with a therapist, Brooke works through her sense of self. She comes out to her parents, who are encouraged to meet with a support group of Christian parents with LGBTQ+ children. Brooke's parents note some improvement in depressive symptoms, and Brooke ends treatment.

LGBTQ+ Youth: Identity Development and Impact of Minority Stress

In order to understand the unique needs of LGBTQ+ youth, we must first understand the basic developmental processes around gender and sexuality and stress that gender and sex development is a universal experience. Everyone develops a gender identity, and everyone develops a sexual identity. In this section, we review the developmental processes for gender identity, sexual behavior, and sexual orientation.

Children first develop a sense of what Lawrence Kohlberg defines as *basic gender identity* by age 2 (Kohlberg 1966). Children are able to define themselves and others as boys or girls, although categories at this age are fluid; that is, a child may say "I am a boy, but when I grow up I will be a mother." Some children who will later grow up to be transgender will identify as their affirmed gender as early as this age, but that is rare, and most of the time a child's declaration at this age will match the gender they were assigned at birth. Around age 4, children reach the stage of gender stability, in which they understand that one's own gender will remain stable over time, although perception of the gender of others remains fluid and by and large determined by gender roles. *Gender role* is defined as the cultural norms around the performance of gender, including but not limited to dress, hair, and toy and play preference. At this age, children understand that their gender is constant—that is, if he is a boy, he will remain a boy whether he is wearing pants or a dress. However, they still perceive others' genders to be fluid—that is, their male friend becomes a girl if he wears dresses. It is not until around age 5 that children reach gender constancy, in which they understand that gender is fixed and independent of gender roles. It is at this age that we often begin to see the tendency toward self-segregation based on gender, and it is at this age that transgender and gender diverse youth often are faced with social exclusion and harassment. For most people, gender development effectively stabilizes at this age, and the developmental process is more focused on the nuanced meaning and expression of gender. However, for transgender individuals, there continues to be an open developmental process that is often expressed in inchoate ways prior to or even after puberty.

Regarding sexual development, anatomic development begins in utero, with all of the parts of the sexual system fully formed by 20 weeks of gestational age; up to 1% of children will have some variability in the appearance of the genitals, representing some kind of intersex condition (Blackless et al. 2000). After birth, babies learn to explore their bodies, including their genitalia; childhood masturbation peaks at age 4–5 before going into quiescence prior to adolescence. Masturbation rates increase with puberty, and sexual behavior rises steadily after that time. Sexual behavior with others is much more common in childhood than most people expect, and clinicians should understand what represents normal exploration (Kellogg and Committee on Child Abuse and Neglect 2009). It is important to note that sexual behavior, particularly in childhood, is often unaligned with later sexual orientation, which is the last to develop (Kellogg and Committee on Child Abuse and Neglect 2009).

Sexual attraction develops for most youth around 2 years prior to the visible signs of puberty (Savin-Williams and Cohen 2004). It is common for people to have some degree of attraction toward both males and females, although there is often a clear and overt stigma around nonheterosexual attractions. It often takes many years for sexual minority youth to come to terms with and understand how to integrate their sexual attractions and behaviors into their identity (Savin-Williams and Cohen 2004).

As mentioned previously, these developmental tasks are universal, not just limited to individuals who identify as LGBTQ+. However, youth who identify as LGBTQ+ often face stigma and bias based on their identity that can be present at home, at school, with peers, and in their communities. A myriad of interconnected processes create a substrate that leads to unique health outcomes seen in LGBTQ+ youth that are often promoted via prejudice, discrimination, bullying, and stigma. As identified by the minority stress model and ongoing clinical research, it is these negative societal stressors that lead to negative physical and mental health via layered cognitive, affective, interpersonal, and physiological responses (Meyer 2003). Link and Phelan (2001) explain this phenomenon concisely through the lens of stigmatization, noting that these youth become "labeled" persons experiencing disapproval, rejection, exclusion, and discrimination, resulting in loss of power, status, and eventually health due to the development of affective disorders, substance use disorders, and suicidality in response to this isolation. Meyer used stigma research to develop the minority stress theory in relation to these negative experiences in youth and adults, noting them to be unique, chronic, and socially based (Hatzenbuehler and Pachankis 2016; Meyer 2003); that is, the LGBTQ+ population is not inherently predisposed to psychological diagnoses due to their sexual orientation or gender identity but rather have higher rates of these illnesses because of the marginalization, stigma, and discrimination they experience targeted to their identities (Meyer 2003).

Approach to Care: Understanding Clinical Needs for LGBTQ+ Youth

LGBTQ+ youth must first be recognized as just that: a youth population. Mental health intervention is often delayed or can be left untreated in any youth population, an important component to recognize for LGBTQ+ youth who may be experiencing elevated risks of depression, anxiety, substance use, suicidality, and other mental illness. This population has specific mental health and developmental needs related inherently to their age but also needs related to their sexual and gender identity. As with all youth, a majority of LGBTQ+ youth may not have mental illness, but a culturally competent provider should know when to intervene when a mental health problem exists.

Clinically, sexual orientation and gender identity can be related and often are placed under the same umbrella, but in practice, they require varying knowledge, skills, and competencies related to everyone's unique experience. Because of the nuances among sex, gender, identity, expression, and attraction, it is important to address the domains of sexual orientation and gender identity separately to capture a youth's clinical needs. Clinicians must be aware of the individual, interpersonal, and structural influences on health in LGBTQ+ youth that predispose this population via minority stress.

Gender Care and Mental Health

The idea of gender care can be divided into several domains, nested from more universal to more individual-specific. On the universal end of the spectrum, everyone develops a gender identity, and everyone negotiates how their interests, appearance, experiences, and peers interface with that identity. These universal developmental processes are then shaped by the structures that children navigate every day—their family; their friends; their school and neighborhood; their cultural, civic, and religious institutions. As providers, we can educate ourselves about gender development and signal in our care (e.g., with badges, stickers, toys of all types for all kids) that diversity of gender identity and expression is welcome in our office, unit, department, and community. We can work to add gender health as a developmental goal for all youth, not just those who experience distress or difference. Supporting and affirming children for who they are, as opposed to who we wish they were, will always improve outcomes.

For children who experience their gender identity as incongruent with their sex assigned at birth, gender care becomes much more tailored to the individual and about how adult parents or caregivers affirm or reject their child's identity. Such care is driven by helping a child come to understand their authentic gender and safely express that gender within their family and community, including access to gender-affirming care, which may or may not include social, medical, or surgical transition. These children often face overt stigma, bias, and threat in the form of rejection, violence, exclusion, and internalized transphobia, or the sense of shame over one's transgender identity. This leads to mental health needs above and beyond the general population that clinicians should be prepared to address.

In general, care for gender diverse youth falls into three domains: assessment, psychotherapy, and transition-related care. Assessment involves a developmentally informed evaluation that helps youth to understand and express their gender in a safe and affirmed way. This entails a review of the child's experience (and other informants' observations) of their identity; their preferences for peers, play, and appearance; and their relationship to their body over time. Particular attention should be paid to the child's experience of puberty because this is often a time of both increased distress and diagnostic clarity for children who experience an incongruence between their sex assigned at birth and their gender identity.

Variability in all of these domains over time is expected, and the goal of the assessment is not to "correctly" identify the child's gender but rather to encourage open exploration led by the child. Psychiatrists can model this openness through simple statements such as "Hi, my name is Dr. X, and I use he/him pronouns. How would you like me to refer to you today?" Most transgender adults recall becoming aware of their identity in childhood but never were asked or felt comfortable disclosing. As psychiatrists, we have an opportunity to destigmatize the process of gender exploration and help our patients reduce the burden of shame in feeling different. Furthermore, no child exists in a vacuum, and any evaluation must also include an assessment of the family and the community. When a child experiences gender dysphoria, the treatment requires the enlistment of family and community. The details of a thorough gender assessment are beyond the scope of this chapter and can be reviewed in other literature (e.g., Coleman et al. 2012; Hembree et al. 2017).

After the assessment, the psychiatrist should sit with the child or adolescent and the family to review options for care. These options should include support around the child's gender de-

TABLE 7–1.   Gender dysphoria: after the assessment

Review goals of patient and specific needs

Discuss family support and needs

Discuss psychiatric needs

Discuss therapy needs (including family therapy)

Identify barriers to care

Make a plan for care with patient and family

velopment as well as any co-occurring psychiatric issues, family concerns, or social barriers that were identified (Table 7–1). Not all transgender youth will meet criteria for gender dysphoria, and not all transgender youth will require or even benefit from ongoing psychotherapy. Psychotherapy should be reserved for those who require additional support to relieve suffering or to treat co-occurring mental illness. Therapy can be individual, family, or group based, depending on the particular needs of the child. It is important to note that transgender youth face tremendous stigma, bias, and rejection and have higher rates of depression, anxiety, suicide attempts, and autism spectrum disorder when compared with the general population (de Vries et al. 2010, 2011a; Janssen et al. 2016). These diagnoses are often difficult to disentangle from the stigma, bias, and rejection the youth have experienced. Psychiatrists engaging in therapeutic work with this population should have ongoing training and supervision about the specifics of gender-affirming care as well as common co-occurring psychiatric conditions (Janssen and Leibowitz 2018).

Treatment specific to gender dysphoria is focused on what is colloquially referred to as *transition*. Transition includes social transition, medical or hormonal transition, and surgical transition. As psychiatrists, we are often asked to help guide the social transition process and to assess for an individual's understanding of the risks, benefits, and alternatives of medical and surgical transition.

Social transition is the process of making steps to live life in one's affirmed gender. This can range from changing one's name, clothes, or hairstyle to changing legal documents such as the gender marker on a passport or a birth certificate. Social transition is a process of asserting one's identity to one's community. It is a completely reversible intervention (i.e., there is nothing permanent about using a new name or different pronouns) that is associated with lower rates of depression and anxiety in prepubertal youth (Olson et al. 2016). Parental support is key because parental rejection of the child's identity is associated with significantly worse outcomes, including increased suicidal ideation and suicide attempts (Bauer et al. 2015).

Medical or hormonal interventions include puberty blockers and gender-affirming hormones. Gonadotropin-releasing hormone (GnRH) agonists, which for years have been used for the treatment of precocious puberty, were first used in 1998 for halting the irreversible effects of puberty for transgender youth in the Netherlands. These treatments have been shown to be highly effective in reducing distress and improving outcomes (de Vries et al. 2011b). Gender-affirming hormones (testosterone for affirmed males, estrogen for affirmed females) are prescribed for adolescents who have gender dysphoria and who can understand the risks, benefits, and alternatives and the partially irreversible nature of these interventions. Specifics for care can be found in the Endocrine Society Guidelines (Hembree et al. 2017). These interventions improve mental health outcomes for transgender youth, as do surgical interventions for those who opt to pursue them (de Vries et al. 2014). Surgical interventions include but are not limited to vaginoplasty, phalloplasty, metoidoplasty, chest reconstruction, breast augmentation, and facial feminization. Some older adolescents will opt for surgery prior to age 18 with familial consent and careful evaluation, but most commonly this is a choice made after reaching adulthood with an interdisciplinary team that includes the patient, the surgeon, one or two evaluating mental health providers, and additional clinical and surgical staff.

Sexuality Care and Mental Health

As with other youth, when providing care, it is important to address the patient on an individual basis to determine the level of care needed (e.g., guidance, screening, inpatient versus outpatient treatment, consultations, crisis services). Often, clinicians may become overly focused on the individual's LGBTQ+ identity with little regard to the patient as a whole person. An important concept to understand in the treatment of these youth recognizes that behavior does not equal complete identity and that many youth want to be treated and accepted just as their peers do, with a full discussion of their life. As with other youth, approach LGBTQ+ youth in an open, nonjudgmental fashion to build rapport and to address any issues that may be present, including those that may be influenced by both their sexual orientation and stressors unrelated to their LGBTQ+ identity.

Many of the mental health symptoms found in LGBTQ+ youth relate to the minority stress model. When evaluating a youth who has identified as lesbian, gay, bisexual, or another sexual minority, it is important to recognize the individual, interpersonal (e.g., relationships, abuse, discrimination), and structural (e.g., laws, policies) variables that may be impacting a particular youth and connect those variables to predictable outcomes that may need to be addressed clinically. Specific to LGBTQ+ youth, it is vital to understand the effects on mental health of internalized homophobia, high rejection sensitivity, and identity concealment due to fears of rejection (Hatzenbuehler and Pachankis 2016; Institute of Medicine Committee on Lesbian, Gay, Bisexual, and Transgender Health Issues and Research Gaps and Opportunities 2011; Lick et al. 2013; Meyer 2003).

Each of these domains can predict negative health outcomes ranging from affective disorders to substance use, suicidality, risky sexual behavior, and disordered eating. As noted previously, LGBTQ+ youth have higher rates of depression and anxiety, along with higher rates of suicidal ideation and attempts. Clinicians should be aware of the likelihood of these specific diagnoses and screen youth accordingly. The higher rate of suicidal ideation and increased suicidality are inherently connected to higher rates of depression, anxiety, and affective disorders. Higher rates of substance use (tobacco, alcohol, marijuana, cocaine, club drugs, methamphetamine, and heroin) compared with heterosexual youth have been noted (Marshal et al. 2008; Weber 2008). Data also support higher levels of bulimic disorders in gay youth, as well as anorexic or disordered eating (The Trevor Project et al. 2018). These diagnoses are also peripherally associated with increased suicidality. There is a clear connection between these diagnoses or outcomes and the experience of being LGBTQ+ through increased levels of hypervigilance or physiological stress responses, anxiety and ruminations, isolation and loneliness, and actual changes to the hypothalamic-pituitary axis secondary to stress responses. When doing any suicide risk assessment, membership within this community should be considered, especially in those children with unsupportive parents.

Individual differences in patients may lead to diverse clinical presentations based on independent resiliency, self-concept and integration, and experiences unique to their life. These nuances can be explored within several sessions with a clear understanding of how to triage youth with respect to these noted higher risks, including assessments of suicide risk and safety at home and school and the need for treatment or intervention. Clinicians should also be cognizant of confidentiality laws and regulations that can vary by state. It is vital to discuss confidentiality early with patients to help them understand how the therapeutic relationship can support open discussions about coming out, sexual behaviors, and health questions the patient may have while also recognizing limitations to their privacy that may exist.

Importantly, without intervention, maladaptive coping skills and/or negative relationship patterns developed during adolescence related to these factors may continue across the life span, promoting negative health effects into adulthood (Downey et al. 1999; Lev-Wiesel et al. 2006). Research also notes that the short-term protective benefits of nonconcealment of sexual identity are associated with negative long-term psychological consequences in affect, self-esteem, and stress (Frable et al. 1998; Frost and Bastone 2008; Pachankis 2007; Pachankis et al. 2015). Further complicating clinical care, providers must also be aware of the interpersonal and structural dynamics (e.g., peer groups, family dynamics, geographical culture) that influence their LGBTQ+ patients, including greater risk of suicidality and substance use, in addition to those factors initiated at the individual level. Clinicians should be familiar with, and screen for, common microaggressions experienced by this cohort, along with overt, hateful actions that may occur (Herek 2009). Researchers have noted not only that the cumulative lifetime burden of microaggressions causes mental and physical health sequelae but also that the LGBTQ+ population is at risk of a higher burden (Nadal et al. 2011). In one cross-sectional study, lesbian, gay, and bisexual youth who lived in areas with laws or policies that discriminated against sexual orientation and gender identity were 20% more likely to attempt suicide than were other lesbian, gay, and bisexual youth (Hatzenbuehler et al. 2010). As noted, in addition to these broader social contexts, LGBTQ+ youth have a higher likelihood of suicide when they are rejected by peers, school, and family (Hatzenbuehler 2014). Supportive environments continue to impart health benefits, an important advocacy component a psychiatrist should promote at the individual and regulatory levels.

Understanding local, community, state, and federal resources is an important aspect of caring for LGBTQ+ youth. Several national organizations, such as the American Psychiatric Association, the American Academy of Child and Adolescent Psychiatry (AACAP), and the American Academy of Pediatrics, have policy statements, treatment recommendations, and support for LGBTQ+ individuals. AACAP recognizes clinical needs and treatment for LGBTQ+ youth via several principles summarized in Table 7–2.

LGBTQ+ Affirming Care

When providing care to LGBTQ+ youth, psychiatrists must be comfortable with and knowledgeable about the terminology and developmental domains of sexuality, gender identity, and

TABLE 7–2. **American Academy of Child and Adolescent Psychiatry mental health principles for treating LGBTQ+ youth**

1.   Complete a full developmentally and age-appropriate psychosexual mental health evaluation
2.   Protect confidentiality and the clinical alliance
3.   Recognize family dynamics, values, and culture
4.   Review circumstances that promote any psychiatric risk
5.   Support healthy development, adaptive functioning, and identity integration
6.   Understand that there is no evidence to support conversion therapy, and the practice is likely harmful to youth
7.   Know treatment guidelines for gender discordance, possible psychopathology, and clinical needs
8.   Liaison with the community via schools, agencies, health care offices, and other local entities to support LGBTQ+ youth
9.   Promote resources, education, and organizations that embrace LGBTQ+ youth and their families

Source.   Adelson et al. 2012.

gender expression and the increased vulnerabilities and resiliencies in LGBTQ+ youth. It is important to note common diagnoses, sources of distress, and preventable outcomes in this population. In addition, familiarity with organizational, local, state, and national resources is of fundamental importance in providing culturally humble care. It is vital to discuss ethical issues such as limits of confidentiality with LGBTQ+ youth to protect them from exploitation and abuse and to support important conversations about sexual health that youth may fear disclosing. Clinicians should strive to promote peer connections, family support, resiliency, and adaptive coping skills. Providing culturally competent care in an open, nonjudgmental, and knowledgeable fashion can help youth who are not ready to divulge and support those who have not yet perceived or identified their sexual orientation or gender identity. Whatever the ultimate identity becomes, "clinicians should be accepting of youth with any expression or disclosure…and foster a clinical relationship characterized by safety and professional support for healthy development" (Adelson et al. 2016, p. 974).

Clinical Vignette *(Continued)*

One year after ending treatment, Brooke returns to the psychiatrist's office and asks that staff use the name Finn and they/them pronouns. Finn is dressed in a manner typical for a 12-year-old boy, and although the psychiatrist honors their requests regarding name and pronoun, their parents continue to use "Brooke" and she/her. Finn's parents express dismay that after coming to terms with what they understood to be their daughter's lesbian identity, they are now confronted with Finn's disclosure of a gender nonbinary and pansexual identity. The parents note that they have been ostracized in their rural community and from their church and are feeling much isolation. Finn, too, endorses some social isolation but notes that their school has created a new social club supportive of LGBTQ+ youth in which they are actively involved.

Intersectionality

Intersectionality is a theoretical framework that recognizes individuals with multiple social or minority identities and their experience of layered, societal-based inequities due to that diverse individuality. Often, the dynamics between these multiple identities interplay to create unique, individual mental health challenges; a culturally humble clinician can appreciate these complex identities and the additive impact of society-influenced health disparities respective to each individual intersection. The list in this section is not exhaustive, but it captures some common key intersections seen in LGBTQ+ youth to provide some insight into cultural complexities experienced by these youth. Although there remains a paucity of literature on the intersections experienced by LGBTQ+ youth, data and research are confirming the important dynamics between patients with a multiple-minority status. Clinicians should be able to navigate these important intersections by understanding the patient's social context and multiple identities; knowing to whom the youth has disclosed their sexual or gender identity; and understanding how youth exist in contentious environments that expose them to discrimination, prejudice, potential abuse, or rejection. Many times, cultural intersections may appear to be a barrier to care, but a diligent clinician will be aware of the protective factors these affiliations may grant in support of LGBTQ+ youth.

Racial- and Ethnic-Based Factors for LGBTQ+ Youth

Race and ethnicity are clear factors in mental health outcomes, and these factors can also impact LGBTQ+ youth. When discussing intersectionality in these groups, there is a distinct need to understand the interplay between racial/ethnic identity, cultural norms, and identifying as a sexual or gender minority youth. Clinicians must recognize the patient's social context in order to elucidate the promotive and protective factors that influence these dynamics.

Understanding the impact of racial and sexual identity on mental health involves clinicians recognizing the health disparities that each separate identity can experience, the additive impact of these barriers, and the effect these identities may have on one another. Racial and ethnic identity is usually the primary identification for an individual, and it creates powerful bonds to community. This identity may be even more significant for self-concept and identification in marginalized or historically oppressed populations, a concept comprehensively discussed in Chapter 2, "The Black Diaspora." Fields et al. (2016) note that "[n]orm compliance and collectivism rather than individualism and self-expression in racial/ethnic minority groups may be more important in the process of sexual identity development in sexual minorities of color than uniform disclosure seen in other groups" (p. 1093).

Research has identified that coming out and affiliation with the LGBTQ+ community may be less relevant in the Black community because of the social context and less interpersonal support for self-expression that contrasts with group norms. The literature also notes that Black youth commonly experience conflict between same-sex attraction or gender nonconformity; internalized and group-promoted homophobia or transphobia; and expectations in gender role, sense of morality, and religious beliefs (Bowleg 2013; Fields et al. 2016). These youth may seek to preserve their primary connection to their racial identity, a community of strength and support, before assuming or embracing an LGBTQ+ identity. In fact, research has shown that during adolescent development, many of these youth may fear rejection and ridicule from their community, choosing to hide their sexual identity in order to stay connected within their racial identity. This is particularly relevant for young Black men because of hypermasculinity/masculinity expectations and for all Black youth because of the roles that religion and morality play in their lives. Notably, nondisclosure of sexual or gender identity and adherence to expected roles may preserve social support but can also cause internalized conflict between culture and sexuality in some youth. This can create a quagmire of poor health outcomes, isolation, and decreased healthy support of sexual or gender identity (Fields et al. 2016).

Similar findings can be found in immigrant populations, ethnicities tied to a dominant religious doctrine, and Native youth (Jamil et al. 2009). Furthermore, the poverty, lower socioeconomic status, segregation, poor or unpromoted assimilation into the prevalent culture, and limited social connectedness often experienced by racial and ethnic minorities may enhance negative outcomes related to the intersectionality of culture and sexual/gender identity (Jamil et al. 2009). Importantly, the protective factors experienced by these youth (e.g., social support from the racial group, religion/spirituality, family connectedness, race centrality) are capable of supporting LGBTQ+ youth in these communities, building resiliency and improving health outcomes. In environments where protective factors are prevalent and the community is supportive of diverse sexual and gender identities, these factors can "buffer the negative effect of existing within multiple marginalized identities" (Fields et al. 2016, p. 1096).

Religion and LGBTQ+ Youth

Religiosity, spirituality, and religious affiliation have been shown to be protective for patients across the life span, imparting physical and mental health benefits; however, in sexual and gender minority youth, some religious affiliations have been implicated in causing mental health pathology. Backed by the minority stress model, religion can create health disparities when it promotes stigma, homophobia or transphobia, discrimination on the basis of sexuality or gender identity, or outright rejection of an individual member because of their identity (Barnes and Meyer 2012; Fields et al. 2016). These experiences often cause LGBTQ+ youth and young adults to migrate away from religion altogether, forgoing even affirmative institutions, in order to avoid stressors within these social environments.

As can be expected, religion often intersects with multiple identities and may even be promoted by memberships within certain populations. As discussed previously, religiosity within Black communities is an important part of group membership and culture. Historically, these churches represented refuge from discrimination and marginalization, but they can harbor negative consequences for youth in these communities who also identify as LGBTQ+. The literature describes the powerful role the church has in the Black community and notes that this institution can be a principal source of homophobic or transphobic perceptions. In addition, the church can cultivate unachievable expectations of individuals who do not ascribe to gender-conforming roles (e.g., gender-nonconforming men unable to meet the religious expectation of masculinity in the church) (Fields et al. 2016). Similar findings have been found within Hispanic or Latin communities of Catholic or Jehovah's Witness faiths (Barnes and Meyer 2012).

Often, when religion is important to a youth's cultural identity, sexual or gender identity may be concealed to avoid prejudice or targeting within these religious spaces. Notably, for youth who have not integrated their identities and sense of self, any negative messages or ideas from a religious institution may manifest as internalized hate and negative mental health outcomes. Affirming churches that offer positive social support, acceptance, and tolerance can offer protective factors for LGBTQ+ youth, decreasing negative health outcomes and increasing social capital that decreases isolation and increases connectedness (Barnes and Meyer 2012; Fields et al. 2016).

Rural LGBTQ+ Youth

Geographic location is another intersecting factor that can impact LGBTQ+ youth. There is a vital need for providers in rural areas to create a culture of acceptance in their offices that can promote self-disclosure and trust to help alleviate disparities seen in youth from these communities (Price-Feeney et al. 2019). In rural communities, LGBTQ+ youth face higher rates of discrimination, prejudice, and bullying, which can be attributed to less racial and ethnic diversity, higher levels of conservative religious fundamentalists, lower socioeconomic and educational levels, and fewer opportunities for peer group socialization compared with urban areas. This is likely due to population homogeneity and fewer "out" youth. Research has shown a higher level of depression in rural female adolescents with same-sex attractions and less feeling of belonging. These female youth also experience higher rates of serious substance use, verbal sexual harassment, and earlier age of first sexual intercourse as compared with urban LGBTQ+ youth. Research also has shown increased rates of suicidal behavior and substance abuse and a higher likelihood of impregnating another youth in LGBTQ+ males from urban areas as compared with youth from rural areas. "Out" rural youth, when compared with "out" urban youth, are more likely to report lower levels of well-being and have lower grade point averages. Rural LGBTQ+ youth also report feeling unsafe at school and in places of worship and are more likely to report substance abuse, depression, and low self-esteem compared with local peers and urban LGBTQ+ youth, likely due to the feelings of rejection, discrimination, and prejudice, real or perceived (Price-Feeney et al. 2019).

Increasing data indicate that the health disparity gaps between rural and urban LGBTQ+ youth may be closing. Online connectivity seems to help build social support in rural LGBTQ+ youth, in addition to changing societal and cultural influencers. Health disparities are also moot when a rural community implements local policies (i.e., school-based, religious-based) that are supportive of LGBTQ+ youth (Paceley et al. 2018). The high levels of social capital available in rural communities can help build resilience and promote adaptive development. These protective factors are unique to small, close-knit communities.

LGBTQ+ Youth and Schools

As noted previously, LGBTQ+ youth can thrive in affirming places, including the institutions of learning where all youth spend most of their time in their formative years. Each school district's policies and environment can hinder or promote growth for LGBTQ+ youth. Unfortunately, the trend in data continues to indicate that many schools are adding to the negative health and social outcomes of this population, despite clear examples of supportive schools helping

LGBTQ+ individuals to thrive with less depression, anxiety, suicidal ideation, and substance use and fewer unexcused absences.

Schools that do not target LGBTQ+ bullying or do not create safe environments increase violence toward this cohort, as observed in reports from the youth themselves. According to the Gay, Lesbian and Straight Education Network (GLSEN; Kosciw et al. 2017), 87% of LGBTQ+ youth reported harassment or assault, with more than 40% reporting some type of physical altercation because of their sexual orientation or gender identity and almost 50% experiencing some type of cyberbullying. Fifty to sixty percent of these youth did not report this violence because they believed there would be no intervention, and 60% of those who did report it received no offer of intervention. LGBTQ+ students are overwhelmingly more likely to skip school because of safety concerns or harassment and have lower GPAs, and they are less likely to finish high school or pursue a college education compared with the national average (Kosciw et al. 2017).

However, there are clear solutions to help mitigate school-based problems for this population. Research has identified that LGBTQ+ youth attending schools with affirming organizations, such as gay-straight alliances, experience reduced depression, missed school days, bullying, and suicide attempts versus youth at schools without these social supports. Schools with policies in place against homophobia and transphobia also mitigate the negative outcomes seen in schools without these regulations. Successful schools implement student-led, tolerant organizations; adopt policies that support sexual and gender minority youth; provide LGBTQ+ training to staff; improve the curriculum to make it more LGBTQ+ inclusive; identify "safe spaces" on campus; and connect with community resources to support LGBTQ+ youth (Johns et al. 2019; Kosciw et al. 2017).

Conclusion

Each youth's trajectory is individual and unique; this holds true for LGBTQ+ youth. Although no individual clinician will ever be able to be truly culturally competent for every individual patient they encounter, we encourage mental health providers to become competent to the extent possible (e.g., through ongoing learning) in the knowledge and skills involved in working with LGBTQ+ youth. As reviewed in this chapter, there are specific mental health, medical, and structural concerns that are unique to LGBTQ+ youth that every clinician should be familiar with. There are stances and techniques that will help psychiatrists to become more skilled at eliciting gender and sexual health histories. However, we encourage mental health providers to recognize that knowledge and skills are meaningless without the recognition that every young person and family has a unique set of life circumstances that we can never hope to fully grasp. We must allow the increased knowledge and skills we acquire to shine a light on what is still left to understand rather than assuming we know everything we need to know. Every patient encounter should be approached with a sense of curiosity and humility.

A clinician who is culturally aware, curious, and willing to learn is likely one who is aware of the dynamics of culture and recognizes knowledge limitations but has a clear, respectful, nonjudgmental attitude and willingness to learn and treat patients from diverse backgrounds. In the treatment of LGBTQ+ youth, clinicians must be aware of the specific mental health needs of this population; evaluate the dynamics of family, peers, and other social experiences of the youth; and recognize the context or intersections of differing and shared values, sense of community, and overarching culture.

Clinical Pearls

- Negative physical and mental health outcomes seen in LGBTQ+ youth are related to the lived experiences of these adolescents. Captured by the minority stress model (Meyer 2003), the discrimination, prejudice, rejection, and stigma too often experienced by LGBTQ+ youth can lead to higher rates of suicide, depression, anxiety, disordered eating, and substance use and can contribute to sociopolitical issues of youth homelessness, increased experiences with law enforcement, and the additive nature of intersectional negative experiences.

- Gender development progresses along a spectrum, beginning with an understanding of basic gender identity, followed by gender stability and gender constancy. For cisgender youth, this developmental process then becomes more focused on the nuanced meaning and expression of gender. However, for transgender individuals, there continues to be an open developmental process that is often expressed in inchoate ways prior to or even after puberty. It is vital for providers to understand that some youth may identify as nonbinary or continue to question gender altogether, so clinical interviews must include an open, nonjudgmental conversation to understand a patient's understanding and labeling of their identity and where they are in their own personal development.

- LGBTQ+ youth do not exist in isolation; every effort must be made to understand the intersectional influences that may be impacting potential health disparities and outcomes in relation to gender identity and sexual orientation.

Self-Assessment Questions

1. What is a gender role?

   A. One's sense of gender, including female, male, nonbinary, or other identities.
   B. Cultural norms around the performance of gender, including but not limited to dress, hair, and toy and play preference.
   C. A person's perception of having a particular gender, which may or may not correspond with their birth sex.
   D. The way in which a person expresses their gender identity, typically through their appearance, dress, and behavior.

2. Developmentally, at what age should a child reach gender constancy?

A. 3 years.
B. 4 years.
C. 5 years.
D. 6 years.

3. The minority stress model has identified clear connections between LGBTQ+ discrimination and health outcomes. This model highlights the need for clinicians to do which of the following?

    A. Recognize the individual, interpersonal, and structural variables that may be impacting a youth and connect those variables to predictable outcomes that may need to be addressed clinically.
    B. Understand that treatment for this youth population can be globalized on the basis of their shared experiences of discrimination.
    C. Recognize that outcomes in LGBTQ+ youth are related to their identity and not their experience.
    D. Focus on sexual and gender identities of youth without regard to intersectional experiences.

Answers

1. B
2. C
3. A

References

Ackard DM, Fedio G, Neumark-Sztainer D, et al: Factors associated with disordered eating among sexually active adolescent males: gender and number of sexual partners. Psychosom Med 70(2):232–238, 2008

Adelson SA; American Academy of Child and Adolescent Psychiatry (AACAP) Committee on Quality Issues (CQI): Practice parameter on gay, lesbian, or bisexual sexual orientation, gender nonconformity, and gender discordance in children and adolescents. J Am Acad Child Adolesc Psychiatry 51(9):957–974, 2012

Adelson SL, Stroeh OM, Ng YKW: Development and mental health of lesbian, gay, bisexual, and transgender youth in pediatric practice. Pediatr Clin North Am 63(3)971–983, 2016

Barnes DM, Meyer IH: Religious affiliation, internalized homophobia, and mental health in lesbians, gay men, and bisexuals. Am J Orthopsychiatry 82(4):505–515, 2012

Bauer GR, Scheim AI, Pyne J, et al: Intervenable factors associated with suicide risk in transgender persons: a respondent driven sampling study in Ontario, Canada. BMC Public Health 15:525, 2015

Blackless M, Charuvastra A, Derryck A, et al: How sexually dimorphic are we? Review and synthesis. Am J Hum Biol 12(2):151–166, 2000

Bowleg L: "Once you've blended the cake, you can't take the parts back to the main ingredients": black gay and bisexual men's descriptions and experiences of intersectionality. Sex Roles 68(11–12):754–767, 2013

Choi SK, Wilson BDM, Shelton J, et al: Serving our youth 2015: the needs and experiences of lesbian, gay, bisexual, transgender, and questioning youth experiencing homelessness. Los Angeles, CA, Williams

Institute, June 2015. Available at: https://nhchc.org/wp-content/uploads/2019/08/true-colors-fund_serving-our-youth-june-2015.pdf. Accessed April 20, 2020.

Coleman E, Bockting W, Botzer M, et al: Standards of Care for the Health of Transsexual, Transgender, and Gender-Nonconforming People, Version 7. Int J Transgender 13(4):165–232, 2012

de Vries ALC, Noens ILJ, Cohen-Kettenis PT, et al: Autism spectrum disorders in gender dysphoric children and adolescents. J Autism Dev Disord 40(8):930–936, 2010

de Vries ALC, Doreleijers TAH, Steensma TD, et al: Psychiatric comorbidity in gender dysphoric adolescents. J Child Psychol Psychiatry 52(11):1195–1202, 2011a

de Vries AL, Steensma TD, Doreleijers TAH, et al: Puberty suppression in adolescents with gender identity disorder: a prospective follow-up study. J Sex Med 8(8):2276–2283, 2011b

de Vries ALC, McGuire JK, Steensma TD, et al: Young adult psychological outcome after puberty suppression and gender reassignment. Pediatrics 134(4):696–704, 2014

Downey G, Bonica C, Rincón C: Rejection sensitivity and adolescent romantic relationships, in The Development of Romantic Relationships in Adolescence. Edited by Furman W, Brown BB, Feiring C. Cambridge, UK, Cambridge University Press, 1999, pp 148–174

Fields E, Morgan A, Sanders RA: The intersection of sociocultural factors and health-related behavior in lesbian, gay, bisexual, and transgender youth: experiences among young black gay males as an example. Pediatr Clin North Am 63(6):1091–1106, 2016

Frable DES, Platt L, Hoey S: Concealable stigmas and positive self-perceptions: feeling better around similar others. J Pers Soc Psychol 74(4):909–922, 1998

Frost DM, Bastone LM: The role of stigma concealment in the retrospective high school experiences of gay, lesbian, and bisexual individuals. J LGBT Youth 5:27–36, 2008

Hatzenbuehler ML: Structural stigma and the health of lesbian, gay, and bisexual populations. Curr Dir Psychol Sci 23(2):127–132, 2014

Hatzenbuehler ML, Pachankis JE: Stigma and minority stress as social determinants of health among lesbian, gay, bisexual, and transgender youth: research evidence and clinical implications. Pediatr Clin North Am 63(6):985–997, 2016

Hatzenbuehler ML, McLaughlin KA, Keyes KM, et al: The impact of institutional discrimination on psychiatric disorders in lesbian, gay, and bisexual populations: a prospective study. Am J Public Health 100(3):452–459, 2010

Hembree WC, Cohen-Kettenis PT, Gooren L, et al: Endocrine treatment of gender-dysphoric/gender-incongruent persons: an Endocrine Society clinical practice guideline. J Clin Endocrinol Metab 102(11):3869–3903, 2017

Herek GM: Hate crimes and stigma-related experiences among sexual minority adults in the United States: prevalence estimates from a national probability sample. J Interpers Violence 24(1):54–74, 2009

Institute of Medicine Committee on Lesbian, Gay, Bisexual, and Transgender Health Issues and Research Gaps and Opportunities: The Health of Lesbian, Gay, Bisexual, and Transgender People: Building a Foundation for Better Understanding. Washington, DC, National Academies Press, 2011. Available at: www.ncbi.nlm.nih.gov/books/NBK64806. Accessed April 20, 2020.

Jamil OB, Harper GW, Fernandez MI: Sexual and ethnic identity development among gay-bisexual-questioning (GBQ) male ethnic minority adolescents. Cultur Divers Ethnic Minor Psychol 15(3):203–214, 2009

Janssen A, Leibowitz S (eds): Affirmative Mental Health Care for Transgender and Gender Diverse Youth: A Clinical Guide. Cham, Switzerland, Springer, 2018

Janssen A, Huang H, Duncan C: Gender variance among youth with autism spectrum disorders: a retrospective chart review. Transgender Health 1(1), 2016

Johns MM, Poteat VP, Horn SS, et al: Strengthening our schools to promote resilience and health among LGBTQ youth: emerging evidence and research priorities from The State of LGBTQ Youth Health and Wellbeing Symposium. LGBT Health 6(4):146–155, 2019

Kann L, O'Malley Olsen E, McManus T, et al: Sexual identity, sex of sexual contacts, and health-related behaviors among students in grades 9–12—youth risk behavior surveillance, selected sites, United States, 2001–2009. MMWR Morb Mortal Wkly Rep Early Release, Vol 60, June 6, 2011. Available at: www.cdc.gov/mmwr/pdf/ss/ss60e0606.pdf. Accessed August 8, 2020.

Kann L, McManus T, Harris WA, et al: Youth risk behavior surveillance—United States, 2017. MMWR Surveill Summ 67(8):1–114, 2018

Kellogg ND; Committee on Child Abuse and Neglect: Clinical report—the evaluation of sexual behaviors in children. Pediatrics 124(3):992–998, 2009

Kohlberg L: A cognitive-developmental analysis of children's sex-role concepts and attitudes, in The Development of Sex Differences. Edited by Maccoby E. London, Tavistock, 1966, pp 82–173

Kosciw JG, Greytak EA, Zongrone AD, et al: The 2017 National School Climate Survey: The Experiences of Lesbian, Gay, Bisexual, Transgender, and Queer Youth in Our Nation's Schools. New York, GLSEN, 2017. Available at: www.glsen.org/sites/default/files/2019-10/GLSEN-2017-National-School-Climate-Survey-NSCS-Full-Report.pdf. Accessed April 20, 2020.

Lev-Wiesel R, Nuttman-Shwartz O, Sternberg R: Peer rejection during adolescence: psychological long-term effects—a brief report. J Loss Trauma 11(2):131–142, 2006

Lick DJ, Durso LE, Johnson KL: Minority stress and physical health among sexual minorities. Perspect Psychol Sci 8(5):521–548, 2013

Link B, Phelan J: Conceptualizing stigma. Ann Rev Sociol 27(1):363–385, 2001

Marshal MP, Friedman MS, Stall R, et al: Sexual orientation and adolescent substance use: a meta-analysis and methodological review. Addiction 103(4):546–556, 2008

Marshal MP, Dietz LJ, Friedman MS, et al: Suicidality and depression disparities between sexual minority and heterosexual youth: a meta-analytic review. J Adolesc Health 49(2):115–123, 2011

Medley G, Lipari RN, Bose J, et al: Sexual Orientation and Estimates of Adult Substance Use and Mental Health: Results From the 2015 National Survey on Drug Use and Health. NSDUH Data Review, October 2016. Available at: https://www.samhsa.gov/data/sites/default/files/NSDUH-SexualOrientation-2015/NSDUH-SexualOrientation-2015/NSDUH-SexualOrientation-2015.htm. Accessed April 20, 2020.

Meyer IH: Prejudice, social stress, and mental health in lesbian, gay, and bisexual populations: conceptual issues and research evidence. Psychol Bull 129(5):674–697, 2003

Mustanski BS, Garafolo R, Emerson EM: Mental health disorders, psychological distress, and suicidality in a diverse sample of lesbian, gay, bisexual, and transgender youths. Am J Public Health 100(12):2426–2432, 2010

Nadal KL, Wong Y, Issa M-A, et al: Sexual orientation microaggressions: processes and coping mechanisms for lesbian, gay, and bisexual individuals. J LGBT Issues Couns 5(1):21–46, 2011

Olson KR, Durwood L, DeMeules M, et al: Mental health of transgender children who are supported in their identities. Pediatrics 137(3):e20153223, 2016

Paceley MS, Thomas MMC, Toole J, et al: "If rainbows were everywhere": nonmetropolitan SGM youth identify factors that make communities supportive. J Community Pract 26(4):429–445, 2018

Pachankis JE: The psychological implications of concealing a stigma: a cognitive-affective-behavioral model. Psychol Bull 133(2):328–345, 2007

Pachankis JE, Cochran SD, Mays VM: The mental health of sexual minority adults in and out of the closet: a population-based study. J Consult Clin Psychol 83(5):890–901, 2015

Price-Feeney M, Ybarra ML, Mitchell KJ: Health indicators of lesbian, gay, bisexual, and other sexual minority (LGB+) youth living in rural communities. J Pediatrics 205:236–243, 2019

Savin-Williams RC, Cohen KM: Homoerotic development during childhood and adolescence. Child Adolesc Psychiatr Clin N Am 13(3):529–549, 2004

The Trevor Project; National Eating Disorders Association; Reasons Eating Disorder Center: Eating disorders among LGBTQ youth: a 2018 national assessment. New York, National Eating Disorders Association, 2018. Available at: www.nationaleatingdisorders.org/sites/default/files/nedaw18/NEDA%20-Trevor%20Project%202018%20Survey%20-%20Full%20Results.pdf. Accessed April 20, 2020.

CHAPTER 8

Religion and Spirituality in Child and Adolescent Cultural Psychiatry

Mary Lynn Dell, M.D., D.Min.
Jonathan J. Shepherd, M.D., FAPA, DFAACAP

In nearly every church, synagogue, and mosque similar things happen. Births are celebrated; children are taught to be virtuous and compassionate; adults learn to enjoy what is beautiful, good, and true; parents grow in wisdom and patience; the hungry are fed; the naked are clothed; and the lonely are redeemed from their isolation. Rabbis, imams, pastors, priests, and lay leaders bless marriages, bury the dead, comfort those who mourn, and challenge their flock with a vision of a more peaceful and just society.

Atwood and Olson 2018

RELIGION, spirituality, and psychiatry share many themes with cultural psychiatry. Religious and spiritual beliefs and practices may transcend many cultures, and one particular culture, ethnicity, geographic region, or nationality may have one or more religious groups, spiritual beliefs, and practices in its midst. Religion and spirituality are important for understanding the history and development of cultures and the contemporary moral, ethical, and political environments in which our patients and their families live. Attitudes and behaviors important for assessment and treatment of psychiatric and medical conditions are influenced by religious and spiritual beliefs and behaviors. Although this topic is usually focused on understanding patients and families in mental health settings, clinicians bring their own broader cultural, religious, and spiritual backgrounds, beliefs, and life experiences into assessment and treatment processes, heightening the relevance of this material in daily practice. In this chapter, we review the continuum of relationships between religion, spirituality, and culture, from the straightforward to the complex. Next, we present key information about major world faith traditions important for mental health clinicians to know. Finally, we offer clinical pearls for working at the intersection of religion, spirituality, and culture in assessment and various treatment modalities.

Key Definitions

Many terms in the area of religion and spirituality are similar. Many overlap in meaning and can be used interchangeably; others are often misunderstood or are ascribed errant definitions. Key definitions and vocabulary for understanding the relationships between culture, religion, and spirituality in clinical work with children and families in the contexts of their communities and cultural backgrounds are listed in Table 8–1.

Relationship Between Culture, Religion, and Spirituality

Culture, religion, and spirituality have a complex relationship. Religion and spirituality may represent one element or a subset of a culture. One culture may encompass many faith traditions and spiritualities not dependent on formal religious communities or affiliations. A single religious orientation or major world faith tradition may transcend or be represented in several different geographically distant cultures and locations. For example, three adults who belong to the same mainline Protestant tradition, such as the United Methodist Church, may interpret the Bible differently, prefer alternative worship styles, and/or prioritize differently the values that inform their views on social issues. These differences may be informed by the number of generations their families have been rooted in Methodism, the denominational makeup of their local communities, their educational and socioeconomic backgrounds, and their experiences in rural or urban settings. Religious affiliation can also be linked to individuals' cultural heritage; many Catholics in America self-identify not only as Catholic but as Irish, German, Italian, or Latinx Catholics. The religious identity of American Jews and the degree of public and private religious observance are influenced by the denomination to which they belong, personal and social connectedness to the communities in which they live, and the individual's spirituality and personal interest in the religious tradition. Certainly, family history may exert significant influence on Jewish identity, especially if touched by the Holocaust or experiences of ancestors who lived in other countries.

    Culture, current events, and prevailing societal beliefs or prejudices influence the extent to which people feel free to express and live out their religion and spirituality in public. In the

TABLE 8-1. Key definitions of religion, spirituality, and culture

Term	Definition
Religion	• Organized system of beliefs, principles, practices, rituals, and symbols that relate individuals to the higher being or God or to the sacred or ultimate truth or reality they believe most important in their lives
	• Includes relationships with others within and outside one's community or immediate social circle who share similar beliefs, practices, and observances
Spirituality	• An individual's search for understanding and relationship with the transcendent, a higher being, the sacred, or whatever holds ultimate meaning in life
	• May or may not include the beliefs and practices of organized religion
Faith	• An integral, centering process more expansive than religious belief yet more tangible and directive than spirituality alone
	• Undergirds formation of beliefs, values, and meanings that foster coherence of competing priorities; connects these abstract concepts to shared trusts and loyalties to others and to local and global religious communities
	• May connect personal and communal ties to a deity or other transcendent frames of reference
	• Facilitates dealing with concrete challenges in life, illness, suffering, and death; ties these experiences to what provides ultimate meaning in life
Worldview	• The belief system, life philosophy, or perspective that directs or explains basic life issues and questions
	• Includes elements influenced by religion and/or spirituality
	• Examples of worldview constructs related to religious or spiritual beliefs include the purpose and meaning of life and the origins of life, suffering, death, and what comprises the good life
	• From Freud's 1933 essay "The Question of a Weltanschauung" (Freud 1933/1962)
Major world faith tradition	• Refers to established world religions in broad and inclusive understandings
	• Examples include, but are not limited to, Judaism, Hinduism, Islam, Buddhism, and Christianity
	• Tradition often understood as less rigid than religion and less prone to historical and cultural biases or inaccuracies
	• Helpful way to inquire about religious/spiritual beliefs and practices in secular contexts of mental health care
Religious or church affiliation	• Church, synagogue, mosque, or formal religious community to which a person belongs or that they claim as their religious or spiritual home
Religious preference	• The faith tradition one prefers to be a part of or associated with
	• Example: when admitted to the hospital, patients often are asked about religious preference; appropriate responses include "Baptist," "Catholic," "Jewish," "none."
Religious or church involvement	• Measurable behaviors such as attendance at religious services and social functions at houses or communities of worship, committee membership, financial support, or contributing to the life and work of the group in other visible, tangible ways

TABLE 8–1. **Key definitions of religion, spirituality, and culture *(continued)***

Term	Definition
Religious beliefs	• Beliefs about the teachings and spiritual truths found in sacred religious texts
Personal religious behaviors	• Actions of a religious nature that can be engaged in alone by individuals • Usually flow from personally held beliefs • Examples include prayer, meditation, fasting, candle lighting, and study of sacred texts

Source. Adapted from Fowler and Dell 2004; Freud 1933/1962; Josephson and Dell 2004; Koenig et al. 2001.

United States, for instance, children and families from majority Christian traditions seldom have worried about security when traveling to and from worship and are able to openly celebrate religious holidays or wear jewelry with crosses or other symbols of faith. However, other groups in American history have not always enjoyed such safety. For example, some nineteenth-century Jewish congregations in the Deep South feared for their safety. To avoid unwanted attention and harm to their members, they adopted the architectural styles of Protestant church buildings for their synagogues, perhaps with a small Star of David in a stained glass window the only exterior indication to the world that a group of Jews were gathered there (Gordon 1986). In the early twenty-first century, influenced significantly by the events of September 11, 2001, Americans have needed to address again in new and different ways the intersection of religious and cultural elements in politics, nationalism, and beliefs about war and peace, to name just a few areas of potential tension.

Sociologist James Davison Hunter has researched religious diversity within historically homogeneous denominations and across world faith traditions. He has observed that although all groups wish for their beliefs, practices, and lifestyles to be respected and tolerated and strive to do the same for other religious groups, there exists nevertheless an "uneasy pluralism" (Hunter 1991). In the presence of increasing religious and cultural diversity, religious tolerance coexists with fears that core aspects of historicity, theology, and group-specific identity are being lost, even sacrificed, for the sake of cultural harmony and peaceful coexistence. Hunter also described an interesting phenomenon regarding family values in contemporary religious and culturally diverse America. His research documented that in Jewish, Protestant, and Catholic communities, individuals of similar ages and education had more in common with families in similar income brackets regarding family values; child-rearing priorities; and views on health care, education, and politics than they did with families of the same religious group but of a different socioeconomic class (Hunter 1991).

These and other observations may be generalizable to the fields of medicine and behavioral health and across other major world faith traditions and cultural groups in North America. Beliefs and practices vary both within and between major world faith traditions and the denominations or smaller groups that comprise them. For instance, Judaism's three largest groups or denominations are Orthodox, Conservative, and Reform. A *continuum of belief and practice* exists whereby the Orthodox group has the most theologically and socially conservative viewpoints and lifestyles and the Reform Jews are theologically liberal and tend to espouse more liberal views on social issues, with Conservative Jews in between their Orthodox and Reform counterparts. Similarly, conservative theological beliefs tend to couple with conservative social views within Protestantism and other major world religious groups. Continua of belief and practice also exist within the same or similar religious groups and those that share religious institutional histories. Within most Protestant denominations, there are individuals who believe that the only family form acceptable to God is the traditional one of a heterosexual couple with children. Others see no theological or cultural reasons for not accepting and embracing nontraditional families such as same-sex couples with children, multiracial families, and various forms of blended families. In other words, individuals with conservative theological worldviews tend to hold conservative positions regarding social and cultural issues, and those with more progressive, liberal, or even no theological beliefs tend to espouse more liberal opinions regarding those same issues (Dell 2016). Certainly, discussions at the intersection of religion, spirituality, and culture have much to inform us about the priorities, moral quandaries, and concerns prominent in societal conversations at any given place and time.

Religion, Spirituality, and Culture in Psychiatric Practice

Almost all areas of life are relevant to the psychiatric care of children and families, and there are very few, if any, aspects of life that are not influenced directly by religious or spiritual belief and practice; these factors have shaped current societal and cultural mores over time (Table 8–2). Religious and spiritual beliefs and practices inform family life, child rearing, education, sexuality and gender concerns, political leanings, and values that influence how families spend their time and money. Religious and spiritual beliefs, sifted through cultural lenses and biases, directly affect attitudes toward medical care, psychiatry, obtaining mental health care, psychotropic medications, and engagement in psychotherapy and other treatment modalities. Religious and cultural backgrounds may dictate decisions in medical ethics quandaries, end-of-life preferences, how bodies are prepared immediately after death, and the timing and location of burials (Josephson and Dell 2004).

The intersection of religion and culture contributes to a fund of knowledge of general and specific importance in health care. Although clinicians cannot be experts in comparative religious studies, several core facts about major world faith traditions can help providers recognize when religious and spiritual concerns are important in the assessment and treatment of children, adolescents, and families. Familiarity with these basic facts can be helpful in single sessions that may be pivotal in therapy or in knowing when to ask the patient to share beliefs and practices in greater detail or when to consult or refer the patient to religious professionals. Memorizing facts about religions is not the goal, but recognizing when this area of life is important and knowing where to obtain additional information and consultation are essential for sound cultural and spiritually sensitive care (Dell 2004, 2016).

Clinicians should be familiar with the names of deities and important figures in a religion's histories, key religious practices, sacred texts, and religious holidays and how they are observed (Table 8–3). For instance, when working with immigrant populations from the Middle East, one should know that Muslims worship Allah, follow the teachings of the prophet Muhammad, observe specific prayer times, read the Qur'an, and fast during the sacred holiday period of Rama-

TABLE 8–2.   Life elements informed or shaped by religion and spirituality

Meaning of life

Justice and fairness

Coping

Afterlife

Blame

Guilt and shame

Diet and exercise

Attitudes toward medical and psychiatric care

Discipline

Corporal punishment

Prejudice

Violence

Psychopathology

Religious education

Abandonment

Gender roles

Peace

Sexuality

Finances and economics

Ecology

Government and politics

dan. Knowing leadership structures and organization of community religious groups is important, such as when working with leaders of African American churches on collaborative projects addressing mental health concerns of urban youth. Clinicians should know the makeup of the religious communities in the geographic locations where they practice and their patients live. After identifying the religious and cultural groups most populous in those areas, clinicians can familiarize themselves with the beliefs and practices that pertain to children, adolescents, and families in general and other religious beliefs relevant to health, wellness, and medical and psychiatric illness (Dell 2016).

Common Major World Faith Traditions and Contemporary American Culture

The core histories, important characters, basic religious beliefs, teachings, and ethical practices of major world faith traditions are established and accepted enough that brief factual summaries are possible, even as interpretations of this information have contributed to disagreement and division. Many helpful texts and resources are available to provide the background in world religions, denominations, religious movements, cults, and other groups that mental health clini-

TABLE 8–3. **Information helpful for clinicians to know about major world faith traditions**

Deity and important historical figures

Core, unique, or defining history, religious beliefs, and practices

Sacred text

Sacred days and observances

Leadership and group structure or institution

How widespread the religion is and its geographic reach

Unique and important beliefs and practices regarding children (e.g., circumcision, rites of passage, gender roles)

Unique or important facts about health and wellness (e.g., diet, exercise, medical care)

Attitudes and practices regarding mental health care (psychopharmacology, psychotherapy)

Attitudes and practices regarding end-of-life care, dying, death, burial customs, mourning rituals

cians should be familiar with in order to understand a general demographic, a group of patients, or a particular family or patient (Al-Mateen and Afzal 2004; Black 2004; Cohen and Numbers 2013; Jeffers et al. 2013; Mathewes 2010; Matlins and Magida 2015; Mercer 2004; Murrell 2004; Partridge 2018; Rube and Kibel 2004). At the same time, American culture is becoming more pluralistic, diverse, and geographically mobile, influenced by assimilation; decades of changing immigration patterns; and shifts in religious and spiritual beliefs, behaviors, and organizational membership.

The Pew Research Center (www.pewresearch.org/about), a nonprofit, nonpartisan, and nonadvocacy fact tank and subsidiary of the Pew Charitable Trusts, conducts demographic research, public opinion polling, and data-driven social science research. In 2007, the Pew Research Center conducted the groundbreaking Religious Landscape Study, which was repeated in 2014. In both studies, 35,000 Americans 18 years and older responded to telephone surveys designed to learn about the religious composition of the United States; specific demographics of religious groups; and the religious beliefs, practices, and social and political leanings of Americans who self-identify with various religious traditions (Pew Research Center 2015). Table 8–4 summarizes facts, beliefs, and ethical priorities of common major world faith traditions, including cultural considerations pertaining to religious and spiritual expression of those who self-identify with these groups in contemporary American society.

Judaism

People of the Jewish faith consider its origin to be more than 3,000 years ago when God, or Yahweh, handed down the Ten Commandments to Moses and the Hebrew people on Mount Sinai. Judaism is both the culture and the religion of the Hebrew descendants that developed in Mesopotamia and surrounding lands in the sixth century B.C.E. It is a monotheistic tradition, or worship of a single deity. Important historical and Biblical figures include Abraham, King David, and prophets Isaiah and Jeremiah. Sacred writings include the Tanakh, the entirety of Hebrew scriptures; the Torah, the first five books of the scriptures attributed to Moses; the Mishnah, the regulations and laws; and the Talmud, teachings and lessons about the contents of the Torah and

TABLE 8–4. Major faith traditions: important facts

Christianity

- Three major groups: Catholic (Roman, others), Orthodox (Greek, Russian, others), Protestant
- 80% of U.S. adults (51% Protestant, 24% Catholic, 0.6% Orthodox, ~3% other)
- Abrahamic, monotheistic, early members from Jewish and non-Jewish backgrounds
- Based on life and teachings of Jesus, Son of God
- Sacred text is the Bible, including Old (Hebrew Scriptures) and New Testaments

Judaism

- 12 million people worldwide
- 6 million in the United States, 1.7% of U.S. adults
- Originated in ancient Mesopotamia; traces heritage to patriarch Abraham
- Can refer to both a religion and an ethnicity
- Defined primarily by practices and ethics found in sacred texts instead of doctrines
- Three major groups in the United States: Orthodox (10%), Conservative (35%), Reform (40%)

Islam (Muslim)

- Second-largest world religion, 20% of world's population (Indonesia, Middle East, Bangladesh, Pakistan, Nigeria)
- 0.6% of U.S. adults, >6 million people, and third-largest religion in the United States
- Abrahamic—shares historical and theological elements with Judaism and Christianity
- Muhammad viewed as last messenger of God (Allah)
- Sacred text is the Qur'an
- Important practices (five pillars): profession of belief, prayer, fasting, charity, pilgrimage to Mecca
- Three major branches: Sunni, Shi'a, Sufi

Buddhism

- Fourth-largest religious tradition in the world (Tibet, Sri Lanka, Thailand, China, Korea, Japan)
- 0.7% of U.S. adults
- Originated in 5th century B.C.E. India with teachings of Siddhartha Gautama, the Buddha
- Three branches: East Asian, Tibetan, Theravada
- Elements include nonextremism (Middle Way), teachings of Buddha (dharma), view of suffering (Four Noble Truths), and state of complete selflessness and dissolution of self's boundaries (nirvana)
- Emphasizes right living, compassion, morality, self-discipline

Hinduism

- 83% of population in India; not widespread in rest of world
- 0.4% of U.S. adults, primarily of Asian Indian lineage
- No clear historical beginning, but roots identifiable as early as 3000 B.C.E.
- Complex system of beliefs, ideals, and practices; God and Truth are one; many gods and goddesses represent truth and divinity
- Key concepts: cycle of birth, death, rebirth in another body (reincarnation); current experiences are fruits of past actions (karma); ethical teachings (dharma); social class system (castes)
- Important duties: personal cleanliness, food preparation and eating habits, marriage and family relationships, quiet meditation

TABLE 8–4.   Major faith traditions: important facts *(continued)*

African American religious traditions

- More African Americans claim formal religious affiliation than all other ethnic groups
- Predominantly Christian, with both predominantly black denominations and black churches in predominantly white denominations
- Two-thirds of historically black Protestant churches in the United States are Baptist
- Centers of community life: education, social justice, social work, culture
- Churches and clergy were leaders in civil rights movement
- Nation of Islam: organized African American Muslim group founded in 1930

American Indian religion and spirituality

- <0.3% U.S. adults
- Nearly as many forms as nations, tribes, and cultures
- Spirituality is a personal relationship connecting the individual's spirit to creation, present world, sense of place, other people, and animals
- Many rituals involving nature, human development, and rites of passage
- Modern expressions may be admixed with traditional aspects of Christianity
- Opposition to majority consumerism, materialism, politics, economics, and environmental abuse and neglect is also attractive to many non–American Indians

Source.   Cutting 2006; Eckel 2003; Esposito 2003; Gill 2003; Johnson 2006; Larson 2003; Neusner 2003; Pew Research Center 2008; Raman 2006; Scarlett 2006. Reprinted from Dell ML: "Cultural and Religious Issues," in *Dulcan's Textbook of Child and Adolescent Psychiatry*, 2nd Edition. Edited by Dulcan MK. Arlington, VA, American Psychiatric Association Publishing, 2016, pp. 565–566. Used with permission.

Mishnah. Worldwide, the history and faith of the Jewish people have been shaped by persecution, movement, and migration even as Jewish people have maintained their religious and cultural identities (Cohen and Numbers 2013; Jeffers et al. 2013; Partridge 2018; Sorajjakool et al. 2010).

There are several recognized denominations within Judaism, defined by their places on the continuum from most to least observant; the three largest are Orthodox, Conservative, and Reform. The percentage of adults who self-identify as Jewish has decreased by 50% since the late 1950s. According to the 2014 Pew Religious Landscape Study, Jews comprise 1.9% of the American population (Pew Research Center 2015). Jewish millennials, or those born between 1980 and the mid-1990s, are more likely than older generations to call themselves Jewish by ancestry, ethnicity, or culture only, with 68% of young Jewish adults believing or practicing the Jewish religion and 32% claiming cultural but not religious connection to their Jewish heritage. Intermarriage with spouses of non-Jewish religions and trends of switching from more to less observant Jewish denominations follow overall trends documented in other non-Jewish faith traditions over the past decade (Pew Research Center 2013).

The Jewish tradition values family, prayer, and regular observance of worship one day a week on the Sabbath. Several holidays are observed yearly both in the community and privately at home, many for remembrance of historically significant events. The Hebrew scriptures pronounce that all of creation is good and that humans are created in God's image; therefore, maintaining health of body, mind, and spirit is desirable and pleasing to God. Attention to mental health is just as valued as caring for one's physical body (Feldman 1986; Flam 2003). Contraception, pregnancy terminations for medical indications, and autopsies are permitted, although more orthodox and conservative groups often consult rabbis in these instances. Many observant Jews keep kosher, the practice of dietary habits that forbids pork, certain fish and fowl items, and mixing milk and meat products (Dayer-Berenson 2011; Spector 2009).

Islam

Islam is the second-largest world religion, representing 20% of the world's population. The Pew Research Center estimated that there were 3.45 million Muslims in the United States in 2017, comprising 1.1% of the U.S. population. There are fewer Muslims than Jews in America, but it is anticipated that the Muslim population will double to 8.1 million by 2050. Muslim communities tend to be larger in some metropolitan areas, such as Washington, D.C., and urban areas in New Jersey. The Muslim population is growing because of immigration to the United States and births within Muslim families. Contrary to popular belief, conversion to Islam is not increasing the numbers of Muslims because the numbers of people leaving the faith are roughly equivalent to the number converting to Islam (Mohamed 2018; Pew Research Center 2015).

Islam is monotheistic and Abrahamic, sharing many historical figures, events, and values with Judaism and Christianity. Similar to Jews and Christians, Muslims revere or greatly respect Noah, Abraham, Moses, and even Jesus. Allah is the name for God, and Muhammad is the principal prophet or messenger of Allah. The sacred text is the Qur'an. Faithful or observant Muslims subscribe to the Five Pillars of Islam, striving to fulfill them if possible. The first tenet of the faith is the *shahadah*, or profession of belief, "There is no god but God, and Muhammad is his prophet." The second pillar is *salat*, or the five ritual prayers Allah instructs to be prayed at designated times every day before the sun rises until late into the evening. The third pillar, *savm*, is fasting during daylight hours during the month of Ramadan. For Muslims, *savm* goes beyond physically abstaining from food, drink, sexual activity, smoking, and other substance use. True fasting means refraining from evil thoughts, words, and deeds. The fourth pillar, *zakat,* is giving charity to those truly in need. The fifth pillar, or *hajj*, is a pilgrimage to the holy city of Mecca in Saudi Arabia, with various ritual observances and tasks to be accomplished along the way.

Great diversity exists in Islam, both worldwide and in North America. Like other major world faith traditions, this diversity exists on a continuum, including beliefs and practices related to health and illness. Clinicians should remember the importance of modesty when examining female patients, inviting another female to be present if possible. Illness is viewed as a time to atone for sins by much prayer. Medications and medical care are permitted, although not for the single purpose of prolonging life. Many patients adjust best to medical and psychiatric hospitalizations if families bring in familiar food prepared according to guidelines of the faith; many Muslims do not eat meat. Muslims permit most medical procedures and medications, including contraception, but disagree with assisted suicide, prolonged time on life support, abortion unless a mother's life is at risk, and autopsies without very clear medical or legal indications (Dayer-Berenson 2011; Sabry and Vohra 2013; Spector 2009).

Al-Mateen and Afzal (2004) have summarized relevant considerations for mental health clinicians working with Muslim youth and their families. For immigrant families whose children straddle American culture at school and outside the home and traditional teachings and practices of Islam and the country of origin at home, adolescence can be especially stressful. Muslim families value obedience, education, and the primacy of family over the individualism of the self. Struggles may arise over dress, gender roles, dating, and sexuality. Stigma may prevent the recognition of psychiatric concerns and seeking appropriate care. Muslim youth are at risk for bullying and abuse and may fear significant physical harm due to prejudice against Muslims in American society. Occasionally, providers will encounter culture-bound syndromes and psychotic symptoms that must be assessed very carefully in order to arrive at an accurate diagnosis. Non-Muslim clinicians may need to be more patient and work harder to earn the trust of Muslim patients. In addition, Muslim families may be from many different countries, introducing additional cultural layers to understanding clinical issues and devising treatment plans. Clinicians' first step when working with Muslim youth and families is to listen as they describe their belief systems, past experiences, and family and cultural backgrounds and how these relate to the concerns that are bringing them to mental health care (Cohen and Numbers 2013; Jeffers et al. 2013; Partridge 2018; Sabry and Vohra 2013; Sorajjakool et al. 2010).

Christianity

Christianity is a broad grouping of faith traditions encompassing 70.6% of Americans according to the 2014 Pew Religious Landscape Survey (Pew Research Center 2015). More than 46% of Americans queried self-identified as Protestant, including evangelical (religiously and culturally conservative), mainline, and historically black denominations. Approximately 21% claimed the Catholic tradition, with Orthodox Christians, Mormons, and Jehovah's Witnesses accounting for a combined 3.3% of survey respondents. Of note, the percentage of adults older than 18 years self-identifying as Christian in 2014 was down by 7.8% from 2007, with decreases seen in all groups comprising Christianity (Pew Research Center 2015).

Like Judaism and Islam, Christianity is monotheistic. The religion is based on the life and teachings of Jesus, the Son of God. The sacred text is the Bible, including the Hebrew Scriptures and the New Testament. Of the Catholic groups, the Roman church is the largest, with a hierarchical organizational structure of pope, cardinals, archbishops, priests, and others. Catholic devotional practices include praying the rosary and the veneration of Mary, mother of Jesus. Catholics may have strong cultural ties going back centuries, including German, Hispanic, Polish, Irish, and Italian roots. Religious orders of men or women, cloistered or community based, have long traditions of service, including the establishment of hospitals, schools, and charities that have championed mental health care (Cohen and Numbers 2013; Jeffers et al. 2013; Partridge 2018; Sorajjakool et al. 2010).

Almost 200 Christian denominations, the overwhelming majority of which are Protestant, are included in the *Handbook of Denominations in the United States* (Olson et al. 2018). The great diversity in religious beliefs and practices and the cultural ramifications discussed in general terms earlier in this chapter apply to American Protestantism. Worship styles range from the formal, liturgical orders of Episcopalians and Lutherans to the informal, spontaneous services of Pentecostal and other charismatic groups. Some groups advocate and initiate ecumenical and community partnerships with other churches, whereas some groups are very independent, even isolative. Just as religious beliefs and practices span a wide range, so too do attitudes and practices regarding medical and psychiatric care, child rearing, education, and all aspects of family life. When questions of a religious or spiritual nature arise in clinical work with Christian families, clinicians are well advised to ask patients directly about their religious and spiritual beliefs pertaining to the clinical concern and to seek consultation with other clinicians and religious professionals to facilitate optimal care.

African American Religious Traditions

No category of religious and spiritual traditions has been shaped by and, in turn, has shaped culture more than those of African Americans. All forms of African American religious traditions—including Christian denominations, Catholicism, African American Judaism, Islam, and spiritual healing traditions—seek explanations for the trials and tribulations of this world while yearning for health, peace, and joy in the future. Religious studies scholar Eddie Glaude Jr. has approached his study of African American religion guided by three core concepts: the practice of freedom, a sign of difference, and an open-ended orientation (Table 8–5) (Glaude 2014). These concepts are helpful for clinicians who wish to appreciate the ways the interdependent relationships influence the lives of their patients and communities.

Today, African American religions are diverse and complex. A minority of African Americans are integrated and worship in predominantly white congregations. Many Protestants belong to denominations that formed after the Civil War and the Great Migration, when people of color moved north and from rural areas to Southern cities. Some denominations, including the African Methodist Episcopal Church, the Christian Methodist Episcopal Church, and the National Baptist Convention, have beliefs that parallel those of white denominations. New Christian denominations grew from the unique historical and urban contexts of African Americans, including the Church of God in Christ, now the fifth-largest Protestant denomination in the United States. Recently, the number of African Americans who have become Sunni Muslims has increased, and other Islam-based traditions have formed, including the Moorish Science Temple and the Nation of Islam (Glaude 2014; Mohamed and Diamant 2019; Olson et al. 2018; Pinn 2013).

The interplay of culture and religion is also illustrated by religious healing practices descended from African traditions that were brought to North and South America centuries ago during the Black Diaspora. Many of these traditions are preserved in South America and the Caribbean, especially Brazil, whereas the majority of Africans and their descendants in the United States became and remained Christians during slavery, emancipation, migration to cities, and the civil rights movement. Voodoo, hoodoo, and conjure are examples of traditions that explained African Americans' experiences of persecution by evil forces, the desire to be kept safe from evil, and the wish to get revenge on those who tortured them. Simplistically, voodoo and hoodoo are traditions descending from Black African magic. Often associated with Haiti, voodoo is an organized religion with a creator God. Followers strive to please spirits (*loas*) to ease life's burdens. Hoodoo incorporates magic practices that defeat evil and bring good luck but does not include any deities (Kuna 1977; Pinn 2013). Hoodoo rituals serve to unite groups of individuals undergoing the same trials (Glaude 2014; Pinn 2013). Candomblé, honed by Africans brought to Brazil and South America, merged religion and culture in response to the denigration and inhumanity of slavery. In Candomblé, one powerful God is served by lesser gods, including deified ancestors who bridge the human and spiritual worlds. Each living person is connected spiritually to an ancestor god who protects them and controls their fate. The faithful

TABLE 8–5.   Three historical concepts of influence in African American religion, spirituality, and culture

Practice of freedom

- Religion has been a vehicle of expression when opportunities have been limited by white supremacy and other historical challenges
- Religion has served to preserve and advance self and community, often with political purpose
- Religion is considered a part of overall African American history

Sign of difference

- Religious practices have been and are being shaped into forms different from those of other cultural groups by specific historical events and cultural contexts
- African American and white churches may use the same Bible, share many theological beliefs, and celebrate the same religious holidays and events, but African American churches view themselves as different from white congregations because of the experiences of slavery and the civil rights movement in the United States

Open-ended orientation

- African American religious traditions, much more so than others in North America and worldwide, are imbued with a sense of "becoming," a belief in a brighter future
- Traditions encourage individuals to dream about the future potentials of themselves, their families, and their communities, unfettered by historical chains and contemporary cultural limitations
- Followers believe that there is more ahead, that "all is not settled"
- Believers keep looking forward with faithful optimism even as they are rooted in their religious beliefs and historical realities

Source.   Adapted from Glaude 2014.

are expected to live out their destinies as guided by their *orixa*, or minor ancestral deity. Religious ceremonies include choreographed dances that unite communities and reinforce cultural continuity. Historically, healing processes were devised for the physical maladies characteristic of colonial life. Over time, practitioners formed political resistance communities such as the Black Power movement and others, advocating for the rights of landless and indigenous Brazilians (DeLoach and Petersen 2010).

Developmental Considerations

Religion and spirituality frame development across cultures and throughout the life span, from conception to death. Some customs, including marriage and funeral ceremonies, are shared by multiple world faith traditions and cultures in the context of religious communities. Many of the practices that originated from faith or religious mandates are also observed because of social benefits for those involved with observing the tradition, regardless of religious or spiritual belief or significance. See Table 8–6 for a list of occasions with both developmental and religious/spiritual significance.

Several theorists have attempted to describe the nature and development of religion and spirituality from birth throughout the life span. Undoubtedly, the most cited of these frameworks is James W. Fowler's *faith development theory*. Fowler, a Protestant theologian steeped in developmental psychology, was influenced heavily by the works of Erik Erikson; Lawrence Kohlberg;

TABLE 8–6. Life cycle events with religious/spiritual significance

Birth and infancy
- Blessings
- Religious services
- Naming of the infant
- Male circumcision (Brit Milah in Judaism)
- Baptisms

Childhood
- Religious education
- Consecrations at the beginning of religious and secular education
- Religious service attendance
- Roles assumed in family life based on gender and birth order
- Participation in extracurricular and group activities
- Baptisms, confirmations, and first communions

Adolescence
- Coming of age observances (e.g., bar and bat mitzvahs)
- Confirmations and first communions
- Assuming adult responsibilities and leadership roles in houses of worship and local faith communities
- Dating and sexuality

Young adulthood
- Decisions about vocation
- Missionary service (e.g., Church of Latter Day Saints)
- Dating and sexuality
- Marriage
- Contraception
- Gender roles
- Dress, hair styles, head coverings
- Childbirth
- Decisions about the religious and spiritual lives of children

Middle adulthood
- Roles as religious leaders and spiritual advisers in the home and in the larger community
- Continuation of parenting responsibilities

Late adulthood
- Roles as spiritual and religious sages
- Prayers and religious/spiritual observances during illness
- Religious/spiritual beliefs and practice at the end of life
- Funerals and burial practices
- Mourning rituals
- Celebrations of life

Jean Piaget; and Wilfred Cantwell Smith, founder of the Institute of Islamic Studies at McGill University in Quebec and later the director of Harvard University's Center for the Study of World Religions. Fowler integrated these existing paradigms with his own empirical research to describe seven distinct stages of an individual's thinking, behaviors, and relationships with the divine and with other humans (Table 8–7). Fowler's work, based on original qualitative research in the 1970s, with expanded studies conducted as late as the 1990s, was innovative and ground-breaking. However, it has been critiqued justifiably, especially by feminist theorists and Black and liberation theologians, for its lack of religious, cultural, ethnic, and socioeconomic diversity in the original work and many of the subsequent study populations. Heinz Streib, Fritz Oser, K.H. Reich, and others have continued and expanded the study of faith development across cultures, with attention to the distinctions between spirituality, formal religious structures, teachings of non-Western societies, and influences in contemporary society. Regardless, Fowler's stages of faith theory remains the best known and most influential work in faith development studies (Fowler 1981; Fowler and Dell 2004, 2006; Hay et al. 2006).

Religion and Spirituality in Cultural Formulation

Psychiatry and mental health care disciplines are making significant strides in embracing the importance and vitality of religion and spirituality, which have been unappreciated—even rejected—during much of the twentieth century. The complexity of the distinct and overlapping elements of culture, religion, and spirituality remains challenging for all clinicians. The inclusion of an entire chapter in DSM-5 on cultural formulation, with attention to religion and spirituality, is evidence that this topic is essential if normal development and its variations, family and community dynamics, various aspects of psychopathology, and treatment resources are to be fully identified and employed in the mental health field (American Psychiatric Association 2013; Whitley 2012).

The DSM-5 Cultural Formulation Interview (CFI) provides valuable background information and explanations of the clinical utility of this instrument when employed in practice (American Psychiatric Association 2013). Indeed, the words *religion* and *spirituality* are quite prominent in the existing tool. For clinical situations in which religion and/or spirituality are hypothesized to factor significantly in assessment, formulation, and treatment planning, clinicians can also envision a variation of the CFI in their own thinking in which they substitute the concept *religious or spiritual* for *cultural*. When applying CFI categories specifically to patients' religious and spiritual lives (religious/spiritual identity, factors or contributors to spiritual and psychological distress, and identification of religious/spiritual mechanisms for coping and resilience), it is especially important for clinicians to listen for relevant information that can foster healing, growth, and future wellness and flourishing. The CFI may be used as written or with appropriate language modifications for adult caregivers and other individuals who are important in the lives of children and adolescents, yielding information helpful to clinicians in order to better understand family dynamics and the immediate day-to-day circumstances of children and adolescents. Clinicians should be mindful of the need to think of these concepts in developmentally appropriate ways, using language and concepts youth can understand according to their

TABLE 8-7.   Stages of faith and selfhood

Primal faith (infancy)
- Occurs before formal language develops
- Infant develops awareness of others
- Development of trust in caregivers eases anxiety when apart

Intuitive-projective faith (early childhood)
- Imagination, perceptions, and feelings are of great importance
- Stories, gestures, and symbols are not yet fully logical
- Child uses imagination, stories, and feelings to deal with protective and threatening powers and influences
- Images, symbols, and feelings created may be long-lasting

Mythic-literal faith (childhood and beyond)
- Logical thinking helps explain the world
- Child has better understanding of cause and effect
- Child is beginning to understand the perspective of others
- Child can explain events and meaning through the use of stories

Synthetic-conventional faith (adolescence and beyond)
- Enhanced ability to engage in mutual perspective taking
- Can integrate different perspectives of oneself and others into a single identity
- Because self-identity is more mature, can unite in solidarity of beliefs and feelings with others

Individuative-reflective faith (young adulthood and beyond)
- Can reflect critically on beliefs and values through third-person perspective taking
- Understands individuals and self as part of greater social order
- Internal locus of control regarding responsibility, orderliness, authority, and lifestyle
- Self-awareness facilitates mature commitments in relationships and vocation

Conjunctive faith (early midlife and beyond)
- Appreciates paradox
- Appreciation of myths, symbols, and metaphors as expressions of truth
- Understands that there are multiple interpretations of reality

Universalizing faith (midlife and beyond)
- Oneness with the individual's being of ultimate power or higher power

Source.   Adapted from Fowler 1981; Fowler and Dell 2004; J.W. Fowler, personal communications, 1991–2008.

cognitive development, experiences, and both imminent and longer-term needs (Aggarwal and Lewis-Fernandez 2015; American Psychiatric Association 2013; Rousseau and Guzder 2015).

Conclusion

Culturally attuned, spiritually and religiously aware clinicians are poised to understand the influences of varied backgrounds and experiences of all children, adolescents, and families, especially those from nonmajority backgrounds. An appreciation of both overt and subtle, unspoken elements of religion and spirituality conveys respect for the patient and an interest in the individual that enhances the therapeutic alliance. Religion and spirituality factor into both patient and family vulnerabilities, as well as resiliency and resources for treatment. Clinicians must be genuinely curious about and inquire into the role of religion and spirituality in the lives of their patients. They should appreciate the roles and authority of clergy, faith leaders, and spiritual advisers in typical family life, traditional medical illnesses, psychiatric illnesses, and treatment.

Religion and spirituality are integral aspects of culture, whether openly acknowledged and embraced by patients and families or expressed privately. Even if individuals do not consider themselves to be spiritual or religious, they nevertheless are part of cultures influenced by faith traditions and institutions. All clinicians will find attention to this vital element of culture helpful in their clinical work with children and families and the communities in which they live.

Religion, Spirituality, Culture, Social Justice, and COVID-19

The events in the United States, North America—indeed the world—in 2020 have underscored as in few other times in history the intricate relationships and complexities of culture, religion, spirituality, and physical and mental health. In the midst of dealing with the novel coronavirus SARS-CoV-2 (COVID-19), the death of George Floyd on May 25, 2020, followed soon by the death of civil rights leader John Lewis on July 17, highlighted not only racial and social justice issues experienced by patients and their families but also the shortcomings of societal institutions such as health care and religious organizations when it comes to preventing, minimizing, and addressing the negative consequences of cultural stereotypes and inequalities.

One way of conceptualizing the entanglements of COVID-19, racial and cultural bias, and religious elements is through the lens of social determinants of health (see Chapter 10, "Social Determinants of Child and Adolescent Mental Health"). The most commonly cited social determinants of health include economic stability, health care, neighborhood and environment, education, and social community and context. Health care, religious communities, and culture, especially race and ethnicity, both inform and are affected by these determinants. Individuals from nonmajority cultures experience economic challenges, often struggle with access to quality health care, are concerned about neighborhood and environmental issues affecting their lives, and seek better educational opportunities, and all these concerns inform societal interactions and activism. Churches, mosques, synagogues, and other religious and spiritual organizations and leaders often give voice to the cultural and political struggles, even as they tend to the personal spiritual needs of the people. Advocacy for cultural and social concerns has been a chief function of religious communities throughout history, always with accompanying failures and successes. The fact that COVID-19 has accentuated the importance of the social determinants of health overlapping with religious ethics and social justice missions of faith communities has brought renewed vitality to these concerns for all, regardless of race, ethnicity, cultural and religious backgrounds, and beliefs.

As mentioned in this chapter, the community aspect of worship in most world faith traditions and the interpersonal relationships and social supports that come from group gatherings comprise elements of religion that can be of tremendous personal and societal value. Certainly, the COVID-19 pandemic has disrupted the traditional ways religious communities worship; care for one another; interact with their neighbors; and provide other services, such as education, childcare and eldercare, food pantries, and ministries to the homeless. As in the fields of education, business, and health care, religious organizations are adapting to new ways of "doing church" that retain what is beneficial, familiar, and comforting, even as the combination of necessity and creativity ushers in new possibilities for the future.

Clinical Pearls

- Religious and spiritual beliefs influence patient attitudes and behaviors regarding health and wellness, illness, seeking medical and psychiatric care, and engaging in psychotherapy or pharmacotherapy.

- Relationships between culture and religion are complex, highly variable, and specific to individual patients and their families.

- It is important for clinicians to take thorough religious and spiritual histories and to ask open-ended, well-timed questions that convey interest and a willingness to listen without coming across to the patient as intrusive or pushy.

- Clinicians should be familiar with basic facts about major world faith traditions common in the geographic area in which they practice but should not make hard and fast assumptions regarding any individual patient and family.

- Intergenerational differences often exist within the same family, especially regarding the specific traditions observed, the degree of piety and personal commitment, and issues such as intermarriage that often exist in immigrant families.

- Local communities of faith play a key role as the bearer and preserver of both religious and secular elements of cultures of origin.

- Clinicians should demonstrate a genuine willingness to include a family's faith leader as a partner in patient care according to the wishes and best interests of the patient and family.

- Elements of the Cultural Formulation Interview can be incorporated into clinical work as a helpful tool for understanding the relationships between culture, religion, and spirituality.

Self-Assessment Questions

1. How might you adjust your current conceptualization of patients to include religion and spirituality?

2. What specific questions might you ask to help you understand the religious and spiritual beliefs and practices of patients and their families?

3. How might additional information about patient spirituality and religiosity inform your future patient care and treatment planning?

References

Aggarwal NH, Lewis-Fernandez R: An introduction to the cultural formulation interview. Focus 13(4):426–431, 2015

Al-Mateen CS, Afzal A: The Muslim child, adolescent, and family. Child Adolesc Psychiatr Clin N Am 13(1):183–200, 2004

American Psychiatric Association: Cultural formulation, in Diagnostic and Statistical Manual of Mental Disorders, 5th Edition. Arlington, VA, American Psychiatric Association, 2013, pp 749–759

Atwood CD, Olson RE: Religion in America, in Handbook of Denominations in the United States, 14th Edition. Edited by Olson RE, Atwood CD, Mead FS, Hill SS. Nashville, TN, Abingdon Press, 2018, pp 1–11

Black N: Hindu and Buddhist children, adolescents, and families. Child Adolesc Psychiatr Clin N Am 13(1):201–220, 2004

Cohen CL, Numbers RL (eds): Gods in America: Religious Pluralism in the United States. New York, Oxford University Press, 2013

Cutting C: Islam, in Encyclopedia of Religious and Spiritual Development. Edited by Dowling EM, Scarlett WG. Thousand Oaks, CA, Sage, 2006, pp 212–217

Dayer-Berenson L: Cultural Competencies for Nurses: Impact on Health and Illness. Sudbury, MA, Jones & Bartlett, 2011

Dell ML: Religious professionals and institutions: untapped resources for clinical care. Child Adolesc Psychiatr Clin N Am 13(1):85–110, 2004

Dell ML: Cultural and religious issues, in Dulcan's Textbook of Child and Adolescent Psychiatry, 2nd Edition. Edited by Dulcan MK. Arlington, VA, American Psychiatric Association Publishing, 2016, pp 559–570

DeLoach CF, Petersen MN: African spiritual methods of healing: the use of Candomblé in traumatic response. J Pan Afr Stud 3(8):40–62, 2010

Eckel MD: Buddhism in the world and in America, in World Religions in America, 3rd Edition. Edited by Neusner J. Louisville, KY, Westminster John Knox, 2003, pp 142–153

Esposito JL: Islam in the world and in America, in World Religions in America, 3rd Edition. Edited by Neusner J. Louisville, KY, Westminster John Knox, 2003, pp 172–185

Feldman DM: Health and Medicine in the Jewish Tradition. New York, Crossroad, 1986

Flam N: Healing of body, healing of spirit, in The Mitzvah of Healing. Edited by Person HE. New York, Women of Reform Judaism/UAHC Press, 2003, pp 53–56

Fowler JW: Stages of Faith. New York, HarperCollins, 1981

Fowler JW, Dell ML: Stages of faith and identity: birth to teens. Child Adolesc Psychiatr Clin N Am 13(1):1–15, 2004

Fowler JW, Dell ML: Stages of faith from infancy through adolescence: reflections on three decades of faith development theory, in The Handbook of Spiritual Development in Childhood and Adolescence.

Edited by Roehlkepartain EC, King PE, Wagener L, Benson PL. Thousand Oaks, CA, Sage, 2006, pp 34–45

Freud S: The question of a weltanschauung (1933), in The Standard Edition of the Complete Psychological Works of Sigmund Freud, Vol 11. Translated and edited by Strachey J. London, Hogarth, 1962, pp 158–167

Gill S: Native Americans and their religions, in World Religions in America, 3rd Edition. Edited by Neusner J. Louisville, KY, Westminster John Knox, 2003, pp 9–23

Glaude ES Jr: African American Religion: A Very Short Introduction. New York, Oxford University Press, 2014

Gordon MW: Rediscovering Jewish infrastructure: the legacy of U.S. 19th century synagogues. American Jewish History 75(4):296–306, 1986

Hay D, Reich KH, Utsch M: Spiritual development: intersections and divergence with religious development, in The Handbook of Spiritual Development in Childhood and Adolescence. Edited by Roehlkepartain EC, King PE, Wagener L, et al. Thousand Oaks, CA, Sage, 2006, pp 46–59

Hunter JD: Culture Wars: The Struggle to Define America. New York, Basic Books, 1991

Jeffers SL, Nelson ME, Barnet V, et al (eds): The Essential Guide to Religious Traditions and Spirituality for Health Care Providers. London, Radcliffe, 2013

Johnson T: Native American Indian spirituality, in Encyclopedia of Religious and Spiritual Development. Edited by Dowling EM, Scarlett WG. Thousand Oaks, CA, Sage, 2006, pp 313–315

Josephson AM, Dell ML: Religion and spirituality in child and adolescent psychiatry: a new frontier. Child Adolesc Psychiatr Clin N Am 13(1):1–15, 2004

Koenig HC, McCullough ME, Larson DB: Handbook of Religion and Health. New York, Oxford University Press, 2001

Kuna RR: Hoodoo: the indigenous medicine and psychiatry of the Black American. Florida Anthropologist 30(4):196–211, 1977

Larson GJ: Hinduism in India and in America, in World Religions in America, 3rd Edition. Edited by Neusner J. Louisville, KY, Westminster John Knox, 2003, pp 121–141

Mathewes C: Understanding Religious Ethics. West Sussex, UK, Wiley-Blackwell, 2010

Matlins SM, Magida AJ (eds): How to Be a Perfect Stranger: The Essential Religious Etiquette Handbook, 6th Edition. Woodstock, VT, SkyLight Paths, 2015

Mercer JA: The Protestant child, adolescent, and family. Child Adolesc Psychiatr Clin N Am 13(1):161–182, 2004

Mohamed B: New estimates show U.S. Muslim population continues to grow. Washington, DC, Pew Research Center, January 3, 2018. Available at: www.pewresearch.org/fact-tank/2018/01/03/new-estimates-show-u-s-muslim-population-continues-to-grow. Accessed November 17, 2019.

Mohamed B, Diamant J: Black Muslims account for a fifth of all U.S. Muslims, and about half are converts to Islam. Washington, DC, Pew Research Center, January 17, 2019. Available at: www.pewresearch.org/fact-tank/2019/01/17/black-muslims-account-for-a-fifth-of-all-u-s-muslims-and-about-half-are-converts-to-islam. Accessed November 17, 2019.

Murrell K: The Catholic child, adolescent, and family. Child Adolesc Psychiatr Clin N Am 13(1):149–160, 2004

Neusner J: Judaism in the world and in America, in World Religions in America, 3rd Edition. Edited by Neusner J. Louisville, KY, Westminster John Knox, 2003, pp 106–123

Olson RE, Atwood CD, Mead FS, et al (eds): Handbook of Denominations in the United States, 14th Edition. Nashville, TN, Abingdon, 2018

Partridge C: Introduction to World Religions, 3rd Edition. Minneapolis, MN, Fortress, 2018

Pew Research Center: U.S. Religious Landscape Survey: religious affiliation. Washington, DC, Pew Research Center, February 1, 2008. Available at: www.pewforum.org/2008/02/01/u-s-religious-landscape-survey-religious-affiliation. Accessed August 21, 2020.

Pew Research Center: A portrait of Jewish Americans: new comprehensive survey examines changing Jewish identity. Washington, DC, Pew Research Center, October 1, 2013. Available at: www.pewforum.org/2013/10/01/a-portrait-of-jewish-americans. Accessed November 17, 2019.

Pew Research Center: America's changing religious landscape. Washington, DC, Pew Research Center, May 12, 2015. Available at: www.pewforum.org/2015/05/12/americas-changing-religious-landscape. Accessed November 17, 2019.

Pinn AB: Introducing African American Religion. New York, Routledge, 2013

Raman VV: Hinduism, in Encyclopedia of Religious and Spiritual Development. Edited by Dowling EM, Scarlett WG. Thousand Oaks, CA, Sage, 2006, pp 199–203

Rousseau C, Guzder J: Supplementary module 9: school-age children and adolescents, in DSM-5 Handbook on the Cultural Formulation Interview. Edited by Lewis-Fernández R, Aggarwal NK, Hinton L, et al. Arlington, VA, American Psychiatric Publishing, 2015, pp 156–164

Rube DM, Kibel N: The Jewish child, adolescent, and family. Child Adolesc Psychiatr Clin N Am 13(1):137–148, 2004

Sabry WM, Vohra A: Role of Islam in the management of psychiatric disorders. Indian J Psychiatry 55 (suppl 2):S205–S214, 2013

Scarlett WG: Buddhism, in Encyclopedia of Religious and Spiritual Development. Edited by Dowling EM, Scarlett WG. Thousand Oaks, CA, Sage, 2006, pp 59–60

Sorajjakool S, Carr MF, Nam JJ: World Religions for Healthcare Professionals. New York, Routledge, 2010

Spector RE: Cultural Diversity in Health and Illness, 7th Edition. Upper Saddle River, NJ, Pearson, 2009

Whitley R: Religious competence as cultural competence. Transcult Psychiatry 49(2):245–260, 2012

CHAPTER 9

Diverse Families and Family Treatment

Neha Sharma, D.O.
John Sargent, M.D.

CHILDREN and adolescents grow and develop in their family and their community. The values and belief systems of the family, influenced by their culture, impact a youth's upbringing, development, dreams, aspirations, and identity. Thus, an individual's presentation of mental illness, definition of mental illness, attitude toward treatment, and ability to seek help are closely tied to family values and family culture. Additionally, family challenges (e.g., poverty, unemployment, marital discord, parental medical and/or psychiatric conditions) can be a source of distress for a child, leading to psychiatric symptoms and somatic complaints. Conversely, a child's condition (e.g., chronic medical illness, psychosis, autism spectrum disorder, intellectual disability, obsessive-compulsive disorder, anxiety, depression) can affect family well-being and be reinforced through enmeshment and/or distancing. In this chapter we focus on strategies to engage distressed families from different cultural, racial, and ethnic backgrounds and highlight approaches that facilitate assessment of the family and family treatment of the youth's condition.

What Is Family?

A family is a group of people (often of multiple generations) who live together, are committed to each other, and share their lives. They can be biologically related or together through adoption, surrogacy, marriage (i.e., stepfamilies), or refugee status, or they can be chosen families.

One primary goal of families is monitoring, supporting, and encouraging the growth and development of the next generation. Families also are a source of historical identity for individuals and for the family as a whole. Thus, families are vehicles of cultural integration and transmission. When individuals live in their home country, their cultural values, identity, and beliefs are reinforced by the larger community. However, when they live in a different country or region where the larger community does not share the same beliefs, the pressure of the family as the sole vehicle for transmitting cultural knowledge and experience is accentuated. This pressure can exacerbate normal family developmental challenges and, at times, can exhaust the strengths of the family, create rifts in relationships, and become a barrier to medical interventions.

Families promote both connection through relationships with caretakers and autonomy to engage in the wider world. Both are necessary for well-being. Families also become the arena for the resolution of conflicts that occur when too much connection threatens autonomy and vice versa. Culture establishes traditions that regulate the balance of connection and autonomy. American culture emphasizes the importance of autonomy, individual success and well-being, and the privacy of the couple and the nuclear family. When families resolve this challenge with love, validation, and acceptance, the duality of connection and independence is simultaneously supported. However, when there is rigidity, inflexibility, and coercion to be on one end of the continuum, family interactions can contribute to mental health issues, rupturing relationships or curtailing individual growth. Often, the work of family therapists is to promote validation while helping the family mitigate extreme reactions of enmeshment, rigidity, punishment, and/or isolation.

Culture and Its Impact on a Family

Culture is a way of living. "Culture has been described as a socially transmitted system of ideas that: shapes behavior, categorizes perceptions, gives names to selected aspects of experience, and is widely shared by members of a particular society or group…" (Hughes 1993, p. 7). It also functions as a framework that coordinates and sanctions behavior and conveys values across the generations. Often, culture defines what is right and wrong, what is acceptable and unacceptable for families, and what affects their everyday actions and interactions.

Culture influences how the members of the family communicate affection, support, and care and how gender roles and responsibilities are assigned. For example, in highly patriarchal communities, such as Asian and Latinx communities, mothers hold the role of showing affection verbally, physically, and by actions. Often, the mother figure may cook elaborate meals or a child's favorite foods to share love and warmth. In contrast, father figures show care predominantly through their actions, such as providing financial or material necessities or by being present at important events and by doing activities with the child. Another way fathers may display care is through setting expectations of respect, discipline, achievements, and participation in household activities. A strict gender-based definition of family roles can be experienced as restrictive and oppressive, especially if male family members expect to exercise power over female family members. Family interactions can subsequently be experienced as authoritarian dictates rather than a reflection of love and protection.

Immigrant families have the additional pressure of acculturating to the host country's culture. Berry et al. (1989) described four models of acculturation: 1) assimilation, 2) integration,

3) marginalization, and 4) separation. Please refer to Figure 1–3 in Chapter 1, "Introduction," for details on how models of acculturation relate to identification with American culture and maintenance of the heritage culture.

These four acculturation processes are on a spectrum of how much the family aligns with their heritage and the culture of the host country. Where the family falls in the acculturation process informs clinicians with regard to parents' expectations, their parenting style, strengths of the parent-child dyad, and potential parent-child conflicts. Keeping the benefits and challenges of these processes in mind can facilitate engagement with families of diverse backgrounds.

Although acceptance of the family's multifaceted experience makes integration the ideal acculturation model, it can also be burdensome to follow and maintain cultural values of two cultures, especially when the cultural values are of opposing nature. At times, having to decide individually which value to uphold can turn into an isolating experience for children and adolescents. On the other hand, if the family promotes making these decisions together, in a collaborative way, the process ends up strengthening the parent-child relationship. This requires the parents to be open and curious to the ways of different cultures as well as to tolerate the discomfort of potentially diluting their own traditional values. Youth are at higher risk of falling into the marginalization group when they feel misunderstood by the family and by the larger society. Frequently, the marginalization process occurs in the context of rigid, inflexible, and authoritarian parenting. The families who are in the separation group may be living in ethnic enclaves and continue to be immersed in their native language, values, food, and art at the cost of limited engagement with the larger host society. Youth who are raised in these households may feel isolated and may experience a lack of confidence when interfacing with the host culture at school and/or when applying for college.

In addition to supporting development, the family encourages adherence to rules and values. Successful immigrant family experience occurs when the parents are able to recognize both cultures and encourage acceptance of values of the traditional and host country cultures. This means that the family is able to promote the value of success in America as well as their cultural values, traditions, and rituals. Parents who are passive about acculturation may fail to get their children to align with one or all elements of their culture. Immigrant families have a multitude of reasons for leaving their home country; some may have migrated because they did not accept the traditional values for themselves. In this case, the family may implicitly convey undervaluing of their own traditions or they may struggle with upholding any rules that they experienced as oppressive. In either case, the acculturation process may be more confusing for youth and can result in a fragmented cultural identity.

Acculturative Stress and Acculturative Family Distancing

The challenge for every diverse family is threefold: to navigate acculturative stress, to assimilate into the mainstream culture without losing their traditional values, and to pass on their cultural values to their children while supporting their success in the mainstream culture. *Acculturative stress* is defined as perceived (psychological, emotional, or health) stress in relation to the process of adapting to a different community. Each individual in the family adapts to the new culture at a different pace depending on the amount and type of exposure to the new community; this leads to different degrees of acculturation among family members. This *acculturation gap* among family members can threaten or weaken family bonds and increase miscommunications, misperceptions, and misunderstandings. If differential gender roles are added to these interactions, it is easy for misunderstandings to escalate into feelings of unfairness, experiences of sexism, and limited communication. The greater the acculturation gap, the higher the intergenerational family conflict and the lower the family cohesion (Hwang et al. 2010). This family distancing due to different degrees of acculturation between parents and youth has been referred to as *acculturative family distancing*. This has been specifically noted in Asian American families and is likely to be present with other immigrant groups as well (Hwang et al. 2010). Furthermore, in the twentieth and twenty-first centuries, scholars have developed the term *transnationalism* (Falicov 2014) to reflect the fact that many immigrant families stay connected to their home countries and family who remain there through technology, including phone calls, video chats, texting, and e-mail. Immigrant families also often send money to family in the home country. These connections can provide significant support to immigrant families and children, but they can also create additional stress through obligations to extended family back home and dilution of attention to members of the immigrant family.

Language and Family Cohesion

Both acculturative stress and acculturative family distancing can contribute to intrafamilial conflicts. In the United States, there are additional factors that can further increase power struggles between youth and immigrant parents as well as between immigrants and the community. One significant factor that enhances power is the ability to speak English and how it impacts the ability to access information. Parents' lack of English proficiency limits their understanding of available resources in the community and their ability to advocate for their child. Children and adolescents also may have access to information that may not be age appropriate. Parents who do not speak English often ask their offspring to translate important information that the youth may either edit or misunderstand. Children's availability to translate and interpret conversations puts them in a position to know financial, medical, marital, and other information that they may not be emotionally or developmentally prepared to process. This privilege can undermine the hierarchical structure of the family by reducing the executive power of the parents, which often makes parents dependent on their children in order to communicate. In addition, the information can burden the child or adolescent and lead to depressive and anxious symptoms. Liu et al. (2009) noted that children of Chinese mothers who spoke English proficiently had fewer depressive symptoms and better academic scores than those whose mothers were not proficient in English. However, bilingual youth were noted to have fewer depressive symptoms, likely due to the fact that communicating via the parent's native language facilitates a stronger bond between the parent and the child (Liu et al. 2009).

Speaking English is a prerequisite for social acceptance and integration in American society (Rothe et al. 2010). Not speaking English or having an accent puts parents at risk of being at the receiving end of discrimination and microaggressions. This may cause youth to feel anger and disrespect toward their parents as well as the larger community. Internalized bias and racism have a deep negative effect on family cohesion and on one's ethnic identity. If children feel ashamed of their parents or do not respect them, then the children are less likely to adhere to their parents' rules and values and might even choose to separate from their ethnic community and not retain their native language. In some impoverished immigrant communities, speaking in one's native language is seen as a reflection of lower status, thus leading caregivers to ask youth not to retain the native language (Portes and Schauffler 1996). Loss of the native language can further limit the youth's ability to communicate with parents and grandparents and decreases shared experiences and meaning making within the family. Youth and parents may feel that they are living in different worlds, further contributing to acculturative family distancing.

Meaning of Success and Its Impact on the Parent-Child Dyad

Every family has its own definition of what success means. For an immigrant family, there is an additional component to consider when defining success: justifying the losses and sacrifices they made to have a life in the "land of opportunity." Families give up relationships with their parents, extended family, and friends and everything that was familiar and associated with important memories. The transnational experience of some immigrant families alleviates to some degree the loss of support, but distance and separation continue to cause stress and distress at different stages of life. Additionally, family members may have to forgo their high status and careers—important aspects of their own identity—in order to start from scratch. One way parents may justify these sacrifices is by focusing excessively on the academic success of their child. This pressure to achieve can make the parent-child relationship more coercive and can affect the emotional well-being of the child; immigrant youth are often very aware that their success has a larger meaning for their family, making it even more burdensome and stressful.

Another component to consider when defining success for an immigrant family is retention of traditional values and culture. Holding on to traditional ways may help families mitigate the sadness of leaving their home country and family members. However, if youth are seen as more "American" rather than accepting of traditional ways, parents may experience guilt about not being able to pass on their traditions. This guilt can result in parents being more rigid regarding their values and less open to their children's perspective. Rigidity may promote more rebellion from the youth, furthering the cycle of guilt, rigidity, and rebellion.

Although all families hope for their children's well-being and want to promote the success of the next generation, specific cultural factors influence family structure and values. These factors are vital to consider when engaging in treatment. In treating immigrant families, the family therapist must be mindful of families' experience of spirituality, oppression, trauma, and events that solidify their identity (Limb and Hodge 2011). For example, African American families are aware of their history of oppression, discrimination, and disruption of family structure due to slavery (Santisteban et al. 1997). The family therapist has to be respectful and open to their notion of spirituality, inclusion of the extended family, and involvement of the church (McCollum 1997). The therapist must appreciate that for some immigrants, as is the case in Latinx families who hold *familismo* as a key value, family goals often may take precedence over individual goals. Another crucial value that therapists working with immigrant families should keep in mind is the respect for elders and parental authority, which in Latinx culture is known as *respeto*. Similarly, Asian American families value reverence to elders while sacrificing oneself for the well-being of the family (Jacob et al. 2011). Asian American families also value opportunities in education and deny psychiatric symptoms that are associated with shame. LGBTQ+ individuals may trust a provider more if the therapist is open to their experience of being a "hidden minority" and their experiences of microaggressions and microrejections by other people, their family, or systems (DeDiego 2016).

The Process of Family Therapy

Families enter mental health treatment for many reasons, including problems with a child's development, challenging behaviors that are difficult to manage, academic failure, communication problems, relationship problems, and adapting to a change in family life. We encourage child and adolescent mental health clinicians to meet with the child's primary caretakers and the child at the onset. This helps the adults appreciate that their concerns and goals are at the center of treatment and helps the child to recognize not only the caretakers' concerns but also their commitment to helping the child through the treatment process. As everyone presents his or her sense of the problem, the therapist listens for what family members want to accomplish or improve through treatment. The therapist then can synthesize the family's goals into a coherent summary that can be shared with the family in order to cooperatively consider which goals can be achieved and which must be modified.

The culture of the family and the degree of acculturation to the host culture play important roles in how the goals of treatment are elaborated and agreed on. Stigma around mental illness within the culture of origin, the degree of trust in mental health care, and a strong desire for the best outcome for the child often influence the family's approach to treatment and their engagement in family therapy. Although parents may expect therapy to change their child for the better, often it improves the interactions of all the family members.

Families may be referred for treatment because of an individual difficulty the child has that makes him or her different from typical children. Children can be experiencing intellectual challenges, challenges in relating and communicating to others (as is the case with autism spectrum disorder), a learning disorder, attentional or emotional regulation challenges (as is the case with ADHD), a problem with obsessionality and compulsions, a mood problem, excessive anxiety, problems with reality testing, or problematic reactions to a traumatic experience. The degree to which these problems can be reduced or eliminated varies, but in most cases, the first step should be acknowledgment of the problem itself, followed by attempts at improving the problem.

In terms of acceptance of the problem, individuals from different cultures can have different reactions and understanding of the reality of the child's experience of being different from typical children. For instance, the child can be seen as an "other" and not a full member of the collective family. If the child's struggles are seen as a sign of poor parenting, a source of shame and embarrassment for the family, the situation can feel like a challenge to their sense of community and belonging. Part of setting the agenda for therapy will always be understanding the family's sense of their child's atypicality and their willingness to live with it as well as make accommodations for the child and themselves that decrease the impact of the difference. Family therapy may promote accommodation to difference by increasing knowledge of and comfort with such difference, which will, in turn, decrease the family's distress. This process may be very challenging for diverse families and requires a patient, compassionate, and collaborative approach, identifying the family's wishes, beliefs, and fears. Integrity, curiosity, and respect on the part of the therapist will always be necessary. Knowing how the family understands the child's difference and honoring their language when describing the situation are part of the keys for successful treatment. The first goal of treatment is always respectful engagement and a willingness to work together regardless of cultural differences.

Clinical Vignette 1

Daniel is a 14-year-old Chinese American male with a history of ADHD, specific learning disorder (impairment in reading and written expression), and conduct disorder referred by his primary care physician to a child psychiatry clinic for a medication evaluation. Daniel speaks English predominantly and only partially understands Cantonese, but at home, his parents speak Cantonese only. The interview was conducted with the assistance of a Cantonese interpreter.

Daniel had been diagnosed with ADHD in third grade and is currently being treated with methylphenidate hydrochloride 40 mg daily and guanfacine 1 mg daily. His mother, Mrs. Luo, described him as impulsive, hyperactive, and distractible. She was not sure the medications were helpful, which was further endorsed by Daniel.

Mrs. Luo expressed concern that Daniel has difficulty regulating his emotions, and he has frequent arguments with his parents that often escalate into aggression. She stated that he does not seem to understand the consequences of his actions. Mrs. Luo is worried about the possibility of losing their housing as a result of Daniel's behaviors and frequent interactions with the police. When the treatment team engaged Daniel alone, he did not see his behavior as problematic but acknowledged that his behaviors were stressful for his parents.

A family meeting was held by a white clinician with an interpreter. Mrs. Luo said she felt that Daniel was a willful child who is oppositional, but her main concern was his limited understanding of the situation. She attributed his behaviors to brain atypicality. Mr. Luo said he did not believe in mental illness, ADHD, or learning issues. He found his son to be mostly oppositional and worried that the family would become homeless if Daniel's behaviors continued to cause more problems with the housing community where they live. Daniel was more focused on his parents not understanding him or supporting him.

The family shared their pattern of managing Daniel's challenges. Usually, Mrs. Luo tried to remind Daniel of the rules and related consequences but struggled to follow through with enforcement of the rules. Mr. Luo, who worked long hours, mostly got involved only after a significant behavioral issue had already occurred. Daniel's engagements with his father often resulted in physical fights that only reinforced Daniel's mistrust of his parents.

The therapist became aware of the importance of seeing the situation through the family's eyes and through the lens of their culture. With the help of the interpreter, the clinician highlighted that the family was under an immense amount of stress and noted that the family wanted to make a positive impression on their neighbors in order to avoid a sense of shame. The clinician presented himself as a partner to the family who understood their worries about Daniel's well-being, their worries about the neighbors' views of them, and their worries about housing. Focus on these three elements became the core of future sessions, and the clinician referred Daniel for in-home weekly individual therapy with a bilingual provider who could also support Mr. and Mrs. Luo.

At times, the request for family therapy is made in response to a traumatic or distressing event. That event can be a normal part of life, such as the birth of a child or death of a loved one, or an unexpected event such as the development of a serious illness or disability, violence or sexual assault, homelessness, moving, loss of employment, or divorce. In each of these instances, there is a process of acceptance, grieving the loss or change, realignment and recovery of relationships, and organization and resoluteness to carry on. Members of a family often have very different reactions to the life-changing event and its cause(s) and impact, as well as differing ideas around the meaning of the event and how to process or cope with it.

Cultural differences lead to varying levels of understanding around the cause of challenging or traumatic events and lead to differences in terms of the best ways of reacting to them. Implicit bias and cultural differences between the family and the clinician can lead to an unrecognized mismatch; power differences between the professional and the family can also interfere with and affect treatment. Professional humility, curiosity, and transparency from the clinician's end as well as openness to learn from the family and acknowledging and apologizing for unconscious bias can lead to successful engagement and effective collaboration. Encouraging the family to share their background story, including hardships, trauma, and experiences of exclusion and discrimination, is very important in early stages of treatment. Respect for the family and appreciation of their values is essential; the therapist will know how to help a family only after getting to know them and becoming familiar with their values and their way of life.

Families often come to a family therapist concerned about parent-child conflict, which can be related to acculturative family distancing. Acculturative family distancing can lead to significant and hurtful conflicts within the family, which, in turn, can lead to defiance and failed attempts at control by parents and other authority figures. This can also lead to adolescents feeling isolated and depressed and parents feeling demoralized and powerless. Hwang et al. (2010) noted that in Chinese American high schoolers, a higher degree of acculturative family distancing was associated with more depressive symptoms and a higher risk of development of clinical depression. Peer discrimination against the culturally diverse adolescent, attempts by authority figures (police, teachers, and parents) to control, and parents' isolation from the host community often worsen these conflicts. By the time these problems are recognized and brought to the therapist's attention, parent-child relationships often have become negatively charged; disrespect is predominant; and the family is filled with feelings of hopelessness, mutual misunderstanding, and hurt. To make matters worse, these problems often have been developing and progressing for some time, leaving family members fixed in their opinions and with limited expectations of change by the time the family seeks help.

Clinical Vignette 2

Sonia is a 17-year-old Mexican American female who was brought to the emergency department by her parents after she ingested 15 acetaminophen tablets. She was hospitalized in the pediatric unit because of concern about acetaminophen toxicity. During the initial interview, it became clear that Sonia had been experiencing significant stress recently. Over the past 2 months, her mother, Mrs. Vargas, had been worried that Sonia was becoming disconnected from the family because of her after-school activities. Sonia had stopped helping her mother with household activities and helping her siblings with homework, and Mrs. Vargas was enraged that Sonia was not contributing to the family and was being "selfish" by focusing only on herself. Sonia was perplexed because she had been working very hard to obtain extracurricular credits so she could get into a good college. Discussion among the family about Sonia's staying after school for extracurricular activities led to an argument in which name calling occurred; Sonia rushed into the bathroom, found the bottle of acetaminophen tablets, and intentionally ingested an excessive number of pills as an over-dose. She then became quite frightened and told her mother that she had taken the pills; Mrs. Vargas called an ambulance, and Sonia was brought to the emergency department.

Sonia talked openly with the clinician about her increasing distress over the past 12 months. She had become increasingly involved with competitive cultural activities while also studying for the SATs and maintaining her grades in Advanced Placement classes. It took her more time and effort to do the same amount of academic work and cultural activities, and she had no time to fulfill family expectations at home. As a result, she felt overwhelmed and irritable and experienced low mood, which resulted in social isolation. Mrs. Vargas reported that Sonia had changed from a happy, upbeat teenager to a surly, irritable child who was very difficult to communicate with.

Sonia lived with her mother, father, and three younger brothers. Her father had migrated to the United States in his 20s in search of opportunities. He struggled with poverty and loss of family support from Mexico and worked three jobs to support his family. Throughout his time in the United States, he had been discriminated against and had to deal with prejudice. Although he and Sonia's mother had been in the United States for more than 20 years, they had chosen to adhere to their cultural values to retain their way of life.

Mr. and Mrs. Vargas valued education as the path to success. They also highly valued obedience, gender roles, family values, and importance of cultural involvement. Sonia had been very close to her father, but as she got older, his expectation that she should help more around the house, be more modest, and take care of the younger brothers increased. She felt isolated and disconnected from her family as she attempted to be successful in the United States while at the same time trying to satisfy her parents' traditional values.

While Sonia was in the hospital, she and her parents were seen by a child psychiatry consultant. Sonia's parents were somewhat defensive, but the clinician understood and empathized with the family's cultural values and supported Sonia's mother and father as they listened to their daughter's difficulties and concerns. Sonia was able to tell her parents that she felt confused and stressed trying to straddle two cultures with opposing expectations for women. The clinician encouraged Mrs. Vargas to listen to her daughter in a nonjudgmental and nonreactive fashion during the hospital stay. In addition, the clinician supported Mr. Vargas by acknowledging the challenges of raising a teenager with Mexican cultural values in America. He encouraged Mr. Vargas to see that healthy Mexican American youth may need more acceptance of their bicultural identity.

After Sonia had been hospitalized for 3 days, the family was referred to an outpatient clinician at the local mental health center, where they were seen 3 days after discharge. Sonia reported improved mood and increased attention from her parents at home, and she returned to school. In future sessions with Sonia, the outpatient therapist focused on her life at school, her schoolwork, and her peer relationships. Sessions that included Sonia and her parents led to enhanced understanding, improved communication, and greater support to manage a bicultural lifestyle.

Family therapists working with adolescents often encounter youth and their families during crisis situations, psychiatric hospitalization, juvenile justice, or in settings of school failure or dropout. The experience of crisis and danger often worsens the experience of isolation and demoralization. The challenge for the family therapist is to gain the respect and affiliation of both the adolescent and the parents. Again, understanding the cultural expectations of the parents, recognizing their fears and their antipathy toward the host culture, and validating their experience of pain around their child's struggles are essential. The family therapist can work successfully with parents by emphasizing their love for their child, respecting that love, and validating their heartache. At the same time, recognizing the adolescent's desire for competence and wish to be accepted as his or her individual self can lead to a therapeutic partnership with the youth. Only when the parents and the youth feel heard and understood by the therapist can reconciliation and repair begin. The therapist can build mutual understanding through elaboration of the narratives of both the parents and the youth. With greater understanding, negotiation and collaboration can be fostered and trust rebuilt. At times, values and expectations may be hardened and reconciliation may seem impossible, but most commonly, the therapist's patient elaboration and recognition of love leads to acceptance and growth.

For more in-depth guidance on ethnicity and family therapy, clinicians can refer to a robust literature, such as the work of McGoldrick et al. (2005), who specifically highlighted cultural factors that influence the assumptions of families and providers. Multiple authors have described adaptations of family therapy to enhance its applicability to different minority groups in the United States. Boyd-Franklin (2006), for example, highlighted the roles of extended family, kin networks, and religion in the lives of African American families. She also described the role that experiences of race and racism play in these families' lives, speaking about some of the work therapists need to engage in by exploring bias and embodying humility. Bigner and Wetchler (2012) described approaches to LGBTQ+ families and couples that appreciate their experience of victimization while celebrating these families and recognizing their resilience. Bernal and Domenech-Rodriguez (2012) have written about cultural adaptations of evidence-based family treatments with Hispanic families, making cultural adaptations to the Oregon Parent Management model, which enhanced engagement of Hispanic families while maintaining the effectiveness of the treatment.

Commonly used models of family therapy emphasize important aspects of family treatment. Narrative family therapy (White 2007) builds cohesiveness and promotes resilience in families. Structural family therapy (Minuchin et al. 2014) pays particular attention to boundaries, hierarchy, and closeness and distance among family members in therapy. The DSM-5 Cultural Formulation Interview and its modules (American Psychiatric Association 2013) also provide helpful direction to family therapists. These approaches can be integrated with curiosity and cultural humility in order to help each family achieve its goals. It is ultimately the respect, honesty, warmth, and advocacy of the therapist that are most valued by diverse families.

Conclusion

Family therapy and Western mental health care do not eliminate individual struggles and cannot undo the disruption and pain associated with traumatic events, developmental change, and the stress of adaptation and acculturation postimmigration or remove the hurt caused by racism or discrimination. Treatment does not eliminate poverty or make difference irrelevant. Family therapy builds on the meaning and importance of family relationships in order to heal wounds, promote acceptance, and proceed with development and change. In the face of cultural difference, it is necessary for the therapist to maintain a curious stance while being willing to recognize unconscious bias, learn from differences, and find comfort in humility and vulnerability. Reframing is helpful; respect is essential.

Family therapy encourages a change in perspective as well as a change in focus. Narrative approaches can lead to this change, altering a story of problems to a story of courage and competence (White 2007). Therapy becomes a shared effort, with the family supplying the details of difference and transition, as well as challenge and struggle, while the therapist shapes the details through listening and highlighting the story elements that reflect resilience. This is especially helpful in situations of unchangeable difference and unavailable change. The goals of therapy are co-created with the family, requiring the therapist's agreement and fostering of achievable goals. The family's satisfaction and the therapist's reinforcement help direct the progression of therapy. The therapist is knowledgeable about child development and mental health problems, and family members are experts on themselves and their culture. The therapist blends his or her expertise with the family's expertise, learning from and about them, and both therapist and family are subsequently changed through their work together.

Most importantly, the therapist participates only in a process with which family members agree, respectfully challenging aspects of the interactions within therapy that are not helpful in resolving the family's problems. Ultimately, therapy is a dialogue across four cultures: the culture of the parents, the culture of the child or adolescent, the culture of the therapist, and the culture of mental health care. Navigating this dialogue is always a creative process that changes everyone involved.

Clinical Pearls

- Openness, curiosity, respect, and humility are necessary qualities for successful engagement with diverse families.

- Awareness of your own biases and how your culture informs your practices helps with minimizing subtle missteps in family therapy with diverse families.

- Therapists should be prepared to respond to significant hurt and distress caused by acculturative family distancing.

- Validation of the family experience and empowering the family's voice are essential aspects of family therapy and diverse families.

- Therapy is a dialogue across four cultures: the culture of the parents, the culture of the child or adolescent, the culture of the therapist, and the culture of mental health care.

Self-Assessment Questions

1. Youth who are proficient in both the native and host language are most likely to do which of the following?

    A. Have poor academic performance.
    B. Experience fewer depressive symptoms.
    C. Feel that parents depend on them excessively to translate.
    D. Experience increased anxiety.

2. Which of the following is *not* advised as an approach to family therapy for diverse families?

    A. Child and adolescent mental health clinicians should meet parents early on in treatment.

    B. Family therapists should build mutual understanding by validating the narratives of both the parents and the youth.

    C. The provider should be aware of and apologize for unconscious bias.

    D. The provider should become an expert on the family's home culture and instruct them on how to maintain their culture's values.

3. What is the purpose of family therapy for diverse families?

    A. Build on the meaning and importance of family relationships in order to promote family development.

    B. Make differences irrelevant in order to avoid family conflict.

    C. Eliminate individual struggles.

    D. Encourage peaceful separation in families experiencing acculturative family distancing.

4. What specific questions will you add to your usual base of interview questions to include content from this chapter?

5. How might you adjust your current rubric for patient conceptualization to include these concepts?

6. As you reflect, how does the information in this chapter inform your future practice?

Answers

1. B
2. D
3. A

References

American Psychiatric Association: Diagnostic and Statistical Manual of Mental Disorders, 5th Edition. Arlington, VA, American Psychiatric Association, 2013

Bernal G, Domenech Rodriguez MM (eds): Cultural Adaptations: Tools for Evidence-Based Practice With Diverse Populations. Washington, DC, American Psychological Association, 2012

Berry JW, Kim U, Power S, et al: Acculturation attitudes in plural societies. Applied Psychology 38(2):185–206, 1989

Bigner JJ, Wetchler JL (eds): Handbook of LGBT-Affirmative Couple and Family Therapy. New York, Routledge, 2012

Boyd-Franklin N: Black Families in Therapy: Understanding the African American Experience. New York, Guilford, 2006

DeDiego AC: A systemic perspective for working with same-sex parents. Counseling Today 59(4):40–44, 2016

Falicov CJ: Latino Families in Therapy, 2nd Edition. New York, Guilford, 2014

Hughes CC: Culture in clinical psychiatry, in Culture, Ethnicity, and Mental Illness. Edited by Gaw AC. Washington, DC, American Psychiatric Press, 1993, pp 3–42

Hwang WC, Wood JJ, Fujimoto K: Acculturative family distancing (AFD) and depression in Chinese American families. J Consult Clin Psychol 78(5):655–667, 2010

Jacob J, Gray B, Johnson A: The Asian American family and mental health: implications for child health professionals. J Pediatr Health Care 27(3):180–188, 2011

Limb GE, Hodge DR: Utilizing spiritual ecograms with Native American families and children to promote cultural competence in family therapy. J Marital Fam Ther 37(1):81–94, 2011

Liu LL, Benner AD, Lau AS, et al: Mother-adolescent language proficiency and adolescent academic and emotional adjustment among Chinese American families. J Youth Adolesc 38(4):572–586, 2009

McCollum VJC: Evolution of the African American family personality: considerations for family therapy. J Multicult Couns Devel 25(3):219–229, 1997

McGoldrick M, Giordana J, Garcia-Preto N (eds): Ethnicity and Family Therapy, 3rd Edition. New York, Guilford, 2005

Minuchin S, Reiter MD, Borda C: The Craft of Family Therapy: Challenging Certainties. New York, Routledge, 2014

Portes A, Schauffler R: Language and the second generation: bilingualism yesterday and today, in The New Second Generation. Edited by Portes A. New York, Russell Sage Foundation, 1996

Rothe EM, Tzuang D, Pumariega AJ: Acculturation, development, and adaptation. Child Adolesc Psychiatr Clin N Am 19(4):681–696, 2010

Santisteban DA, Coatsworth JD, Perez-Vidal A, et al: Brief structural/strategic family therapy with African and Hispanic high-risk youth. J Community Psychol 25(5):453–471, 1997

White M: Maps of Narrative Practice. New York, WW Norton, 2007

PART III
External Influences

CHAPTER 10

Social Determinants of Child and Adolescent Mental Health

Phillip Murray, M.D., M.P.H.
Kamille Williams, M.D.
Sarah Y. Vinson, M.D.

If you came with no preconceptions about the purpose of the child welfare system, you would have to conclude that it is an institution designed to monitor, regulate and punish poor families of color.

Dorothy Roberts,
Shattered Bonds: The Color of Child Welfare (Roberts 2002)

THE child and adolescent population is uniquely impacted by the social determinants of mental health. Children are utterly reliant on their family of origin, adoptive parents, or agents of the child welfare system to ensure that their basic needs are met. Children are physically, cognitively, and emotionally immature, rendering them susceptible to abuse and exploitation, limiting their means to support themselves financially, and undercutting their ability to skillfully navigate social situations and societal structures. Finally, they are often subject to compulsory education, meaning that most children spend most of their waking hours during the week in a school setting.

TABLE 10–1. Social determinants of mental health for youth

Societal values and community dynamics related to gender, sexual orientation, other characteristics of the child

Community systems (e.g., juvenile justice, social services, educational institutions, developmental disabilities programs)

Access to medical care

Access to mental health care

Access to substance abuse treatment services

Employment opportunities

Adverse childhood experiences

Family dynamics

Gender

Geographic location

Housing quality

Income level

Race/ethnicity

Social support

Immigration

It was not without controversy that British physician Thomas McKeown introduced the concept of social medicine into the western medical literature (Link and Phelan 2002). In the 1950s, he examined the causes for the reduction in mortality for British society over the past several centuries. He acknowledged some medical progress but highlighted improved social and economic opportunities as deserving most of the credit. These social and economic factors were precursors to the concept of social determinants of health.

Fast forward several decades, and the concept of social determinants of health is more well defined and broadly accepted (Braveman and Gottleib 2014). According to the World Health Organization, social determinants of health are "the conditions in which people are born, grow, live, work and age" (World Health Organization 2020). These conditions are shaped by the distribution of money, power, and resources at local, national, and global levels (Table 10–1). It is the social determinants of health, not the medical system with its cures and treatments, that are mostly responsible for health inequities. Not only are these inequities unfair and avoidable (Braveman and Gottleib 2014; Centers for Disease Control and Prevention 2018; World Health Organization 2020); they also further contribute to the ongoing cycle of poverty, illness, and social inequality.

The social determinants perspective is starting to permeate the financially unsustainable U.S. health care system. The United States has not been getting its money's worth, spending more than 10 of the highest-income countries but with the lowest life expectancy, higher infant mortality, and higher rates of obesity (Pecora et al. 2009). The U.S. government initiative Healthy People 2020 acknowledges that social determinants impact a wide range of health, functioning, and quality-of-life outcomes and risks (HealthyPeople.Gov 2020). Health inequity in the United States is rooted not in inept providers or out-of-date practices but in environments supported by societal structures that fail to provide a milieu conducive to the healthy existence,

TABLE 10–2.   Same symptoms, different diagnoses

Both Jason and John have PTSD symptoms.

For Jason, the psychiatrist uses the 10-question Adverse Childhood Experience (ACE) questionnaire and identifies abuse by Jason's stepfather. A diagnosis of PTSD is given, and appropriate interventions for that diagnosis are put in place.

For John, the psychiatrist uses the 10-question ACE questionnaire, which was negative. This leads to missing John's trauma, which was from sustained, significant neighborhood and community violence. Not recognizing the trauma symptoms results in misdiagnosis of oppositional defiant disorder, a stigmatizing disorder that leaves the child's actual problem unaddressed.

growth, and development of substantial subsets of the population (Braveman and Gottleib 2014; Centers for Disease Control and Prevention 2018).

For many years, the health implications of individual and structural racism, sexism, ableism, and discrimination against sexual minorities were not widely recognized or explored within the medical community. Neither were such issues as trauma, income inequality, poverty, housing shortages, educational disparities, and food insecurity. These topics were thought of as best addressed in their social and structural contexts. It is now clear that these factors can directly affect both the physical and mental health of the population. There are correlations between education, income levels, health outcomes, life expectancy, and quality of life—for however long that life may be (Arias et al. 2018; Evans et al. 2000, 2003; Hummer and Hernandez 2013).

When social determinants adversely impact mental health, they can do so synergistically, resulting in significant distress and impairment and a limiting of the individual's coping mechanisms. Furthermore, individuals who are negatively impacted by social determinants of health are simultaneously at a higher risk for mental health problems such as depression, anxiety, and PTSD. They are also less likely to seek or stay engaged in care. This lack of treatment engagement is, in part, due to structural issues that limit health care access. Additionally, within mental health, these factors can directly impact how people are diagnosed and treated. Patients can present with similar symptoms but receive different diagnoses (DelBello et al. 2001; Pumariega 2010; Schwartz and Blankenship 2014) (Table 10–2). Any of these factors can lead to a disproportionate burden of treatable mental health conditions within the general population.

Because the impact of social determinants of mental health on both illness and treatment is substantial and well beyond the control of any single child or family, a thorough understanding of children's mental health must acknowledge social and structural factors. In this chapter, we focus on four systems—family, child welfare, education, and juvenile and criminal justice—where disparities have a profound impact on many children. Mental health inequities are the result of our current systems of governance and a reflection of societal values. In the following sections, we explore how these systems work for the healthy mental development of some children while posing barriers to the healthy mental development of others.

Families and the Social Safety Net

Family is the most important system with which children will interact. Families provide practical resources to sustain a child's life and lead to appropriate growth. Families are where children learn coping strategies, value systems, how to deal with conflict, and how to navigate life in general. Raising children is demanding and a stressor for any family system. This is compounded when families do not have ready access to resources.

Although the conceptualization of resources is often focused on material resources, we must include emotional and social resources. In fact, material, emotional, and social resources are directly related. This is illustrated through the fact that women without adequate monetary resources are at higher risk for maternal depression, which puts their children at risk for negative mental health outcomes (Center on the Developing Child at Harvard University 2009). Maternal depression, which has higher rates in low-income families, is associated with unhealthy parenting practices and negative behavioral consequences for children (Chenven 2010). These early experiences also impact brain development, leading to hyperactive stress centers. Maternal depression is one of many possible adverse childhood experiences (ACEs) that children in poor families are vulnerable to experiencing (Merrick et al. 2018). The Centers for Disease Control and Prevention (2019) define ACEs as "all types of abuse, neglect, and other potentially traumatic experiences that occur to people under the age of 18."

Families in societies with frayed social safety nets are under the constant threat of financial insecurity. Although this can negatively impact children directly, it can also negatively impact parents and their ability to provide care. There are also additional forms of insecurity, including housing and food (Bernard et al. 2018; Braveman and Gottlieb 2014; Evans et al. 2000, 2003). Evidence supports that instability in either of these areas can lead to increases in externalizing behaviors (Merrick et al. 2018; Park et al. 2011), which can lead to a damaging feedback loop in which children act out, thus further stressing parents who likely have limited resources and may have limited coping mechanisms themselves. This cycle can negatively impact interactions with external entities, such as child protective services, juvenile justice, or school systems, further compromising the family's ability to interact with safety net institutions that are usually underfunded and characterized by red tape and regulations.

To complicate things further, current political and sociological realities show a trend toward limiting access to these resources in the name of increasing personal responsibility and decreasing dependency. Although these are noble goals, they can be at best shortsighted and at worst cruel when policies fail to account for the limited agency many children and families have had in determining their current circumstances. They also fail to account for historical context and current systemic drivers of poverty (National Fair Housing Alliance 2018; Turner et al. 2016). For example, historical (and current) lending practices have led to segregated and under-resourced neighborhoods. Children born into these neighborhoods will not have home equity or houses passed on to them and are less likely to attend schools that prepare them to enter a competitive job market, perpetuating the disproportionate allocation of wealth. The narrative that they are simply not working hard enough is incomplete. When money does move into these neighborhoods via gentrification, it has been shown to have significant negative effects on the health of the original inhabitants of these spaces. These individuals, usually vulnerable populations such as people of color or of low socioeconomic status, are displaced from their homes because of the upsurge in cost and have worsening health conditions that result in more emergency department visits and hospitalizations (Lim et al. 2017; Mehdipanah et al. 2018). The promises and benefits of urban renewal all too often lead to new resources for a neighborhood's new occupants at the literal expense of its old residents (Lim et al. 2017; Mehdipanah et al. 2018).

Child Protective Services and Youth in State Custody

Although the stated purpose of child protective services is to shield youth and help them heal from traumatic experiences, outcomes data indicate that youth who have been in foster placement are more likely to experience mental illness, including PTSD, as adults (Côté et al. 2018; Pecora et al. 2009). At the time of its creation, child welfare was the result of social and legal shifts reflecting beliefs about children, who previously were viewed as sources of labor and were readily exploited as such (Chenven 2010; Hart 1991). Children exist primarily within their family system but typically interact with health care and education systems at regular intervals. Professionals in these areas are mandated to report any instances where there is reasonable suspicion of a child or adolescent experiencing abuse or neglect. The report is supposed to trigger an investigation, with the goal of improving support for the family system or, if necessary for the child's safety, removal from the home. Tragically, over time, in some cases, the system has evolved to be more punitive for parents perceived as inadequate rather than supportive for families in need of help.

Most children served by child welfare do remain with their family of origin; however, a substantial proportion do not. Child welfare interventions can lead to the reality-based fear that families will be separated. This separation does not ensure a safe or better environment, nor does it reliably provide built-in supports to address the abrupt transition some children can face. When youth are removed from their families, the separation from loved ones can be traumatic in and of itself (Merrick et al. 2018; Murray et al. 2012; Teicher 2018). Additionally, removal from family may result in placement in a new community where youth do not have access to community supports, a familiar school district, fictive kin, or, when applicable, their current mental health providers. Tragically, youth may also experience additional traumas while in state care, including multiple placement disruptions, neglect, and/or abuse. Research clearly demonstrates that the best homes for children are stable, supportive family settings rather than a system with multiple placements. Although federal law requires that the children be placed in the least restrictive (most family-like) environment, the majority of these children are in group or congregate care (Child Trends 2018; McMurtry and Lie 1992; U.S. Department of Health and Human Services 2013; World Health Organization 2020).

Youth from distressed environments are at higher risk of maladaptive coping mechanisms and subsequent externalizing disorders and behaviors (Merrick et al. 2018; Murray et al. 2012; Park et al. 2011). Furthermore, the traumas experienced also increase the risk of internalizing disorders, which can then jeopardize their ability to integrate into a new environment, rendering them subject to disrupted placements. In many cases, children can adjust appropriately. When they cannot, they are inevitably brought into the mental health system to aid in adjusting to this change. Their symptoms are a result of the intersection of multiple factors that will take significant time and resources to adequately treat. This is an example of the adverse synergism mentioned earlier in the chapter.

Access to high-quality treatment that includes psychosocial therapeutic interventions or care by child and adolescent psychiatrists is often quite limited for children with public insurance (Alegria et al. 2015; Olfson et al. 2014; Owens et al. 2002). This leaves a high-risk, developmentally immature group that is vulnerable to mental illness because of a myriad of factors—family genetic loading, trauma, ongoing psychosocial stressors—subject to a critical discrepancy between what is readily available and what is clinically indicated. Too often, this means that clinicians who do not have specialized training in children's mental health are prescribing psychotropic medications and are doing so without having the appropriate corresponding psychosocial interventions in place (Anderson et al. 2015; Cama et al. 2017; Menahem 2009; Olfson et al. 2014).

Understandably, alarms have been raised about prescribing practices for children in these circumstances given the lack of appropriate intervention and the exposure to potential medication side effects (Crystal et al. 2016; Olfson et al. 2014; Vanderwerker et al. 2014). Additionally, there are concerns about sedation for the ease of caregivers or even profiteering as motives for increasing prescription of psychotropic medication in this population. This comes at the youth's expense—both mentally and physically. Take, for example, an instance in which an antipsychotic medication is prescribed to improve impulse control in a child with dangerous externalizing behaviors. The medication can be immediately effective but could lead to short- and long-term side effects such as sedation, emotional muting or numbing, obesity, increased blood sugar, and other metabolic side effects. Furthermore, receiving an inaccurate diagnosis of a severe mental illness during a critical developmental period could have negative implications for youth's perception of their autonomy and/or their personal identity. That said, many of these children and adolescents do struggle with legitimate mental illness that warrants mental health treatment, which in numerous cases may justifiably include medications. Many are primarily in need of intensive psychotherapy.

The child welfare system disproportionately involves families in poverty as well as children who are African American, those who identify as two or more races, and American Indian/Alaskan Native youth, as described by the U.S. Department of Health and Human Services (2013). However, the fact that these racial groups are disproportionately impacted by poverty alone does not explain their overrepresentation in the system. Bias on the part of child welfare workers and institutional racism have been identified as additional possible contributors (U.S. Department of Health and Human Services 2013). Tragically, vulnerable families are mandated to participate in a child welfare system that does not reliably promote mental wellness or equity and is chronically underfunded and intertwined with many other systems that contain rampant inequities (see Table 10–1).

The Educational System

Although home certainly continues to be their base, school-age children spend most of their waking hours within the educational system. The structure, mores, and expectations there interact with the children's ability (or inability) to conform and greatly impact academic and occupational trajectories. For some children, school is a reprieve from unstable or unsafe home environments. For others, it is an environment with academic and/or social demands that are challenging to meet. As mandated reporters with frequent access to youth, school personnel are key drivers in referrals to child protective services. They are also well positioned to identify youth who may be in need of mental health services who have flown under the radar of stressed family systems. Additionally, a school system's policies can play a critical role in either stemming or feeding the *school-to-prison pipeline*, the phenomenon in which racial inequities in school disciplinary actions place youth at increased risk for juvenile justice system involvement) (American Academy of Pediatrics Committee on School Health 2003; Heitzeg 2009; NAACP Legal Defense and Educational Fund 2020).

There is a clear correlation between high school completion and overall life as an adult (Hummer and Hernandez 2013). Inequitable resource allocation for education provides greater opportunities for those who already are at an advantage because of family income or neighborhood. The cumulative effect of the social determinants of health renders children in impoverished school districts even more reliant on the appropriate resources being readily accessible in the school setting. Unfortunately, all too often, these schools are not equipped with the necessary tools to provide the proverbial "way out" of the neighborhood.

Distressed households usually manifest as having difficulty adjusting to educational settings. The special education process provides a road map and legal accountability so that all children, including those with disabling symptoms due to mental illness, have access to a free and appropriate education; however, at times, the indicated services are not easily obtained from often overwhelmed and under-resourced schools. If parents are not well versed in the resources to which they are entitled within the educational system, they may require coaching and support in exercising their rights to evaluation and support in the classroom. This is significantly more difficult for children and families from diverse backgrounds (Tamzarian et al. 2012).

In addition to book-based learning, the educational system also plays a vital role in socialization. The behaviors modeled and reinforced in this controlled environment impact a youth's understanding of the larger world. School is a place where typical and atypical development is identified and possibly addressed. Regrettably, it is also a setting where distress from home environments or symptoms from unaddressed mental illness can come pouring out, imperiling academic progress. For example, in a study of children in an urban public school district, it was found that those exposed to maternal interpersonal violence and child abuse were almost twice as likely to have been suspended from school during the study period—even after adjusting for confounders (Kernic et al. 2002).

Teachers and administrators have to juggle the demands of managing behavioral issues with providing the instructional environment needed for pupils to attain educational benchmarks and requirements. Although school personnel can recommend that families seek mental health evaluations or professional help, this may be in the context of variable levels of support within, and between, public, charter, and private schools. Parents with low incomes or poor medical coverage can face tremendous barriers to following through on the school's recommendations. Given the shortage of providers trained in children's mental health, obtaining the appropriate treatment may pose a challenge even to families with solid resources (American Academy of Child and Adolescent Psychiatry 2019; Cama et al. 2017). The persistence of untreated symptoms in the school setting can lead to a tense relationship between parents and school personnel. These situations can leave parents at a disadvantage due to societal power dynamics and may have undue consequences on the youngster's future.

Families with limited resources may be judged and punished instead of receiving the extra support they need as school personnel become burned out and have less patience for disturbing or externalizing behavior. This punitive approach can lead to disciplinary interactions that slow a child's educational development and lead to internalizing feelings of being inadequate. Maladaptive behaviors continue, leading to increasing severity in consequences. Zero-tolerance school discipline policies, which automatically expel students for certain conduct infractions, are a prime example. Although the policies are intended to preserve educational opportunities and safety for most children, the consequences for children from under-resourced backgrounds can be devastating. Even after controlling for the type of problematic behavior as well as income and racial disparities, the most severe punishments are still prevalent for children with limited resources. Not only are youth who experience suspensions and expulsions missing out on educational opportunities, some are set along a devastating path to juvenile justice and eventual criminal justice system involvement (American Academy of Pediatrics Committee on School Health 2003; NAACP Legal Defense and Educational Fund 2020).

Juvenile Justice and Criminal Justice Systems

A true catchall, the juvenile and criminal justice systems are the tragic end point for many youth who have cycled through familial instability; child welfare systems; and inadequately resourced, punitive school environments. Both the juvenile justice and the criminal justice systems can significantly impact children's mental health on a population level, particularly in communities that have had disproportionate contact with them. Minority and impoverished populations are overrepresented at every phase of the legal process in both the juvenile and criminal justice systems, and overrepresentation in one can impact overrepresentation in the other (U.S. Department of Health and Human Services 2013). The school-to-prison pipeline funnels vulnerable youth into the juvenile and/or criminal justice systems, and communities and families destabilized by mass incarceration are less able to provide an environment that has the level of supervision needed to support healthy development (Murray et al. 2012; NAACP Legal Defense and Educational Fund 2020).

Incarceration rates increased after the United States took an aggressive stance toward prosecuting drug offenses in the 1980s (Pecora et al. 2009; Pumariega et al. 2003). The articulated goal was to dissuade illicit substance use—despite the United States' history of failed drug policies based on punishment (e.g., Prohibition) and other countries' success with more rehabilitative models (Drug Policy Alliance 2015; Marlowe 2003). Opinions are slowly changing around approaches to individuals with substance use disorders, with state-level movements to decriminalize marijuana as well as more public support for people with opioid use disorders. The rise of opioid use has been characterized as a medical epidemic rather than a moral failing, and this conceptualization has benefited from the narrative of the origin of the epidemic in overprescribing by the medical establishment. However, although this more treatment-oriented and empathetic approach toward people with substance use disorders is laudable and overdue, it will not likely benefit individuals who are currently incarcerated. Furthermore, it has not been extended consistently to individuals who use other substances such as cocaine or methamphetamines that are more prevalent in marginalized communities such as hypersegregated urban neighborhoods or rural communities.

Mass incarceration removes parents, and other significant adults, from families and communities. Individuals without significant financial resources are not only reliant on an overextended public defender system for legal representation but also may be unable to post bail. Cash bail is particularly burdensome for individuals impacted by poverty, is discriminatorily applied to Blacks even when accounting for income, and is a key driver of incarceration rates (Arnold et al. 2017; Liu et al. 2018). In fact, despite the fact that both violent and property crime have fallen since the mid-1990s, the number of people in jail who have not been convicted of a crime has more than doubled (U.S. Sentencing Commission 2011, 2017). Even though this might only represent a brief period of time in the eyes of the court system, for parents, this means time away from their children during critical developmental windows, an inability to work or pay bills, and the risk of interruptions in medical coverage. Parental incarceration leads to further stress on the family system (Murray et al. 2012). There is the practical loss of income, companionship, and emotional resources to navigate the demanding task of raising children. Adults who are unaccustomed to taking on these roles may step in but do so with varying levels of preparation and support.

If family members are fortunate enough to be reunited after incarceration, this introduces a new set of challenges as formerly incarcerated people face difficulties obtaining the resources needed for them to thrive on reentry. Relief from the emotional burden of separation can give way to the stress of reintegration into both the family and the larger community. There may even be further economic burden because another person who struggles to find employment is being introduced into the family system. The situation is further complicated if there are ongoing issues of substance use or episodes of reoffense. There is the issue of heavy policing in some communities. Disproportionate interactions with law enforcement can lead to community distress, even if residents are not directly involved with the police (DeVylder et al. 2018).

Naturally, minority and low-income children who are part of families and communities overrepresented in the criminal justice system experience an unreasonable burden and exposure to that system. Parental incarceration leads to multiple negative outcomes, including both internalizing and externalizing consequences (Murray et al. 2012). Children are more likely to experience internal feelings of anxiety, loneliness, and depression. The result of these family stressors can also manifest externally as maladaptive behaviors and substance use (Murray et al. 2012).

Youth may, in turn, find themselves involved in the juvenile or, depending on the charge and the jurisdiction, the adult justice systems. Although not all youth with an incarcerated parent end up in the juvenile justice system, those who have one are clearly at higher risk. After entry into the juvenile justice system, detention all too often does not serve the stated purpose of rehabilitation. Youth chances of criminal justice system involvement as adults are higher for those who have experienced the incarceration of adult caregivers (Murray et al. 2012). Detaining youth can have the unintended consequence of reinforcing maladaptive behaviors, promoting socialization with a delinquent peer group, and strengthening an impressionable person's self-identification with delinquency. Following involvement in these systems, it is difficult for youth to realign to developmental norms or to reintegrate into societal systems without substantial support. Poor, Black, Hispanic, Native, and sexual minority youth are at greater risk for involvement with the juvenile justice system (NAACP Legal Defense and Educational Fund 2020).

Implications for Mental Health Professionals

Mental health professionals should be aware of social determinants of health that directly impact mental health. Youth often lack the emotional vocabulary to articulate their experiences, whether external or internal, or the interplay between the two. Treating children without the proper context can lead to gross mismanagement and unintended consequences. Simply put, taking these factors into account is a requirement for appropriate diagnoses and treatments. Social determinants shape every system and context in which children think, feel, and act. It is imperative, and becoming more urgent, that providers invest time in understanding patients' communities in order to understand ongoing challenges and barriers.

Public discourse and understanding are rapidly changing around some of these issues because of key events. At the time of this writing, the United States continues to have the highest number of cases and deaths from an ongoing pandemic that has disrupted daily functioning and disproportionately impacts minority communities (Centers for Disease Control and Prevention 2020). Disruptions to income, extended shelter-in-place orders, and school closings are some of the factors that risk exacerbating negative impacts from existing social determinants of health and worsened mental health outcomes (Fegert et al. 2020; Golberstein et al. 2020). Public protests in response to police killings of unarmed African Americans have brought more conversations about the impacts of white supremacy and institutional racism to the mainstream. Providers should be prepared to address this in the treatment context. As there is a need for providers to exercise cultural humility to best serve patients, so too is there a need for them to exercise structural humility.

Providers should educate themselves around the historical context for current risk factors, protective factors, and engagement within the various social systems. This will help to reinforce the magnitude of structural limitations patients and families can face and place their decisions and actions in the proper context. This perspective will also demonstrate that individual willpower alone is often far from enough. The development and implementation of appropriate treatment goals and plans may very well require the incorporation of resources and/or interventions outside the traditional mental health care system context.

Conclusion

It is understandable that families and communities who have been on the wrong end of inequities that abound in every other major societal structure may be reluctant to engage with the mental health care system. Not only do they have a history of having their personal agency undermined, but on the basis of their experiences, they may also have difficulty believing that they will be treated fairly. It is imperative that providers advocate for patients and families in a way that promotes structural change because that is the best way to ensure lasting interventions. Many times, patient and family voices from the most vulnerable communities are muted by political realities, power dynamics, and marginalization. Mental health providers, by virtue of their subject matter expertise and privilege, should use their platform to amplify those voices. Doing so may provide an intervention that is just as, if not more valuable than, individual treatment interventions.

Without a common language to identify the social determinants of children's mental health and a basic understanding of them by both mental health professionals and the larger society, families are forced to fend for themselves when psychopathology is attributed to genetic predispositions; family dynamics; or, even worse, individual failures. The myriad mental health ramifications of structural shortcomings that go beyond individuals are a result of the intersection of multiple decisions we have collectively made as a society.

Vignette

It is 5:00 A.M. on Thursday, and 16-year-old Nicholas has just woken up to prepare for the day. He lives with his mother, grandmother, younger brother, and younger sister in a one-bedroom apartment in Peachville, Georgia, a small, poor community within metropolitan Atlanta. Every morning, he helps his younger siblings wake up and get ready, walks them to school, administers his grandmother's morning medications, and catches public transportation to his school across town. His family had to move during the school year and has not yet registered him in the new district. Nicholas's mother works two jobs because one job does not provide enough for her to pay their rent, utility, and food bills, and usually she does not arrive home from work until 7 A.M.

Nicholas is particularly exhausted this morning because the neighbors were fighting again, which led to the police being called out for the third time in the past 2 weeks. He really wants to stay home so that he can rest before his after-school job, but he knows his mother would not approve. He drops off his siblings at school and heads toward the nearest bus stop. Some guys who attend his school approach, and he hurriedly ducks behind some bushes to avoid being seen. Nicholas gets picked on a lot because his clothes are old and he has no name-brand shoes. Money is tight for his mother because their food stamp budget was recently decreased and his father has stopped sending money. Nicholas hopes to be able to afford to buy some new clothes soon with his new job. Currently, he is wearing a shirt that he wore earlier in the week.

The guys keep walking by, narrowly avoiding Nicholas. The bus approaches moments later, and Nicholas gets on. He realizes that he does not have any more money on his bus card and will need to figure out a plan to catch the bus home, or he will end up walking 5 miles, which he hates. Exhausted, Nicholas dozes off on the bus and ends up missing his stop. He wakes up an hour later and is frantic when he sees on the bus's clock that it is 9 A.M. School began 90 minutes ago, and his school has a "zero tolerance" policy for consecutive tardiness. Nicholas has been late several times over the past month, and after the last instance, Principal Shelby told him that he would be suspended if he were late again. Nicholas rushes off the bus at the next stop and runs for 15 minutes to get to school. He hopes he can sneak into school before the next period begins to avoid being caught by the administration.

Nicholas barely makes it to school before the next bell rings. Unfortunately, Principal Shelby is in the hallway and sees him. "Remember what I said last time about being late, Nicholas," he says. "Follow me to my office. We need to call your mom to pick you up because you are suspended for tardiness." Dreading the next couple of hours, Nicholas follows Principal Shelby down the hallway.

In this vignette, we see how Nicholas's family's challenges with poverty, housing insecurity, and food insecurity force him to take on more responsibility and stress than is expected of his more fortunate peers. Nicholas has made sincere efforts to support his family and balance the pressures that come with typical adolescent development. Unfortunately, others can see only his deficits, causing his school experience to contribute further to his distress. Nicholas has to deal with being bullied and the consequences of the school's zero tolerance policy, which cause him to fall further behind, thus limiting his future prospects for elevating himself and his family. It is clear that Nicholas is going above and beyond, but the principal sees him as undisciplined and not putting forth enough effort. Nicholas's situation is the logical outcome of several circumstances outside his control. Social determinants do not occur in isolation, and people do not always volunteer that they are having challenges with them. Without this context, Nicholas will continue to be punished for something that is far beyond his ability to change, and he will be denied the assistance he needs to overcome these barriers.

TABLE 10-3.   Social determinants of health screening sample questions for parents or adolescents

Are you worried that you may not have stable housing in the next 2 months?

Are there any problems with your house or apartment? (Do you have heat/air conditioning? Do you have lead paint or pipes? Are you able to cook in your home? Is your water working? Is there mold? Are there bugs?)

Do you always have enough money for food?

Do you put off or avoid doctor visits because of transportation problems or distance?

Have any services been cut off in your home in the past 12 months (electricity, heat, oil, water, Internet)?

Is obtaining child care a problem?

Do you have a job?

Have you graduated high school?

Do you always have enough money to pay your bills?

Source.   Adapted from American Academy of Family Physicians 2019.

Clinical Pearls

- Social determinants of health are the result of larger societal policies that are not easily overcome through sheer effort. Lasting changes can come only from systems-based interventions.

- Social determinants of health rarely happen in isolation but usually intersect and can compound deficits for children and families.

- Difficulties with social determinants of health can interfere with treatment. It is important to address them in order to eliminate potential barriers to treatment.

- Clinicians should normalize asking about potential challenges during initial assessments to tailor interventions and avoid labeling under-resourced families as noncompliant. For sample questions, see Table 10–3.

- Clinicians should educate themselves about local community-level difficulties to provide further context for presenting complaints and appropriate interventions.

- Clinicians should also learn about available resources for social determinants of health because it can be difficult to address them during the clinical encounter. Clinicians can use their health care organization resources, available social work services, or online resources such as Aunt Bertha (www.auntbertha.com).

Self-Assessment Questions

1. What are key social determinants that one should routinely consider when assessing youth with atypical mental health development?

2. Zach is a 14-year-old male, the oldest of three, who lives with his father, grandfather, siblings, and two cousins in a two-bedroom apartment. His father is currently unemployed. Zach works two part-time jobs to support his family and help make ends meet. What social determinants are present that will impact Zach's health?

3. Judge Tomato is a newly appointed judge of Snaketon, Mississippi, an impoverished and segregated community that is known for harshly using minimum sentencing requirements for drug possession charges. What social determinant(s) factor into the mental health of the child and adolescent population there?

4. Of the social determinants described in Table 10–1, which determinants impact the youth you see the most?

5. As you reflect, how does the information in this chapter inform your future practice?

Answers

1. Families and the social safety net, child protective services and youth in state custody, the educational system, juvenile justice and criminal justice systems
2. Family, overcrowded apartment, no mother present, father was incarcerated, housing and food insecurity, father is unemployed, Zach is working two jobs
3. Mass incarceration, poverty, family unemployment

References

Alegria M, Green JG, McLaughlin KA, et al: Disparities in child and adolescent mental health and mental health services in the U.S. New York, William T. Grant Foundation, March 2015. Available at: https://wtgrantfoundation.org/library/uploads/2015/09/Disparities-in-Child-and-Adolescent-Mental-Health.pdf. Accessed April 23, 2020.

American Academy of Child and Adolescent Psychiatry: Workforce issues. Washington, DC, American Academy of Child and Adolescent Psychiatry, April 2019. Available at: www.aacap.org/AACAP/Resources_for_Primary_Care/Workforce_Issues.aspx. Accessed December 20, 2019.

American Academy of Family Physicians: Social Needs Screening Tool. Leawood, KS, American Academy of Family Physicians, 2019. Available at: www.aafp.org/dam/AAFP/documents/patient_care/everyone_project/hops19-physician-form-sdoh.pdf. Accessed, September 15, 2020.

American Academy of Pediatrics Committee on School Health: Out-of-school suspension and expulsion. American Academy of Pediatrics Committee on School Health. Pediatrics 112(5):1206–1209, 2003

Anderson EL, Chen ML, Perrin JM, et al: Outpatient visits and medication prescribing for US children with mental health conditions. Pediatrics 136(5):e1178–e1185, 2015

Arias E, Escobedo LA, Kennedy J, et al: U.S. Small-Area Life Expectancy Estimates Project: methodology and results summary. National Center for Health Statistics. Vital Health Stat 2(181), 2018

Arnold D, Dobbie W, Yang CS: Racial bias in bail decisions. Working Paper 23421. Cambridge, MA, National Bureau of Economic Research, 2017. Available at: www.nber.org/papers/w23421.pdf. Accessed April 23, 2020.

Bernard R, Hammarlund R, Bouquet M, et al: Parent and child reports of food insecurity and mental health: divergent perspectives. Ochsner J 18(4):318–325, 2018

Braveman P, Gottlieb L: The social determinants of health: it's time to consider the causes of the causes. Public Health Rep 129(suppl 2):19–31, 2014

Cama S, Malowney M, Smith AJB, et al: Availability of outpatient mental health care by pediatricians and child psychiatrists in five U.S. cities. Int J Health Serv 47(4):621–635, 2017

Center on the Developing Child at Harvard University: Maternal Depression Can Undermine the Development of Young Children. Working Paper No 8. Cambridge, MA, Center on the Developing Child at Harvard University, 2009

Centers for Disease Control and Prevention: Sources of data for social determinants of health, in Social Determinants of Health: Know What Affects Health. Atlanta, GA, Centers for Disease Control and Prevention, February 15, 2018. Available at: www.cdc.gov/socialdeterminants/data/index.htm. Accessed July 25, 2019.

Centers for Disease Control and Prevention: Adverse childhood experiences (ACEs). Atlanta, GA, Centers for Disease Control and Prevention, 2019. Available at: https://www.cdc.gov/violenceprevention/childabuseandneglect/acestudy/aboutace.html. Accessed August 14, 2020.

Centers for Disease Control and Prevention: Health equity considerations and racial and ethnic minority groups. Atlanta, GA, Centers for Disease Control and Prevention, 2020. Available at: www.cdc.gov/coronavirus/2019-ncov/community/health-equity/race-ethnicity.html. Accessed August 15, 2020.

Chenven M: Community systems of care for children's mental health. Child Adolesc Psychiatr Clin N Am 19(1):163–174, 2010

Child Trends: Foster care. Bethesda, MD, Child Trends, May 2018. Available at: www.childtrends.org/indicators/foster-care. Accessed December 19, 2019.

Côté S, Orri M, Marttila M, et al: Out-of-home placement in early childhood and psychiatric diagnoses and criminal convictions in young adulthood: a population-based propensity score-matched study. Lancet Child Adolesc Health 2(9):647–653, 2018

Crystal S, Mackie T, Fenton MC, et al: Rapid growth of antipsychotic prescriptions for children who are publicly insured has ceased, but concerns remain. Health Aff (Millwood) 35(6):974–982, 2016

DelBello M, Lopez-Larson MP, Soutullo CA, et al: Effects of race on psychiatric diagnosis of hospitalized adolescents: a retrospective chart review. J Child Adolesc Psychopharmacol 11(1):95–103, 2001

DeVylder JE, Jun H-J, Fedina L, et al: Association of exposure to police violence with prevalence of mental health symptoms among urban residents in the United States. JAMA Netw Open 1(7), e184945, 2018

Drug Policy Alliance: Drug decriminalization in Portugal: a health-centered approach. February 4, 2015. Available at: www.drugpolicy.org/resource/drug-decriminalization-portugal-health-centered-approach-englishspanish. Accessed April 23, 2020.

Evans G, Wells N, Chan H-Y, et al: Housing quality and mental health. J Consult Clin Psychol 68(3):526–530, 2000

Evans G, Wells N, Moch A: Housing and mental health: a review of the evidence and a methodological and conceptual critique. J Soc Issues 59(3):475–500, 2003

Fegert JM, Vitiello B, Plener PL, Clemens V: Challenges and burden of the coronavirus 2019 (COVID-19) pandemic for child and adolescent mental health: a narrative review to highlight clinical and research needs in the acute phase and the long return to normality. Child Adolesc Psychiatry Ment Health 14:20, 2020

Golberstein E, Wen H, Miller BF: Coronavirus disease 2019 (COVID-19) and mental health for children and adolescents. JAMA Pediatr April 14, 2020 Epub ahead of print

Hart SN: From property to person status: historical perspective on children's rights. Am Psychol 46(1):53–59, 1991

HealthyPeople.Gov: Social determinants of health. Washington, DC, U.S. Department of Health and Human Services, 2020. Available at: www.healthypeople.gov/2020/topics-objectives/topic/social-determinants-of-health. Accessed December 19, 2019.

Heitzeg NA: Education or incarceration: zero tolerance policies and the school to prison pipeline. Forum on Public Policy, 2009. Available at: https://files.eric.ed.gov/fulltext/EJ870076.pdf. Accessed August 14, 2020.

Hummer RA, Hernandez EM: The effect of educational attainment on adult mortality in the United States. Popul Bull 68(1):1–16, 2013

Kernic MA, Holt VL, Wolf ME, et al: Academic and school health issues among children exposed to maternal intimate partner abuse. Arch Pediatr Adolesc Med 156(6):549–555, 2002

Lim S, Chan PY, Walters S, et al: Impact of residential displacement on healthcare access and mental health among original residents of gentrifying neighborhoods in New York City. PLoS One 12(12):e0190139, 2017

Link BG, Phelan JC: McKeown and the idea that social conditions are fundamental causes of disease. Am J Public Health 92(5):730–732, 2002

Liu P, Nunn R, Shambaugh J: The economics of bail and pretrial detention. Economic Analysis. Washington, DC, The Hamilton Project, Brookings Institution, December 2018. Available at: www.hamilton-project.org/assets/files/BailFineReform_EA_121818_6PM.pdf. Accessed: August 14, 2020.

Marlowe DB: Integrating substance abuse treatment and criminal justice supervision. Sci Pract Perspect 2(1):4–14, 2003

McMurtry S, Lie G-Y: Differential exit rates of minority children in foster care. Soc Work Res Abstr 28(11), 1992

Mehdipanah R, Marra G, Melis G, et al: Urban renewal, gentrification and health equity: a realist perspective. Eur J Public Health 28(2):243–248, 2018

Menahem S: Pediatricians' role in providing mental health care for children and adolescents. J Dev Behav Pediatr 30(1):104, 2009

Merrick MT, Ford DC, Ports KA, et al: Prevalence of adverse childhood experiences from the 2011–2014 Behavioral Risk Factor Surveillance System in 23 states. JAMA Pediatr 172(11):1038–1044, 2018

Murray J, Farrington DP, Sekol I: Children's antisocial behavior, mental health, drug use, and educational performance after parental incarceration: a systematic review and meta-analysis. Psychol Bull 138(2):175–210, 2012

NAACP Legal Defense and Educational Fund: Dismantling the school to prison pipeline. New York, NAACP Legal Defense and Educational Fund, 2020. Available at: www.naacpldf.org/wp-content/uploads/Dismantling_the_School_to_Prison_Pipeline__Criminal-Justice__.pdf. Accessed August 14, 2020.

National Fair Housing Alliance: Making every neighborhood a place of opportunity: 2018 fair housing trends report. Washington, DC, National Fair Housing Alliance, 2018. Available at: https://nationalfairhousing.org/wp-content/uploads/2018/04/NFHA-2018-Fair-Housing-Trends-Report_4-30-18.pdf. Accessed November 28, 2019.

Olfson M, Blanco C, Wang S, et al: National trends in the mental health care of children, adolescents, and adults by office-based physicians. JAMA Psychiatry 71(1):81–90, 2014

Owens P, Hoagwood K, Horwitz K, et al: Barriers to children's mental health services. J Am Acad Child Adolesc Psychiatry 41(6):731–738, 2002

Park JM, Fertig AR, Allison PD: Physical and mental health, cognitive development, and health care use by housing status of low-income young children in 20 American cities: a prospective cohort study. Am J Public Health 101(suppl 1):S255–S261, 2011

Pecora PJ, Jensen PS, Romanelli LH, et al: Mental health services for children placed in foster care: an overview of current challenges. Child Welfare 88(1):5–26, 2009

Pumariega AJ: Children and adolescents, in Disparities in Psychiatric Care: Clinical and Cross-Cultural Perspectives. Edited by Ruiz P, Prim A. Philadelphia, Lippincott Williams & Wilkins, 2010, pp 117–126

Pumariega AJ, Winters NC, Huffine C: The evolution of systems of care for children's mental health: forty years of community child and adolescent psychiatry. Community Ment Health J 39(5):399–425, 2003

Roberts DE: Shattered Bonds: The Color of Child Welfare. New York, Basic Books, 2002

Schwartz RC, Blankenship DM: Racial disparities in psychotic disorder diagnosis: a review of empirical literature. World J Psychiatry 4(4):133–140, 2014

Tamzarian A, Menzies HM, Ricci L: Barriers to full participation in the individualized education program for culturally and linguistically diverse parents. Journal of Special Education Apprenticeship 1(2):1–11, 2012

Teicher MH: Childhood trauma and the enduring consequences of forcibly separating children from parents at the United States border. BMC Med 16(1):146, 2018

Turner MA, Santos R, Levy DK, et al: Housing Discrimination Against Racial and Ethnic Minorities 2012: Full Report. Washington, DC, Urban Institute, 2016

U.S. Department of Health and Human Services: Recent demographic trends in foster care. Data Brief 2013-1. Washington, DC, Office of Data, Analysis, Research, and Evaluation, Administration of Children, Youth and Families, September 2013. Available at: www.acf.hhs.gov/sites/default/files/cb/data_brief_foster_care_trends1.pdf. Accessed June 29, 2019.

U.S. Sentencing Commission: Mandatory minimum penalties for drug offenses in the federal system. Washington, DC, U.S. Sentencing Commission, October 2017. Available at: www.ussc.gov/research/research-reports/mandatory-minimum-penalties-drug-offenses-federal-system. Accessed December 20, 2019.

U.S. Sentencing Commission: 2011 report to Congress: mandatory minimum penalties in the federal criminal justice system. Washington, DC, U.S. Sentencing Commission, 2011. Available at: www.ussc.gov/research/congressional-reports/2011-report-congress-mandatory-minimum-penalties-federal-criminal-justice-system. Accessed December 20, 2019.

Vanderwerker L, Akincigil A, Olfson M, et al: Foster care, externalizing disorders, and antipsychotic use among Medicaid-enrolled youth. Psychiatr Serv 65(10):1281–1284, 2014

World Health Organization: About social determinants of health. Geneva, Switzerland, World Health Organization, 2020. Available at: www.who.int/social_determinants/sdh_definition/en. Accessed January 20, 2020.

CHAPTER 11

Aliens, Illegals, Deportees

Children, Migration, and Mental Health

Schuyler W. Henderson, M.D., M.P.H.
Maria Baez, M.D.

THROUGHOUT history and across the globe, people have migrated. Today, the numbers of migrants across the world remain vast. According to the United Nations, there were 258 million migrants in 2017, including 68 million forcibly displaced persons (25 million refugees, 3 million asylum seekers, and more than 40 million internally displaced persons) (United Nations 2019). Of these migrants, the United Nations identified 36.1 million children and 4.8 million international students. Approximately 44 million people who were born in another country reside in the United States (Batalova and Aperin 2018).

As a global phenomenon, migration has been and continues to be a controversial topic, and a host of fears surrounds migrants, including fear of disease and fear of upsetting national identities and cultures. There is also a fear of exploiting local resources, ranging from taking away jobs to sneaking into the country in order to obtain health care. Mental health providers, caregivers, advocates, educators, and researchers should develop a cautious, careful approach when

---

This chapter has been informed by Henderson SW, Sung D, Baily C: "The diverse migrant: families, children, migration and acculturation," in *Cultural Sensitivity in Child and Adolescent Mental Health*. Edited by Parekh RI, Gorrindo T, Rubin TH. Boston, MA, MGH Psychiatry Academy Press, 2015, pp. 239–263.

encountering migrants, recognizing this patchwork background of resentment and hostility that can influence the therapeutic relationship. It is worth noting that mental health professionals are not infrequently migrants themselves. When discussing cultural competency, mental health, and migration, it is therefore important to consider the cultural competency of all involved.

After becoming aware of this complex and controversial sociopolitical background, the culturally competent care provider can approach migration positively, with sensitivity to the experiences of bias and bigotry the patient may have faced (Schouler-Ocak et al. 2019). In addition, the care provider should consider patients' bona fide concerns for safety—their own and that of their families as potential targets for bias. To approach the topic of migration, the mental health provider first and foremost needs to consider any legal ramifications to asking about migration history or status (such as in cases where the provider may be compelled to disclose this information). The provider must also consider the extent to which migration can or should be documented in records. This also pertains to asking about family. It is not uncommon to meet a youth whose status is documented ("legal") but who has relatives, including parents, who are undocumented ("illegal"). Knowing your legal obligations as a health care professional and the standards and practices of any institution for which you are working is a prerequisite to approaching this topic.

It is also important to inform patients and their family of any potential repercussions of confiding their migration status. Once mental health caregivers have established for themselves the extent to which they can ask about migration history, they must inform the family the extent to which it is safe for them to discuss migration. The provider can begin with an introduction such as "I want to ask about your history and past, and I can keep all the information you tell me confidential, even about your migration." Migration history can then be taken. Some of the many reasons for asking about migration history are listed in Table 11–1.

There are three key concepts that mental health providers should bear in mind at the outset of any discussion of migration and cultural competency. The first is that every person's migration experience is unique, although some aspects of it may be common to the experiences of other migrants. The second is that migration is a fluid experience; when you encounter individuals with a migration history, their journey may not yet have ended. Migration is rarely, if ever, a completed process. There may be ongoing involvement between migrants and their homeland, including communication with friends and family, and continued sharing of the culture. The third is that migration reflects intersectionality. Immigration cannot be understood without recognizing the ways in which race, religion, class, gender, sexual orientation, and other demographic and social identities interact. These factors often play a role in decisions regarding whether and how to immigrate as well as in individuals' perception of and adaptation to their experiences during migration and settlement.

The DSM-5 Outline for Cultural Formulation (OCF; American Psychiatric Association 2013), which is described in more depth in Chapter 21, "DSM-5 Outline for Cultural Formulation and Cultural Formulation Interview," can help guide how clinicians think about and interact with immigrant and refugee children and families. The OCF, which first appeared in DSM-IV (American Psychiatric Association 1994), creates a framework that can be used to provide reliability and validity when assessing cultural identity, illness representation, cultural stressors, and other culturally informed concepts. At the same time, the OCF facilitates inclusion of the patient in treatment planning.

Also available in DSM-5 is the Cultural Formulation Interview (CFI), which has three components: a 16-item core questionnaire, the CFI informant version, and 12 supplementary modules related to different domains of a patient's environment and culture (American Psychiatric

TABLE 11–1. Importance of migration history

Elucidates prior exposures (e.g., to trauma or illnesses)

Elicits current stressors and strengths

Clarifies current plans and whether long-term treatment is feasible (e.g., if the family is planning to move on)

Identifies current resources and supports

Ensures that recommended services are available or accessible (e.g., when an undocumented family cannot avail themselves of certain social supports)

Establishes rapport

Lets the patient know that disclosures around migration are a "safe" topic

Association 2013). The CFI, including the supplementary modules, may be especially helpful when providing mental health care for immigrants and refugees. By the time immigrants or refugees have made it to a new destination (see the clinical vignette in the following section), they often have had many adverse experiences with authority figures. They may be reluctant to speak openly with a clinician and may be suspicious of a clinician's intentions and recommendations. The CFI approach encourages the clinician to understand what is most important to the patient about his or her background and identity and how it relates to the current clinical encounter, in a standardized way, without necessarily invoking migration. The content helps the clinician appreciate that immigrants and refugees may view their challenges in a much different way than the clinician does, and this culturally informed approach strives to help the clinician figure out how the patient views his or her problem.

In this chapter, we explore the complex experience of immigrants and describe how mental health professionals can best care for this vulnerable patient population. These patients deserve our most thoughtful approaches.

Understanding the Journey
Clinical Vignette

Angelica is a 14-year-old girl from Guatemala whose foster parents brought her to meet a psychiatrist for an evaluation because she was refusing to go to school, was complaining of constipation and stomach pains, and was saying she wished she were dead. During the meeting with Angelica, the psychiatrist asked why she had come to the United States. Angelica said her life in Guatemala was chaotic because of poverty, poor social supports, and violence, and she talked about her history of being sexually and physically abused by male cousins. Prior to fleeing Guatemala, she was being actively recruited to join the gangs, which prompted her mother to hire a *coyote* to take her to the United States. Angelica said she had heard of the United States prior to her immigration, and although she now knew people in the United States and wanted to be safe, she missed her mother and her younger sisters.

It is important to allow space for understanding a patient's reasons for migration without assuming one particular reason. In fact, most people will make the difficult decision to migrate for multiple reasons. These may include wanting to be in a new country, going to a new school, joining relatives, escaping persecution, or getting a job. The list of reasons for migration are extensive, and although people may have one particularly important reason, they may have others as well. Some people may want to share a reason that they think their listener will find particularly important. For example, one of the authors (S.W.H.) previously presented a case report in which a young woman's doctors thought she was not a refugee because she told them she had come to the United States to go to school (Suardi et al. 2010). In fact, she was a refugee and had been terribly persecuted, but when she was discussing her situation with a group of people fairly close to her own age, she wanted to foreground that she was a proud and ambitious student. In other situations, as in the case of Angelica, the individual's family may have encouraged migration, even if that individual was uncertain about leaving.

Migration can be considered to be either voluntary or involuntary/forced, categories that have social and legal ramifications. For example, someone who is designated a refugee may have more access to services and supports than someone who has come to the United States as a seasonal farm worker. However, these overarching categories are not always clear. For example, some people who appear to be making a voluntary decision to come to another country to seek work may have been facing extensive marginalization, persecution, poverty, or inequality, rendering their decision less volitional than it may seem.

In order to get beyond the "voluntary forced" construct and to recognize the multiple reasons for migration, the mental health caregiver can ask about push and pull factors. The former are the factors that compel someone to leave a country, such as unemployment, persecution, structural violence, or the desire for a better education. The latter are those that draw someone into a new country, such as family reunification, a familiar language, or a familiar history. These reasons are different for each patient and help inform the cultural formulation. For Angelica, the push factors were a chaotic life due to poverty, poor social supports, and violence, and the pull factors were her hopes for safety and new opportunities.

Clinical Vignette *(continued)*

During her month-long journey to the United States, Angelica had many challenging experiences, including prolonged periods of time in a truck with many other people and limited food and water. The *coyote* gave her medications to prevent her from needing to go to the bathroom. At the border, Angelica was detained and removed from the truck, along with 15 other people, and held overnight in a camp where she had to share a cot with another girl. After being interviewed by federal agents, she was identified as an unaccompanied minor and was flown to New York City— her first time in an airplane. In New York, Angelica was met by officers who took her to a foster agency. This period of detainment was a source of high anxiety for her because she was provided with little information about what was happening to her.

Premigration stressors typically precipitate the migration and can include structural violence, targeted violence, domestic violence, commercial exploitation, famine, environmental disasters, dangerous communities, warfare, and gang violence. Migration stressors can include exposure to further violence and exploitation, dangerous travel arrangements, isolation, loneliness, and fear (Bhabha and Schmidt 2008; Fazel and Stein 2002).

When thinking about migration, the journey can be divided up into three phases: premigration, migration, and postmigration. Although migration can be a positive, exciting, and well-planned process, each step can involve stressors. These stressors may be cumulative and have compounding effects on postmigration vulnerabilities and mental health; therefore, it is important

TABLE 11–2. Sample questions about migration

Tell me about the reasons you left your home country. What are the things that compelled you to leave? What are the things that attracted you to coming here?

What happened prior to departure?

Tell me about your journey here and any challenges you might have had along the way.

How did you get to where you are now?

Did your whole family come at the same time, or were you separated? For how long? How was that separation for you?

Tell me about the family and friends you left behind. How do you keep in touch with them? Do they plan to come join you?

Describe any concerns about your life right now. What are you most happy about? What are your plans looking ahead?

Do you plan to return to your home country?

Who is still back in the country you came from? How do you connect with them?

Source. Adapted from Henderson SW, Sung D, Baily C: Table 8.1, "The diverse migrant: families, children, migration and acculturation," in *Cultural Sensitivity in Child and Adolescent Mental Health.* Edited by Parekh RI, Gorrindo T, Rubin TH. Boston, MA, MGH Psychiatry Academy Press, 2015, p. 245.

to discuss these stressors and challenges with patients because this discussion can provide more insight into trauma, resources, resilience, needs, and adaptation (Courtois 2008; Pumariega et al. 2005; Robjant et al. 2009).

Postmigration stressors can include detention, isolation, family separation, further violence and exploitation, and ongoing discomfort due to the uncertainties of the migrant's life in the new country (Suárez-Orozco et al. 2002). Often, very vulnerable populations may not be receiving medical or mental health treatment, or the postmigration treatment they do receive may be exacerbating existing vulnerabilities (Mares and Jureidini 2004; Mares et al. 2002; Silove et al. 2007; Sultan and O'Sullivan 2001). In addition, postmigration stressors can include fear of deportation (including being deported back to the very circumstances that precipitated migration) as well as ongoing debts and vulnerabilities. For example, some Fuzhounese migrants working in restaurants in the northeast United States owe many thousands of dollars to the "snakeheads" who smuggled them in (Lai et al. 2013). Relationships in the country of origin may be sources of strength, but they can also pose problems, such as when migrant children are recruited for terrorism (Weine et al. 2013). Table 11–2 provides sample questions that may be helpful in clarifying the cultural formulation when asking about a patient's journey.

Where Are We Now?

Clinical Vignette *(continued)*

The foster agency placed Angelica in a home with two parents and two older boys. All of them treated her nicely. She struggled with anxiety about her future and about her family back home, whom she was unable to contact. She went to school at the foster agency, and even though the teachers and support staff were supportive there as well, she was reluctant to connect with anyone.

She did not want to learn English. Several students made fun of her for being shy. Eventually, she opted to just stay at home and refused to go to school. She confided to one of the older boys in the home that she was feeling depressed and suicidal. He alerted the foster parents, and together with staff at the foster agency, they took her to see a psychiatrist.

In terms of understanding children in the context of migration, a family perspective will always be required. This introduces complexity to such already multifaceted topics as integration into the new country and parenting.

There are many ways in which migrants can integrate into their new country. One of these ways is *assimilation*, in which "the culture of origin is rejected and the host culture largely adopted, with the loss of language and customs of origin" (Pumariega et al. 2013, p. 1107). In *acculturation*, people, families, and communities change as they enter and learn about a new culture, engaging partly or in whole with the new culture while often retaining aspects of the cultures from which they came. A similar concept is *biculturality*, in which migrants are "rooted in their culture of origin" but have "the necessary knowledge and interpersonal skills to navigate the mainstream culture (i.e., a hyphenated identity)" (Pumariega et al. 2013, p. 1107). These models can be somewhat useful to explore, but there are a number of challenges in doing so, including *intersectionality*. For example, what culture does a person come from if the immigrant is, say, a Muslim woman from Xinjiang or a Jewish man from Wyoming or a gender fluid Christian from Buenos Aires? Similarly, there may be transgenerational differences; parents, for example, may be more bicultural, whereas their children may be more assimilated.

Migration is often described as a process of significant risk, including posttraumatic sequelae; the effects of dislocation on psychological resilience; and the amplification of vulnerabilities through isolation, bias, and stigma. Migration can also reflect resilience, strength, optimism, and global connection that transcends national boundaries. It is worth keeping in mind that migration often bears the stigma of sickness and morbidity. For the cultural formulation to be meaningful, it requires not only a capacity for rapport and eliciting histories but an understanding of the significance of the cultural interaction. Language poses a particular challenge, and professional interpretation should be emphasized, in concert with thoughtful and engaged communication practices (Clarke et al. 2019). Table 11–3 contains a list of questions to ask parents or other caregivers that may be helpful in understanding the degree of integration and family roles. Of note, psychiatric symptoms are stigmatized globally. The caregiver should not make assumptions about whether they are more or less stigmatized in the country of origin.

Trauma

Clinical Vignette *(continued)*

Angelica experienced sleep disturbance, nightmares, and flashbacks and was diagnosed with PTSD. She was open to treatment, especially when it was revealed that she would have a Spanish-speaking psychiatrist. During treatment, she began to open up about her multiple physical and sexual traumas. Angelica discussed how these traumas prevented her from feeling safe in her new country. She believed her constipation and stomach pains were related to her traumas and feared that there was something permanently "wrong" with her.

TABLE 11–3.   How to ask about integration and family roles

What languages are spoken at home?

How well do your family members speak [the home language]?

How well do your family members speak [the language of the destination country]?

How do parents and other adults communicate with children in [the home country]? What differences have you found in [the destination country]?

What sort of activities did you do with your children in [the home country]? How have the activities changed?

What do you and your children agree about? Disagree about?

Are your children (or parents) embracing the values of the new culture more than your home culture? Is this causing problems?

Do you worry that some people in the family are not retaining enough of their native culture?

How are children expected to behave in [the home country] and how do they behave here?

How are children expected to perform in school? What role do adults—teachers and parents—play, and how is that different here?

What are the differences in the way kids are raised?

What do adults do in [the home country] to punish children? What happens here?

Do you and your child share beliefs about gender roles, freedom, autonomy, professional goals, and romantic relationships?

Source.   Henderson SW, Sung D, Baily C: "The diverse migrant: families, children, migration and acculturation," in *Cultural Sensitivity in Child and Adolescent Mental Health.* Edited by Parekh RI, Gorrindo T, Rubin TH. Boston, MA, MGH Psychiatry Academy Press, 2015, pp. 239–263.

The association between migration and trauma has been studied extensively, and a consistent finding is that increased trauma is related to increased vulnerabilities, lack of resources, and traumatic events (Fazel et al. 2005; Schweitzer et al. 2006; Silove et al. 1997). The trauma experienced by Angelica is quite clear, but other types of trauma may be less apparent. For example, consider the case of 15-year-old Jasmine, who came from Kenya to live with her father after not seeing him for more than 10 years in order to attend high school in New York City. She found herself frequently home alone while her father worked, isolated at school from her peers, and frightened by the sights and sounds of the big city. She soon became depressed and had frequent nightmares, and her father decided to send her back to Kenya without seeking any formal mental health treatment for her. Although Jasmine was never physically harmed, she left the United States feeling traumatized and unwell.

Advocacy

Advocacy for child patients and their families is a part of practicing mental health care, and it is most effective when the advocate recognizes the multiple determinants of refugee mental health, including psychological, social, biomedical, historical, cultural, and economic dimensions (Kirmayer et al. 2018). On a larger scale, groups such as the Global Mental Health and Psychiatry Caucus of the American Psychiatric Association (APA) have clearly communicated the need for providers to be active against policies that harm immigrants, especially those that have separated young immigrant children from their families (Mahmoud et al. 2019). The APA discusses the need for everyone—from government agencies to psychiatrists to the public—to partner together to develop comprehensive strategies to combat problematic policies and to engage in widespread educational activities about the harms of these policies (Mahmoud et al. 2019). As clinicians, we must continue to further study how to best care for immigrants and learn more about the many different barriers to care (Gómez and O'Leary 2019).

For each individual immigrant patient, the clinician should do more than just treat the child's psychiatric disorders; it is challenging to address a patient's psychiatric conditions without helping the child and family figure out how to navigate their complicated social situation. Children and their families often need help connecting to local resources so that they can learn their rights; have access to proper medical care (Dave 2019), schooling, and other resources; and understand their legal situation.

Conclusion

Home remains one of the most important human psychosocial constructs. It is

> a place of belonging, a personal history, a space infused with familiarity, expectation, and intuition; it is where customs and rituals begin; and it is where the lived realities of culture are learned, adopted, absorbed, and changed, generation by generation. A home is where we come from. Migration complicates and challenges simplified notions of home. With migration, we may have multiple homes, multiple places we come from, multiple cultures and societies in our backgrounds, shifting and changing and developing and intermingling. (Henderson et al. 2015, p. 259)

Cultural competency with migrants requires a sensitive, thoughtful discussion around and about the home. Because migration is such an essential human experience, however stigmatized or politically controversial, it should be met with welcoming and familiarity, not with hostility or difference.

Clinical Pearls

- Migration is a complex phenomenon with many different contributing factors.
- Addressing migration requires a willingness to listen to the patient's entire story and an ability to ask about different stages of the migration, including the next stage: What comes next?
- The DSM-5 Outline for Cultural Formulation and Cultural Formulation Interview can help guide psychiatrists in their thinking about and interactions with immigrant and refugee children and families.
- Letting patients know that it is safe (and when it is not safe) to talk about their migration with you is critical.

Self-Assessment Questions

1. When assessing a patient's migration history, it is important to do which of the following?

    A. Figure out the single most important reason for migration.
    B. Avoid speaking about connections to the country of origin for fear of alienating the migrant.
    C. Wait until later interviews to ask about family members left behind because it may be traumatizing to do so.
    D. Ask about connections to the country of origin.
    E. Insist that the migration story be told in the language of the country of origin.

2. Which of the following areas of discussion should be avoided?

    A. Differences between parents and children in how they relate to their country of origin.
    B. Difference in cultural practices for raising children between the host country and the country of origin.
    C. Which languages are used in the home and when they are used.
    D. The patient's hopes and plans for connections with the country of origin.
    E. None of the above.

3. Which of the following is *not* a clinical reason for eliciting a migration history?

    A. A migration history may be helpful in determining what current resources are available.
    B. Eliciting a migration history can help establish rapport.
    C. The migration history lets you know when you have to inform the authorities about a family's migration status.
    D. A migration history may provide information about the patient's prior trauma, exposures, and vulnerabilities and his or her potential resources, resilience, and strength.

Answers

1. D
2. E
3. C

References

American Psychiatric Association: Diagnostic and Statistical Manual of Mental Disorders, 4th Edition. Washington, DC, American Psychiatric Association, 1994

American Psychiatric Association: Diagnostic and Statistical Manual of Mental Disorders, 5th Edition. Arlington, VA, American Psychiatric Association, 2013

Batalova J, Aperin E: Immigrants in the U.S. states with the fastest-growing foreign-born populations. Washington, DC, Migration Policy Institute, July 10, 2018. Available at: www.migrationpolicy.org/article/immigrants-us-states-fastest-growing-foreign-born-populations. Accessed April 25, 2019.

Bhabha J, Schmidt S: Seeking asylum alone: unaccompanied and separated children and refugee protection in the U.S. J Hist Child Youth 1:127–138, 2008

Clarke SK, Jaffe J, Mutch R: Overcoming communication barriers in refugee health care. Pediatr Clin North Am 66(3):669–686, 2019

Courtois CA: Complex trauma, complex reactions: assessment and treatment. Psychol Trauma1:86–100, 2008

Dave A: The need for cultural competency and healthcare literacy with refugees. J Natl Med Assoc 111(1):101–102, 2019

Fazel M, Stein A: The mental health of refugee children. Arch Dis Child 87(5):366–370, 2002

Fazel M, Wheeler J, Danesh J: Prevalence of serious mental disorder in 7000 refugees resettled in western countries: a systematic review. Lancet 365(9467):1309–1314, 2005

Gómez S, O'Leary AO: "On edge all the time": mixed-status households navigating health care post Arizona's most stringent anti-immigrant law. Front Public Health 6:383, 2019

Henderson SW, Sung D, Baily C: The diverse migrant: families, children, migration and acculturation, in Cultural Sensitivity in Child and Adolescent Mental Health. Edited by Parekh RI, Gorrindo T, Rubin TH. Boston, MA, MGH Psychiatry Academy Press, 2015, pp 239–263

Kirmayer LJ, Kronick R, Rousseau C: Advocacy as key to structural competency in psychiatry. JAMA Psychiatry 75(2):119–120, 2018

Lai GY-C, Lo G, Ngo H, et al: Migration, socio-cultural factors, and local cultural worlds among Fuzhounese Chinese immigrants: implications for mental health interventions. Int J Cult Ment Health 6(2):141–155, 2013

Mahmoud H, Fleming JL, Halbreich U, et al: Grave concerns expressed by psychiatrists over current immigration policies. J Am Acad Child Adolesc Psychiatry 58(1):140–141, 2019

Mares S, Jureidini J: Psychiatric assessment of children and families in immigration detention—clinical, administrative and ethical issues. Aust N Z J Public Health 28:520–526, 2004

Mares S, Newman L, Dudley M, et al: Seeking refuge, losing hope: parents and children in immigration detention. Australas Psychiatry 10:91–96, 2002

Pumariega AJ, Rothe E, Pumariega JB: Mental health of immigrants and refugees. Community Ment Health J 41(5):581–597, 2005

Pumariega AJ, Rothe E, Mian A, et al: Practice parameter for cultural competence in child and adolescent psychiatric practice. J Am Acad Child Adolesc Psychiatry 52(10):1101–1115, 2013

Robjant K, Hassan R, Katona C: Mental health implications of detaining asylum seekers: systematic review. Br J Psychiatry 194(4):306–312, 2009

Schouler-Ocak M, Laban CJ, Bäärnhielm S, et al: Transcultural psychiatry: refugee, asylum seeker and immigrant patients over the globe, in Advances in Psychiatry, Vol 4. Edited by Javed A, Fountoulakis KN. Cham, Switzerland, Springer, 2019, pp 637–655

Schweitzer R, Melville F, Steel Z, et al: Trauma, post-migration living difficulties, and social support as predictors of psychological adjustment in resettled Sudanese refugees. Aust N Z J Psychiatry 40(2):179–187, 2006

Silove D, Sinnerbrink I, Field V, et al: Anxiety, depression and PTSD in asylum-seekers: associations with pre-migration trauma and post-migration stressors. Br J Psychiatry 170:351–357, 1997

Silove D, Austin P, Steel Z: No refuge from terror: the impact of detention on the mental health of trauma-affected refugees seeking asylum in Australia. Transcult Psychiatry 44(3):359–393, 2007

Suardi E, Mishkin A, Henderson SW: Female genital mutilation in a young refugee: a case report and review. J Child Adolesc Trauma 3:234–242, 2010

Suárez-Orozco C, Todorova ILG, Louie J: Making up for lost time: the experience of separation and reunification among immigrant families. Fam Process 41(4):625–643, 2002

Sultan A, O'Sullivan K: Psychological disturbances in asylum seekers held in long-term detention: a participant-observer account. Med J Aust 175(11–12):593–596, 2001

United Nations: Migration. 2019. Available at: www.un.org/en/sections/issues-depth/migration/index.html. Accessed August 2, 2019.

Weine S, Henderson S, Shanfield S, et al: Building community resilience to counter violent extremism. Democracy and Security 9(4):327–333, 2013

CHAPTER 12

Clinical Strategies to Address the Mental Health of Forcibly Displaced Children (Refugees, Asylum Seekers, and Unaccompanied Minors)

The Role of Silence, Family, and Socioecological Resilience

Suzan Song, M.D., M.P.H., Ph.D.

THE forced displacement and mass migration of children and communities due to disruptions caused by economic and political instability; natural and man-made disasters; war and armed conflict; and chronic, pervasive interpersonal and community violence have surged to crisis levels around the world. Approximately half of the world's refugees are younger than 18 years. At the end of 2017, nearly 31 million children were forcibly displaced from their homes: 13 million child or adolescent refugees, 936,000 asylum-seeking children, and 17 million children internally displaced by armed conflict and violence (United Nations Children's Fund 2018). Historically, the United States was one of the largest countries of resettlement for forcibly displaced children until the 2016 Trump administration, which emphasized stringent immigration policies (Table 12–1). These policies resulted in more stressful family conditions (e.g., full-time supervision of children, stigma and consequent hiding of children to avoid deportation) due to increased

TABLE 12–1.   Immigration policies during the Trump administration

Banned nationals of eight mostly Muslim-majority countries from entering the United States

Reduced refugee admissions to the lowest level since the creation of the 1980 resettlement program (~22,000 from an average of 75,000 in the previous decade)

Canceled the Deferred Action for Childhood Arrivals (DACA) program that provided work authorization and temporary relief from deportation to 690,000 unauthorized immigrants who came to the United States as children

Instituted a "zero tolerance" policy that called for every illegal entry case across the border to be prosecuted, which separated children who could not be prosecuted with their parents

Source.   Adapted from Rush N: The U.S. Refugee Admissions Program Under the Trump Administration. Center for Immigration Studies, April 1, 2019. Available at: https://cis.org/Rush/US-Refugee-Admissions-Program-under-Trump-Administration. Accessed April 28, 2020.

difficulties in accessing humanitarian aid, support, and supplies. In April 2018, the Department of Justice instituted an "iron triangle" of deterrence, detention, and deportation aimed at unaccompanied minors crossing the U.S. border. Because of these policies, the United States now has the world's largest immigration detention system (Global Detention Project 2018).

It is important to consider how individuals come to the United States because each immigrant or refugee faces different struggles and has different social, political, and moral entailments (Table 12–2).

Once refugees arrive in the United States, voluntary agencies provide resettlement services (food, housing, medical care, employment training, clothing) during the first 90 days. Refugees are eligible for cash assistance and Medicaid for 8 months after arrival and can receive federally funded public benefits for 5 years unless they obtain U.S. citizenship. After 1 year of residence in the United States, refugees and asylees can apply for legal permanent residence (green card), then finally U.S. citizenship after 5 years.

For ease of discussion, in this chapter, the term *forcibly displaced child* includes child and adolescent refugees, asylum seekers, and unaccompanied minors or those separated from their caretaker(s). The terms *child/adolescent* and *child* are used interchangeably in this chapter to follow the United Nations definition of a child as age 0–18 years and a youth as 5–24 years old, highlighting the concept that *childhood* is largely a social construct with local and cultural underpinnings. This chapter is not intended to be a comprehensive approach to the assessment or care of forcibly displaced children; rather, I highlight clinical issues for mental health professionals without experience working with this population.

Mental Health and Forced Displacement and Migration

Forced Displacement and Children

The experience of forcibly displaced children is varied. Some have endured chronic pervasive exposure to interpersonal and community violence, uncertainty of the future, personal or family

TABLE 12–2. **Examples of forcibly displaced children and adolescents**

Term	Definition
Refugees	Individuals seeking a safe haven because of a well-founded fear of persecution due to race, religion, nationality, or membership in a particular social group or political opinion (United Nations High Commissioner for Refugees 1951); legal permission to resettle in the United States is given prior to arrival
Asylum seekers	Individuals with a well-founded fear of persecution who seek legal immigration status while in a host country
Internally displaced persons	Individuals who flee their homes because of armed conflict, community violence, human rights violations, or disasters but have not crossed an internationally recognized state border
Unaccompanied and separated minors	Youth fleeing interpersonal and community violence who arrive in a new country without a parent or caretaker (unaccompanied) or apart from their caretaker (separated) and may seek asylum for safety

persecution, violent loss of loved ones, and an insecure environment. Others have experienced a shorter exposure to high violence such as active war. Some children come from areas of armed conflict and war and have been conscripted into the armed forces as child soldiers, and other children flee with intact families. The migration experience for children forcibly displaced from their homes to the United States is also varied. Refugee and asylum-seeking children may travel by plane or train without exposure to violence or danger if they have resources. Others have long migration journeys across multiple countries that include hiding; exposure to physical and sexual assault; separation from loved ones or caretakers; and lack of basic needs such as food, clean water, and the ability to maintain personal hygiene. Often, forcibly displaced children must abruptly leave all belongings except only the most necessary and must quickly say goodbye to loved ones who may be unable to join them. They do not necessarily want to leave the home environment and culture in which they were raised. These children lose not only material resources such as housing, education, access to food and water, and security, but also social relationships and cultural supports.

Once they reach the United States, children and their families often face multiple postmigration stressors, including poverty, insecure housing, unemployment, multiple moves with changes in neighborhoods, difficulty in establishing peer and family supports, and lack of supervision and support (DeJong et al. 2017; Goosen et al. 2014). Daily life stressors, such as isolation, stressful legal issues, poor access to services, and general disadvantage in the host country, can all adversely impact mental health (Miller and Rasmussen 2017; Morgan et al. 2017).

Current studies on the mental health course of forcibly displaced children focus on PTSD, depression, and anxiety, with a review of child/adolescent refugee mental health showing a 5% prevalence of depression and 11% prevalence of PTSD (Fazel et al. 2005). Studies have shown a 20% or more risk of PTSD for children living in refugee camps (Ceri et al. 2016; Eruyar et al. 2018), with the prevalence of PTSD symptoms higher among refugees than among same-age nonrefugee peers. Although PTSD and depression symptoms have been shown to decrease over time, particularly if there are low postmigration stressors (Betancourt et al. 2013; Oppedal and Idsoe 2015), some children continue to have significant mental health problems (Beiser and

Wickrama 2004; Rothe et al. 2002). However, the exact disability burden is unknown because many studies do not capture functional impairment (Steel et al. 2009).

PTSD, depression, and anxiety do not provide the full scope of emotional issues that many conflict-affected persons face. Survivors of forced dislocation can also struggle with existential crises and grief-related disorders (Fazel et al. 2005; Martens 2007), depending on the length of the relocation process, their language proficiency and social supports; acceptance by the new country; employment and educational opportunities; and similarity between the home and host cultures (Bhugra and Becker 2005). Although a child may not meet the full criteria for major psychiatric disorders, he or she may be dealing with issues related to traumatic loss, complicated grief, complex trauma, despair, isolation, anger, lack of trust, cultural bereavement, and acculturative stress.

Dimensional Approaches to Mental Health

Many forcibly displaced children have normal reactions to abnormal situations. Children should not be forcibly taken from their loved ones nor have to witness the rape and murder of their neighbors. War is not conducive to a supportive environment for development. We therefore need to better understand the distinction between situational forms of distress and a clear mental disorder by focusing attention on the interplay between past exposures, current daily stressors, and the core social systems in which the child lives (Hodes and Vostanis 2019). Exposure to trauma itself does not necessarily lead to a mental health disorder, and understanding which factors can promote well-being and protect against development of adverse mental health is imperative. When considering the burden of adverse experiences on forcibly displaced children, it is critical to consider not only premigration persecution or exposure to traumatic events but also the stress associated with the transition to a new society and new daily life changes (Miller and Rasmussen 2017; Song et al. 2015).

Taking a dimensional, staged approach to mental health diagnosis can be a useful framework for forcibly displaced children (Patel et al. 2018). The symptom checklists used to define categories of mental disorders may undervalue the complexities of children's experiences; in contrast, a staged approach can help clinicians evaluate the dimensions of mental distress at various stages (e.g., prodromal) or symptoms that are reactive and transient. Such an approach emphasizes the importance of prevention. For example, a diagnosis may not be helpful for a child with nonspecific psychological distress, but increased monitoring, support, and engagement may assist with early intervention if the distress worsens.

Mental Health Treatment Gap for Children and Families of Forced Displacement

The increase in children forcibly displaced to the United States can create mental health needs that pose unique challenges for clinicians. Despite the mental burden in survivors of forced displacement, children rarely interface with formal mental health services, in part because of scarcity of appropriate services and stigma against mental health care (Satinsky et al. 2019). The mental health treatment gap for refugee children is therefore large, with an estimated 92% of refugees (and immigrants) either not receiving needed services (Ellis et al. 2011) or using the emergency department as a first point of contact for mental health care (Saunders et al. 2018). Routine health care providers and agencies may therefore feel overwhelmed and uncertain about how to best address the nuanced mental health needs of this population. Although necessary, culturally appropriate care is often difficult to provide (Rousseau and Frounfelker 2019). Such care includes an understanding of the patient's cultural traditions and norms (Osterman and de Jong 2007); different explanatory models for mental distress in children and families that may relate emotional problems to nonbiomedical causes such as spirits, supranatural forces, nature, or daily life; and a flexible adaptation to different cultural explanations and perceived ways of healing (Ventevogel et al. 2013).

Forcibly displaced children also may not receive mental health services because of distrust of authority or health systems, language and cultural barriers, stigma, or other daily life stressors taking priority over mental health care (Ellis et al. 2011). Children who are forcibly displaced from their homes often are fleeing an abuse of power by an (adult) authority figure, which can contribute to a lack of trust in disclosing personal and emotional information. Families may develop a fear of authorities because of persecution and a family and community experience of government-sanctioned violence (Scuglik et al. 2017). Distrust can be transmitted across generations, with children and families using silence as a way of coping (Song and de Jong 2014).

Relative to the rest of the world, the United States has more formal mental health care than many low-resource countries (for example, 185.2 mental health professionals per 100,000 people in the United States versus 0.62 in the Democratic Republic of the Congo) (World Health Organization 2017). However, having a high number of mental health providers does not in itself lessen the mental health treatment gap for forcibly displaced children. Children who come from low-income countries may not be acquainted with psychiatrists or the formality of the American mental health system and may seek care primarily from their families, religious or spiritual figures, or healers. Because all children develop in interaction with their environment, building community resilience and interweaving individual and family resilience may be effective in addressing the mental health needs of forcibly displaced children (United Nations Children's Fund 2019).

Clinical Strategies to Address the Mental Health Distress of Forcibly Displaced Children

The experiences of persecution that children may have faced in their country of origin can be harrowing, and the inexperienced clinician may focus solely on the extreme experiences or violence. However, a full assessment and evaluation should also incorporate an understanding of risk and resilience at the ecosocial levels (individual, family, peer, community) that helped promote well-being for the child prior to, during, and after the adverse experiences (Song and Ventevogel 2020a). In addition to general mental health assessment and treatment approaches, including a developmental history, assessment of academic and social functioning, and family influences (Thapar et al. 2015), careful attention should be paid to the child's current presentation, which can be seen as a product of his or her environment and experiences (Di Nicola and Song, in press). Approaches that pay attention to the roles of silence and distrust, are family centered, and emphasize ecosocial resilience can assist mental health professionals in building an alliance with forcibly displaced children and engaging them in mental health services.

Recognize the Roles of Silence and Distrust

Many persecuted children and families who have experienced chronic threats to life and liberties may feel uncomfortable disclosing information to clinicians. In the past, information they revealed may have been used against them. Some have been told that if they disclose specific information, they or their family will be harmed (United Nations High Commissioner for Refugees 2013). For many children and families, authorities have not been able to maintain their safety, leaving them distrustful of authorities and their ability to help. Therefore, children who have experienced displacement and traumatic experiences may have learned to use silence for various survival reasons (Song et al. 2014). Silence may be perpetuated by symptoms related to war trauma: feeling emotionally numb, detached from others, distrustful, and alert to perceived threats. The use of silence as a means of coping and surviving can prevent children from discussing traumatic events, resulting in amplified destructive feelings such as loneliness, isolation, and mistrust. Silence, therefore, can become a restrictive coping style because the child may desire to talk with someone about hardships (Song and de Jong 2014). Distrust builds when the child believes others are not genuine in their desire to understand him or her. These feelings of distrust and silence contribute to the perpetuation of isolation and low self-worth.

Clinicians should recognize the difference between *being silenced* and *being silent* (Fivush 2010). The difference is in who holds the power. Some forcibly displaced children may use silence to manage stigma-related shame or confusion. They may be silent because they feel demoralized or hopeless. When children feel powerless, they may feel there is nothing else they can control except when to speak and what they say. By withholding speech, these children can marginalize or anger others, withhold love, and attempt to hide.

Understanding the use of silence in interpersonal relationships can facilitate an understanding of the psychological consequences of discrimination, marginalization, and the effects of traumatic experiences. Therefore, silence and the role it plays in interpersonal relationships is an important element to include in the mental health and psychosocial rehabilitation of forcibly displaced children. Clinicians can show respect for children and build the therapeutic alliance by allowing children to use silence and disclosure at their own pace. Contextualizing a child's distress as common and understandable can be an important first step to helping him or her gain a sense of coherence and make meaning out of difficult experiences.

Clinical Vignette

Joseph, a 16-year-old Congolese boy, arrived in the United States by way of Tanzania, where he had been in a refugee camp with his four siblings. He has limited English proficiency and is withdrawn, quiet, and shy. His peers and teachers report that he is socially awkward. When Joseph was 12 years old, his family was targeted by local government authorities, and when he was 14 years old, he witnessed his father's murder. Since then, he had moved from city to city throughout the Democratic Republic of Congo, Rwanda, and Tanzania, with limited access to food, clean water, and shelter. He knew he could not trust local authorities and was taught to not speak to anyone he did not know well. After living in a refugee camp, Joseph was eventually given approval to enter the United States as an unaccompanied refugee minor. When he arrived, he felt ashamed, embarrassed, and angry at himself for not being a better son. His teachers said he did not participate in class or engage with peers.

Joseph met with a psychiatrist who validated his experiences and allowed large portions of the sessions to be conducted in silence. Over time, Joseph began to trust the psychiatrist and to disclose minimal information, which then grew into longer conversations. The psychiatrist showed interest in Joseph's early childhood and the role of sports and family in his life and followed the boy's lead in how much and which topics to discuss. Joseph began to feel more comfortable speaking, and soon his peer relationships developed. His social isolation slowly lifted, and with two new friends with whom he felt a sense of kinship, his depression, social isolation, and sleep all improved.

Engage the Family

Family is often the most proximal source of support and stress for children, and many forcibly displaced children come from cultures that have a "being" orientation in which identity is described through interpersonal relationships and group membership versus achievement and independence. Therefore, engaging the family can be a critical step in understanding and caring for these children (Song and Ventevogel 2020a). Understanding the structure and functioning of the family prior to migration and currently is important in identifying available resources to promote well-being and prevent emotional distress. Clinicians should define families from the child's perspective, with the awareness that non–blood relatives or extended family may be perceived as critical family relationships. Clinicians can ask whether all family members are present. Is anyone missing? Are all family members safe? If a family member is missing, the clinician can query how the family roles have changed. Is a primary caretaker or financial supporter missing? Who is filling that role presently? As in the previous subsection about respecting and understanding the roles of silence and expression, identifying the communication style of the family can be useful in understanding how to engage the family. Just as individual children can have fragmented identities due to past traumatic events, families also can have fragmented stories and incoherent identities (Neimeyer 2001). Clinicians can therefore be a moral witness to children and their families (Weingarten 2004). By allowing families to tell their own stories, we as clinicians can help actively construct meaning out of their experiences.

Family-centered approaches can be used by clinicians who do not have formal training in family therapy (Sederer 2013) (for some tips, see Table 12–3). Clinicians can engage and support the family during every encounter with children and their families. They can ask questions regarding the family's cultural values and which values they want to maintain and which values they want to adopt from the mainstream culture. Because parents may be overwhelmed with past experiences and current stressors, linking children and families with community resources can expand the child's helping network.

By assisting parents in raising awareness of their child's distress reactions or how to engage in positive parenting, clinicians can support caregiver well-being to allow parents to be poten-

TABLE 12–3. Practical tips for engaging a refugee family

Approach the family with curiosity

Allow the child and family to teach you about their culture, values, and beliefs

Provide psychoeducation to the parents on the developmental effects of stress in order to help build capacity of parents or caregivers

Provide strategies to support developmental stages

Bolster parents' perceived competence in parenting

Identify ways parents can engage with their child's school (e.g., parent-teacher conferences, sports, extracurricular or other events) and safe spaces where the children can play (e.g., parks, clubs, recreation centers)

Link children and families with community resources

Encourage the family to build a sense of family belonging with rituals, such as a scheduled weekend dinner meal as a family or nighttime routines unique to the family

tially more available to their children. It is important to recognize that if the parent feels a deep-rooted sense of being rejected, unloved, and undervalued in the past or present, it may be hard for that parent to tolerate a wide range of emotions and to engage with the child's pain in order to provide an empathic response (Fraiberg et al. 1975). Therefore, families may need help developing patience for each family member's different coping, decision-making, and grief processes. Helping families build the capacity to listen to and understand each other can help the family actively participate in shared meaning making of past exposure to potentially traumatic experiences in order to build family coherence and identity.

Promote Resilience

Resilience is often regarded as the capacity of the individual to maintain good mental and physical health despite adversity (Ungar 2005). There is growing interest in researching the concept of resilience among forcibly displaced children—why and how are the majority of children who are exposed to war and potentially traumatic events such as community violence and forced separation from loved ones able to function and remain on track developmentally (Panter-Brick and Leckman 2013)? Scholars have shown that resilience is a dynamic process, as opposed to a static trait or factor that one does or does not possess (Luthar et al. 2000). This is important because it means that resilience is something we can learn and build on. Resilience is also context-dependent, meaning a youth can be resilient in one area of life (e.g., school) but not another (e.g., family) (Goldstein and Brooks 2012), and time-dependent, meaning it is a process that unfolds over the course of the child's development (Fergus and Zimmerman 2005).

Individual-Level Resilience

Incorporating resilience into a clinical approach can be complementary to the traditional problem- or deficit-focused approach in the biomedical sciences, moving attention away from problems and risks and toward capacity and well-being. Clinicians can assist the shift from research on resilience into practice by taking an ecosocial resilience approach to the mental health assessment of forcibly displaced children (Song and Ventevogel 2020b). Such an approach em-

TABLE 12–4. **Practical tips for supporting family resilience**

Ask children to define who they consider their family to be

Ask children to define their communities and sources of support past and present

Encourage families to clarify their understanding of the political and social contexts of the past and present

Identify sources of stress and support that can strengthen the cohesion of the family unit

Invite family members to discuss neutral topics such as their culture or goals instead of leading with discussion about traumatic events

Build narratives to make meaning of adversity

Facilitate active coping

phasizes the connectivity between the individual, family, and community levels in influencing mental health and well-being. An assessment of the child's past mental health and developmental history should also incorporate an assessment of the child's longitudinal resilience. Children may have been exposed to adversity prior to the war, conflict, or disaster that led them to seek refuge elsewhere. Understanding the context in which children managed through these adversities and the processes that facilitated well-being can be critical in understanding a child's innate way of coping. This can be useful for helping the child build coping strategies that can be embraced thoroughly and can be easy to call up in the face of future adversity. Moreover, fostering resilience may be more accepted by children because it may be less shaming than a traditional query into their problems. Some resilience-building psychotherapeutic approaches such as strength-based cognitive-behavioral therapy (Padesky and Mooney 2012) and positive psychology (Conoley et al. 2015) hold promise for working with this group of children.

Family-Level Resilience

Among war-affected families living in low- and middle-income countries, family-level variables, such as parenting and support, are shown to have the strongest level of impact on promoting mental health for children (Tol et al. 2013). Therefore, emphasizing a family resilience approach is a promising method of fostering well-being for forcibly displaced children while they are in the United States. To build family resilience, clinicians can assist families in connectedness, meaning making, and collaborative problem-solving (Walsh 2017). After multiple potentially traumatic experiences, loss of culture and community, and migration to a new way of living, forcibly displaced children (and their families) will need someone to rely on for safety and emotional comfort. Table 12–4 offers practical tips for clinicians that should be considered when working with refugee children.

Caregivers and children may each have wide-ranging and fluctuating emotions due to different experiences past and present. Many parents may have experienced extremely traumatic events, but relaying details of past traumas may be developmentally inappropriate for all family members. However, silence about traumatic events does not necessitate general silence. Children can be encouraged to listen to their parents discuss values important to them, and the parents can listen to how their child feels being immersed in multiple seemingly conflicting cultures. Resilience is supported when clinicians help families shift from avoidant coping toward a sense of connectedness. Helping families build narratives to make meaning of adversity can begin a healing process by restoring order and purpose that is otherwise lost (Neimeyer 2001). Discussion of discrimination, social violence, and exploitation may help counter social silence and allow individuals and families to expand their voice and identity to facilitate active coping.

Community-Level Resilience

Resilience also can be strengthened by increasing positive supports for forcibly displaced children when the family's capacity to help may be limited. Communities are a wealth of knowledge; not only can they identify people who may be in need, but they also may be prepared to refer people to appropriate resources. Outsourcing needs to the community can help children identify other resources to turn to if parents cannot give guidance. Prosocial engagement in the community also may help to improve social skills and self-esteem. A clinical community-level resilience approach can strengthen resources in the child's defined community, make use of community knowledge and capacity, and engage communities in all phases of care (United Nations Children's Fund 2019). Forcibly displaced children can be asked to define their communities—where they feel a sense of belonging and can turn to for support if needed. Mental health professionals can assist with engaging the child's cultural community by building partnerships with key stakeholders and including communities of forcibly displaced children in the development of services through parent outreach programs and community advisory boards (Ellis et al. 2011). Clinicians can support communities by engaging with both the formal systems of care for forcibly displaced children and informal systems, such as religious figures and community organizations.

Conclusion

Forcibly displaced children have varied experiences with regard to exposure to potentially traumatic events, migration, and resettlement in the United States. Because of the potential lack of access to basic needs such as security, housing, clean water, and food at any point of their lives, it is unsurprising that many forcibly displaced children have higher rates of PTSD, depression, anxiety, and general emotional distress than the general population, in addition to complicated grief, cultural bereavement, isolation, and existential stress. Although some children are stretched beyond their capacity to cope, many of them are able to maintain positive mental and developmental health. Mental health professionals can therefore take a dimensional and developmental approach to emotional and behavioral distress. In addition, clinicians can emphasize building trust, understanding the role of silence, and using a family-centered approach to care, whether or not they have been formally trained in family therapy or whether family members are present or absent. Incorporating a socioecological resilience approach emphasizes the dynamic processes at various levels that impact children's lives, that promote well-being, and that protect against developing or worsening emotional and behavioral distress.

Clinical Pearls

- Mental health professionals can foster well-being for forcibly displaced children by building trust and understanding the role of silence.

- A family-centered approach to working with this population includes assessing the structure and functioning of the family, addressing ambiguous loss of loved ones, and strengthening cohesion by facilitating moral witnessing among family members.

- Incorporating socioecological resilience into assessment and treatment highlights the dynamic processes that promote well-being and protect against the development of mental health disorders.

Self-Assessment Questions

1. When working with forcibly displaced youth, which of the following can be useful to evaluate during a mental health assessment?

   A. Premigration attachments and relationships.
   B. Migration experience.
   C. Postmigration environment.
   D. Experiences of resiliency.
   E. All of the above.

2. Which of the following is a practical tip to use when engaging with a refugee family?

   A. Read about the cultural background of the family.
   B. Use rituals to build a sense of family belonging.
   C. Separate children from the community so they must rely only on their families.
   D. Explain to parents how their actions are negatively affecting their children.

Answers

1. E
2. B

References

Beiser M, Wickrama KAS: Trauma, time and mental health: a study of temporal reintegration and depressive disorder among Southeast Asian refugees. Psychol Med 34(5):899–910, 2004

Betancourt TS, Borisova I, Williams TP, et al: Psychosocial adjustment and mental health in former child soldiers—systematic review of the literature and recommendations for future research. J Child Psychol Psychiatry 54(1):17–36, 2013

Bhugra D, Becker MA: Migration, cultural bereavement and cultural identity. World Psychiatry 4(1):18–24, 2005

Ceri V, Özlö-Erkilic Z, Özer U, et al: Psychiatric symptoms and disorders among Yazidi children and adolescents immediately after forced migration following ISIS attacks. Neuropsychiatr 30(3):145–150, 2016

Conoley CW, Pontrelli ME, Oromendia MF, et al: Positive empathy: a therapeutic skill inspired by positive psychology. J Clin Psychol 71(6):575–583, 2015

DeJong J, Sbeity F, Schlecht J, et al: Young lives disrupted: gender and well-being among adolescent Syrian refugees in Lebanon. Confl Health 11(suppl 1):23, 2017

Di Nicola V, Song S: Family matters: the family as a resource for the mental, social, and relational well-being of migrants, asylum seekers, and other displaced populations, in Social and Cultural Psychiatry. Edited by Gogineni R, Pumariega A, Kallivayalil R, et al., in press

Ellis H, Miller A, Baldwin H, et al: New direction in refugee child mental health services: overcoming barriers to engagement. J Child Adolesc Trauma 4(1):69–85, 2011

Eruyar S, Maltby J, Vostanis P: Mental health problems of Syrian refugee children: the role of parental factors. Eur Child Adolesc Psychiatry 27(4):401–409, 2018

Fazel M, Wheeler J, Danesh J: Prevalence of serious mental disorder in 7000 refugees resettled in western countries: a systematic review. Lancet 365(9467):1309–1314, 2005

Fergus S, Zimmerman MA: Adolescent resilience: a framework for understanding healthy development in the face of risk. Annu Rev Public Health 26:399–419, 2005

Fivush R: Speaking silence: the social construction of silence in autobiographical and cultural narratives. Memory 18(2):88–98, 2010

Fraiberg S, Adelson E, Shapiro V: Ghosts in the nursery: a psychoanalytic approach to the problems of impaired infant-mother relationships. J Am Acad Child Psychiatry 14(3):387–421, 1975

Global Detention Project: Global detention project annual report 2018. Geneva, Switzerland, Global Detention Project, 2018. Available at: www.globaldetentionproject.org/global-detention-project-annual-report-2018. Accessed April 28, 2020.

Goldstein S, Brooks RB (eds): Handbook of Resilience in Children, 2nd Edition. New York, Springer, 2012

Goosen S, Stronks K, Kunst A: Frequent relocations between asylum-seeker centres are associated with mental distress in asylum-seeking children: a longitudinal medical record study. Int J Epidemiol 43:94–104, 2014

Hodes M, Vostanis P: Practitioner review: mental health problems of refugee children and adolescents and their management. J Child Psychol Psychiatry 60(7):716–731, 2019

Luthar SS, Cicchetti D, Becker B: The construct of resilience: a critical evaluation and guidelines for future work. Child Dev 71(3):543–562, 2000

Martens M: Prevalence of depression in various ethnic groups of immigrants and refugees: suggestions for prevention and intervention Int J Ment Health Promot 9(1):25–33, 2007

Miller K, Rasmussen A: The mental health of civilians displaced by armed conflict: an ecological model of refugee distress. Epidemiol Psychiatr Sci 26(2):129–138, 2017

Morgan G, Melluish S, Welham A: Exploring the relationship between post-migratory stressors and mental health for asylum seekers and refused asylum seekers in the UK. Transcult Psychiatry 54(5–6):653–674, 2017

Neimeyer RA (ed): Meaning Reconstruction and the Experience of Loss. Washington, DC, American Psychological Association, 2001

Oppedal B, Idsoe T: The role of social support in the acculturation and mental health of unaccompanied minor asylum seekers. Scand J Psychol 56:203–211, 2015

Osterman JE, de Jong JTVM: Cultural issues and trauma, in Handbook of PTSD: Science and Practice. Edited by Friedman J, Keane TM, Resick PA. New York, Guilford, 2007, pp 425–446

Padesky CA, Mooney KA: Strengths-based cognitive-behavioural therapy: a four-step model to build resilience. Clin Psychol Psychother 19(4):283–290, 2012

Panter-Brick C, Leckman JF: Editorial commentary: resilience in child development—interconnected pathways to wellbeing. J Child Psychol Psychiatry 54(4):333–336, 2013

Patel V, Saxena S, Lund C, et al: The Lancet Commission on Global Mental Health and Sustainable Development. Lancet 392(10157):1553–1598, 2018

Rothe E, Lewis J, Castillo-Matos H, et al: Posttraumatic stress disorder among Cuban children and adolescents after release from a refugee camp. Psychiatr Serv 53(8):970–976, 2002

Rousseau C, Frounfelker RL: Mental health needs and services for migrants: an overview for primary care providers. J Travel Med 26(2), 2019

Satinsky E, Fuhr D, Woodward A, et al: Mental health care utilisation and access among refugees and asylum seekers in Europe: a systematic review. Health Policy 123(9):851–863, 2019

Saunders N, Gill P, Holder L, et al: Use of the emergency department as a first point of contact for mental health care by immigrant child in Canada: a population-based study. Can Med Assoc J 190(40):E1183–E1191, 2018

Scuglik D, Alarcon R, Lapeyre A, et al: When the poetry no longer rhymes: mental health issues among Somali immigrants in the U.S.A. Transcult Psychiatry 44(4):581–595, 2017

Sederer L: The Family Guide to Mental Health Care. New York, WW Norton, 2013

Song SJ, de Jong J: The role of silence in Burundian former child soldiers. Int J Adv Counsel 36(1):84–95, 2014

Song SJ, Ventevogel P: Bridging the humanitarian, academic, and clinical fields towards the mental health of child and adolescent refugees, in Child, Adolescent and Family Refugee Mental Health: A Global Perspective. Edited by Song SJ, Ventevogel P. Cham, Switzerland, Springer International, 2020a, pp 3–12

Song SJ, Ventevogel P: Practical considerations in the mental health assessment for refugee children and adolescents, in Child, Adolescent and Family Refugee Mental Health: A Global Perspective. Edited by Song SJ, Ventevogel P. Cham, Switzerland, Springer International, 2020b, pp 69–79

Song SJ, Kaplan C, Tol W: Psychological distress in torture survivors: pre- and post-migration risk factors in a U.S. sample. Soc Psychiatry Psychiatr Epidemiol 50(4):549–560, 2015

Steel Z, Chey T, Silove D: Association of torture and other potentially traumatic events with mental health outcomes among populations exposed to mass conflict and displacement: a systematic review and meta-analysis. JAMA 302(5):537–549, 2009

Thapar A, Pine DS, Leckman JF, et al: Rutter's Child and Adolescent Psychiatry, 6th Edition. Chichester, UK, Wiley-Blackwell, 2015

Tol W, Song SJ, Jordans M: Annual research review: resilience and mental health in children and adolescents living in areas of armed conflict—a systematic review of findings in low- and middle-income countries. J Child Psychol Psychiatr 54(4):445–460, 2013

Ungar M (ed): Handbook for Working With Children and Youth: Pathways to Resilience Across Cultures and Contexts. Thousand Oaks, CA, Sage, 2005

United Nations Children's Fund: Child displacement: refugees and internally displaced persons. December 28, 2018. Available at: https://data.unicef.org/topic/child-migration-and-displacement/displacement. Accessed April 28, 2020.

United Nations Children's Fund: Operational guidelines: community-based mental health and psychosocial support in humanitarian settings: three-tiered support for children and families, field test version. New York, UNICEF, 2019. Available at: www.unicef.org/media/52171/file/Mental%20health%20and%20psychosocial%20support%20guidelines%202019%20.pdf. Accessed April 28, 2020.

United Nations High Commissioner for Refugees: Convention and protocol relating to the status of refugees. Geneva, Switzerland, United Nations High Commissioner for Refugees, 1951. Available at: www.unhcr.org/en-us/3b66c2aa10. Accessed April 28, 2020.

United Nations High Commissioner for Refugees: The issue of "trust" or "mistrust" in research with refugees: choices caveats, and considerations for researchers. New Issues in Refugee Research Working Paper No 98. Geneva, Switzerland, United Nations High Commissioner for Refugees, 2013. Available at: www.unhcr.org/3fcb5cee1.pdf. Accessed April 28, 2020.

Ventevogel P, Jordans M, Reis R, et al: Madness or sadness? Local concepts of mental illness in four conflict-affected African communities. Confl Health 7(1):3, 2013

Walsh F: Traumatic loss and major disasters: strengthening family and community resilience. Fam Process 46(2):207–227, 2017

Weingarten K: Witnessing the effects of political violence in families: mechanisms of intergenerational transmission of trauma and clinical interventions. J Marital Fam Ther 30(1):45–59, 2004

World Health Organization: Mental Health Atlas–2017 country profiles. Geneva, Switzerland, World Health Organization, 2017. Available at: www.who.int/mental_health/evidence/atlas/profiles-2017/en/#D. Accessed April 28, 2020.

CHAPTER 13

The Global State of Child and Adolescent Mental Health

Ayesha Irshad Mian, M.D., DFAACAP, SFHEA
Aisha Sanober Chachar, MBBS, FCPS

GLOBAL child and adolescent mental health (G-CAMH) is a field of research and practice that prioritizes excellence and promotes equity in health care services for the world's child and adolescent population (Koplan et al. 2009). The concept of G-CAMH derives from the contemporary concept of global health, which includes any health-related concern that is affected by transnational social determinants. It deals with the scope rather than the geography of the problem and encompasses complex interactions between societies and cultures (Koplan et al. 2009). Contrary to the common perception that it is the practice of international aid, technologies, and interventions flowing from wealthier countries to poorer countries, global health is a more nuanced and contemporary approach that emphasizes interdependence and recognizes the contributions of both resource-rich and resource-scarce nations. In 2001, the World Health Organization (WHO) issued a report focusing on the growing concerns of global mental health (World Health Organization 2001) and suggested solutions, the application of which can safely be extended to G-CAMH (Table 13–1).

G-CAMH has taken center stage in global health conversations, specifically in the past 10–15 years, given the increasing burden of mental health disorders and the severe shortage of trained practitioners who can respond to the growing need. Global figures indicate that 20% of children and adolescents have a mental illness, and the first onset of mental disorders usually

TABLE 13–1. **Proposed solutions to the growing concerns of global mental health**

Integration and provision of treatment in primary care

Ensuring the availability of psychotropic medications

Community-based care

Public awareness and psychoeducation

A holistic approach involving communities, families, and patients

National policies and legislation

Increasing mental health workforce through training and increasing skills of the existing workforce

Multisectoral approach

Promotion of community mental health

Source. Adapted from World Health Organization 2001.

occurs in childhood or adolescence (Kessler et al. 2007). Despite these high numbers, efforts toward early recognition and management are suboptimal, and most children and adolescents remain untreated or suffer because of delayed treatments (MacDonald et al. 2018). This burden speaks to the need for an expanded role for child and adolescent psychiatrists as these professionals find themselves having responsibilities as leaders and advocates who can create innovative and impactful solutions to manage the G-CAMH crisis (see Table 13–1). As such, the lens of global health becomes pertinent and applicable to both individual providers and organized child and adolescent mental health across countries and continents.

This chapter is divided into the larger headings of "History of Global Child and Adolescent Mental Health," "Epidemiology," "Landscape of G-CAMH," "Challenges," and "Call for Action." We conclude by discussing future directions and a need for innovative and sustainable solutions to deal with this urgent concern. For the purpose of this chapter, the geographic regions will be described on the basis of the World Bank's classification of four income groupings: low-income countries (LICs), middle-income countries—subdivided into upper-middle-income countries (UMICs) and lower-middle-income countries (LMICs)—and high-income countries (HICs). This classification is based on the generated income measured by using gross national income per capita in U.S. dollars, as converted from the local currency (Figure 13–1).

History of Global Child and Adolescent Mental Health

CAMH disorders existed long before there were CAMH professionals. The earliest reference to CAMH disorders is found in eighteenth-century medical writings focused mainly on sleep disturbances, stuttering, sibling rivalry, and epilepsy. The prevailing view, based on the observation that children were not institutionalized, was that "insanity" did not occur before puberty (Parry-Jones 1989). Some historians have dated the beginnings of child psychiatry to 1899, when the United States established the first juvenile court in Chicago (Schowalter 2003). Around the same time, Maudsley (1895) published a book with a chapter on "Insanity of Early Life," modeled after work that acknowledged mania and melancholia in children (Griesinger 1845/1867).

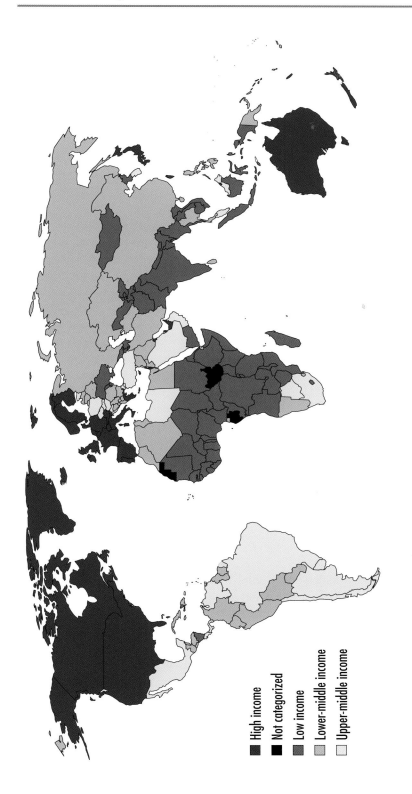

FIGURE 13–1. World Bank income groups.

Income classifications are split into four categories determined by the gross national income per capita in U.S. dollars. The link below shows data for the period 1987–2016.

Source.   Reprinted from World Bank 2016.

TABLE 13–2. CAMH advocacy initiatives

Initiative	Inaugural year
Child guidance movement	1920
International Association for Child and Adolescent Psychiatry and Allied Professions (IACAPAP)	1937
American Academy of Child and Adolescent Psychiatry (AACAP)	1953
European Society for Child and Adolescent Psychiatry (ESCAP)	1954

Source. Rey et al. 2015.

The twentieth century has been called "the Century of the Child" (Key 1909), and it was during the twentieth century that child and adolescent psychiatry became a medical discipline. Epidemiological work began in the earlier part of the century; the first prevalence study of parent-reported problems in children ages 6–12 was published in 1958 (Lapouse and Monk 1958), followed by the Isle of Wight series of epidemiological studies that investigated educational, psychiatric, and physical disorders in 9- to 11-year-old children (Rutter et al. 1976) and introduced new classification systems (Rutter et al. 1970). During the later decades, there was a remarkable proliferation in scholarship on the interaction between genetics, environment, developmental psychology, and psychopathology. A burgeoning literature emerged in the areas of epidemiological research and agendas for policy, research, rights, and provision of services, leading to the roles of current-day child and adolescent psychiatry.

The first evidence of service development comes from 1906, when William Healy, a neurologist, started a movement for the prevention of juvenile delinquency (Levy 1968). This movement led to the creation of child guidance clinics, which followed a robust multidisciplinary ethos. Soon after, Healy's model was recognized and adopted internationally, starting with Britain and then the Scandinavian region, India, and, subsequently, Ireland. Organized child and adolescent psychiatry also took root in the twentieth century; Table 13–2 shows the time line of major CAMH advocacy initiatives.

Epidemiology

Children and adolescents constitute almost a third of the world's population, approximately 2.2 billion, of which almost 90% live in lower- and middle-income countries (LAMICs). Population-based studies from LAMICs and HICs estimate that 10%–20% of children and adolescents have at least one diagnosable mental health disorder (Kieling et al. 2011). Fifty percent of mental health disorders begin by age 14 and 75% by age 24 (Table 13–3) (Kessler et al. 2007). Differences found in the prevalence of various CAMH disorders across the globe have been attributed to distinctions in the regional sociocultural context, epidemiological methodology, rigor, strategy, design, and culturally adapted instruments used for the data collection.

A meta-analysis from 41 studies conducted in 27 countries from every world region reported a 13.4% prevalence of CAMH disorders (Polanczyk et al. 2015). The global prevalence of anxiety disorder was 6.5%, prevalence of depressive disorder was 2.6%, prevalence of ADHD was 3.4%, and prevalence of disruptive disorder was 5.7% (Polanczyk et al. 2015). A landmark ep-

TABLE 13–3. **Age at onset distributions of commonly occurring disorders**

Disorder	Median age at onset distribution (years)
ADHD	7–9
Oppositional defiant disorder	7–15
Conduct disorder	9–14
Intermittent explosive disorder	13–21
Specific phobias and separation anxiety disorder	7–14
Panic disorder, generalized anxiety disorder, and PTSD	25–53
Mood disorders	25–45
Substance use disorders	18–29
Psychotic disorders	15–17
Schizophrenia	15–35

Note. Distributions are based on a comparative analysis across 16 countries and 5 continents (see www.hcp.med. harvard.edu/wmh). For mood disorders, there was a wide range across countries (Thomsen 1996).
Source. Kessler et al. 2007.

idemiological study conducted by WHO in 2016 showed that suicide is one of the top five causes of mortality among children ages 10–14 years in the European region, with the highest mortality rate in Kazakhstan, and numbers are higher in marginalized populations—minorities and migrants (Kyu et al. 2018). Erskine et al. (2017) evaluated data from the series of systematic reviews conducted for the Global Burden of Disease (GBD) project in 2010 and 2013. This study looked at the mean global coverage of prevalence data for six CAMH disorders. Coverage refers to the proportion of the target population (in this case, ages 5–17 years) represented by the available data. This epidemiological approach is useful for identifying strengths, limitations, and gaps in the available data to direct future investment in research effectively. According to the GBD study, mean global coverage of prevalence data for CAMH disorders (ages 5–17 years) is 6.7%, including conduct disorder (5%), ADHD (5.5%), autism spectrum disorders (16.1%), eating disorders (4.4%), depression (6.2%), and anxiety disorders (3.2%).

Over the past decade, there has been a 20.9% increase in childhood disability secondary to developmental or mental health conditions, and at the same time, the prevalence of disability attributable to physical health conditions declined by 11.85% (Houtrow et al. 2014). As shown in Figure 13–2, CAMH disorders account for 15%–30% of the disability-adjusted life years (DALYs) lost during the first three decades of life (Murray and Lopez 1994).

Landscape of Global Child and Adolescent Mental Health Services

In light of the epidemiology mentioned in the previous subsection, the concepts of treatment gap and pathway of care demand special consideration. *Treatment gap* is the difference between the population with mental health disorders requiring care and the population with access to appropriate services (Kohn et al. 2018). *Pathway to care* is a "sequence of contacts with individuals

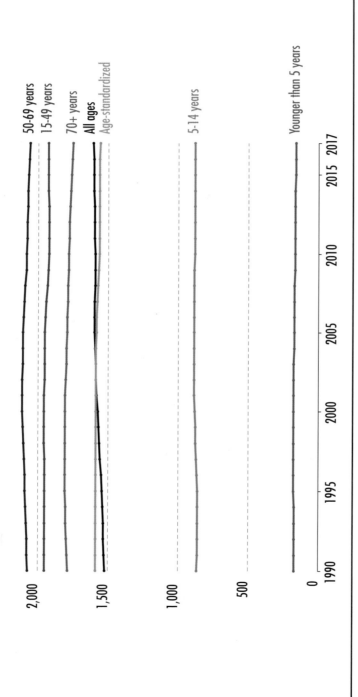

FIGURE 13–2. Disability-adjusted life years (DALYs) from substance use and other mental disorders per 100,000 population.

DALYs are used to measure the total burden of disease from both years of life lost and years lived with a disability. One DALY equals 1 lost year of healthy life.

Source. Institute for Health Metrics and Evaluation: Global Burden of Disease Study 2016 (Degenhardt et al. 2018).

TABLE 13–4.   Key findings from the WHO *Mental Health Atlas* Project

There is a lack of program development in low-income countries

Low-income countries generally lack health policies, and both low- and high-income countries lack specific comprehensive child and adolescent mental health policy

Low-income countries lack data-gathering capacity, including for country-level epidemiology and services outcomes

Low-income countries are characterized by failure to provide social services, lack of a continuum of care, and universal barriers to access

Source.   Adapted from World Health Organization 2018.

and organizations prompted by the distressed person's efforts, and those of his or her significant others to seek help, as well as the help delivered in response to such efforts" (Rogler and Cortes 1993, p. 555). Understanding these concepts can facilitate the successful application of epidemiological knowledge in order to plan, organize, evaluate, and fund CAMH-based services for the prevention of disorders and the promotion of health (Ford 2008).

The latest version of the WHO *Mental Health Atlas* details information on the availability of resources across the world (World Health Organization 2018). It is evident that countries differ widely in terms of awareness, willingness, and preparedness to take action on CAMH services. According to the *Atlas*, only 46% of 78 countries reported having a plan or strategy for CAMH. Taking our lead from the key findings of the *Atlas* (Table 13–4), in the following section, we focus on services (including access), the workforce and training, and research.

CAMH Services

The treatment gap with regard to CAMH is wide in LAMICs (Vikram et al. 2008). In the United States, a HIC, it ranges from 64% to 86% (Kohn et al. 2018). This gap is wider in Sub-Saharan Africa; some countries, such as Sierra Leone, have a treatment gap as high as 98.8% (Yoder et al. 2016).

Morris et al. (2011) evaluated CAMH services in 42 LAMICs. Their findings showed that the child and adolescent population is underserved, with a treated prevalence of 159 per 100,000 compared with 664 per 100,000 for the adult population. The child and adolescent population makes up 12% of the patient population in mental health outpatient facilities, 5% of day treatment, and 6% of community-based psychiatric inpatients. Less than 1% of beds in inpatient facilities are reserved for children and adolescents. Similar discrepancies have been reported in the WHO *Mental Health Atlas* project (World Health Organization 2018). Notably, HICs reported having eight times more child and adolescent beds per 100,000 population than did LICs. The number of visits to CAMH outpatient facilities is far higher in HICs (1,609 visits per 100,000 population) than LICs (11 visits per 100,000 population).

Access to CAMH Services

The pathway from the first signs of illness to receiving CAMH care includes emergency departments, social services, criminal justice systems, school counselors and administrations, and religious institutions (MacDonald et al. 2018). Populations in regions with well-developed CAMH services experience direct routes from the community to professional care. However, in areas with inadequate services, the population experiences a variety of pathways, which may include traditional and faith healers (Sheikh and Furnham 2000). Stigma is a pervasive barrier to treatment access. Other reasons for delays in seeking appropriate help differ from region to region, but common factors include sociodemographic and cultural values, mental health literacy, the attitudes of family and society, fear of discrimination against both the individual and the family, accessibility of psychiatric services, and referral patterns (Cullins and Mian 2015; Trivedi and Jilani 2011).

The impact of CAMH disorders is felt not only by the affected children and adolescents worldwide but also by caregiving families. This is important to consider because the impact of CAMH disorders on caregivers is another essential factor that determines barriers of access to care (Karp and Tanarugsachock 2000). A complex interplay of these factors leads to delayed detection, long waitlists, and multiple help-seeking contacts before proper professional care is reached (MacDonald et al. 2018), making it harder to access specialized care on time (Sheikh and Furnham 2000). These factors become even more pronounced for vulnerable groups such as refugee and street children, homeless families, young offenders, gender-nonconforming youth, victims of war and violence, and youth facing social and economic disadvantages (Vostanis 2017).

Workforce and Training

The global shortage of child and adolescent psychiatrists is a well-established fact and has significant implications worldwide (World Health Organization 2018). Although the field of child and adolescent psychiatry has now been formally and firmly established in academic medicine for more than 50 years, the demand for child and adolescent psychiatrists continues to outstrip the supply. There are approximately 8,000 practicing child and adolescent psychiatrists in the United States, with a ratio ranging by state from 1 to 60 per 100,000 children. There is also a shortage of developmental and behavioral pediatricians and adolescent mental health specialists (Findling and Stepanova 2018). These shortages led to the development of policy statements from the American Academy of Pediatrics that focus on prevention; early detection; and management of behavioral, developmental, and social problems as the central part of the scope of pediatric practice (Coleman et al. 2009). The discrepancy between demand and supply is magnified manifold in LAMICs. The scarcity of professionals in LAMICs and HICs is shown in Figure 13–3. In HICs, the number of child and adolescent psychiatrists is 1.19 per 100,000 youth, but in LAMICs, the number is less than 0.1 per 100,000 youth (World Health Organization 2018).

This workforce scarcity is partially attributed to limited training sites. CAMH training provided for mental health professionals is minimal, with less than 1% receiving refresher training, and many developing countries do not formally offer fellowship and training programs. Data from the Middle East region have shown that despite the recognition of child and adolescent psychiatry as a specialty in a majority of the countries (11 of 15), only 6 countries have established a designated child and adolescent psychiatry training program (Clausen et al. 2020). In Far East Asia, 12 of 18 countries offer a separate child and adolescent psychiatry training program for specialists (Hirota et al. 2015). In Europe, 32 of 38 countries recognize child and ad-

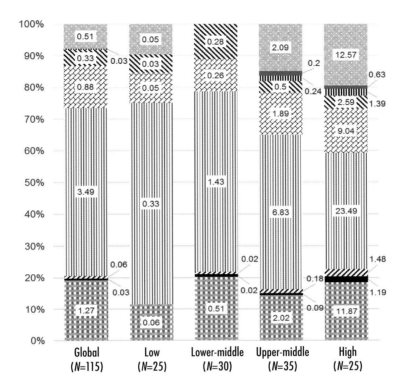

FIGURE 13-3. Mental health workforce per 100,000 population, by World Bank income group.

Source. Reprinted from World Health Organization: *Mental Health Atlas 2017.* Geneva, Switzerland, World Health Organization, 2018, p. 33. Available at: https://apps.who.int/iris/handle/10665/272735. Accessed April 30, 2020.

olescent psychiatry as a distinct specialty or subspecialty (Barrett et al. 2020). Data from most LAMICs have reported that in the absence of formal fellowship programs, these countries have ongoing CAMH training via short educational courses (Morris et al. 2011).

Research

The dearth of research is evident in the numbers: of the 1,521 global mental health studies carried out worldwide in 2007, only about one-tenth of them were conducted in LAMICs, with only 1% of research trials focusing on children and adolescents. Hence, less than 0.1% of the global trials in mental health focus on children and adolescents in LAMICs. In another example, the GBD study showed that out of 187 countries studied, 124 had no data for any CAMH disorder. The lack of data was more striking for LAMICs; for example, no region in sub-Saharan Africa had more than 2% coverage for any disorder (Erskine et al. 2017). Similarly, among studies on CAMH indexed in the Web of Science database over the past decade, about 90% authorship was from HICs (Patel et al. 2013). Authorship from UMICs, LMICs, and LICs occurred in only 7.79%, 1.19%, and 0.33% of the studies, respectively.

Challenges

As highlighted in the section "Landscape of Global Child and Adolescent Mental Health Services," G-CAMH is currently faced with myriad demands that stem from significant sociocultural determinants, spanning lack of awareness, mental health literacy, funding, and more, at the primary health care level to a dearth of trained child and adolescent psychiatrists at the tertiary end. Implementation of CAMH services is an ongoing challenge, mainly because of the structural barriers marked by health disparities; the geopolitical situation; ineffective health policies, practices, and interventions; the stresses of the inadequate systems of the registry; an economy under pressure; and unequal distribution of funds (Dubicka and Bullock 2017).

The current novel coronavirus SARS-CoV-2 (COVID-19) pandemic has imposed multifaceted burdens on children and adolescents, affecting them individually and in their micro and macro systems. Social isolation, contact restrictions, economic shutdown, closure of schools, and limited or absent out-of-home co-curricular and leisure time activities are some of the challenges facing children and adolescents. Families are also spread thin as parents are being asked to support children with home schooling while working from home, with external support from other family members and social support systems withering away. All the above stressors are being cited as causes of increasing emotional distress, mental health problems, and familial violence, including child abuse (Fegert et al. 2020). Individuals who have been known to CAMH services are facing a double disadvantage due to interruption of ongoing services, particularly in the areas of speech, occupational, and play therapy, and at times routine physician visits where telehealth is unavailable.

Health Disparities

Over the past decade, evidence of mental health disparities has grown rapidly. Researchers are making efforts to quantify the extent of the problem, identify causal mechanisms, and develop

TABLE 13–5. Mitigation of early childhood inequities

Adverse life experiences	Protective and mitigating experiences
Early-life adversity measurably impairs functioning in later childhood and adolescence and includes the following: • Nutritional deprivation • Infections or exposure to toxins • Child abuse	Interventions are more effective earlier in life rather than later and include the following: • Iodine supplementation • Early childhood parenting support • Wealth transfers • Family group conferencing

Source. Adapted from Engle et al. 2011; Walker et al. 2011.

interventions to eliminate specific mental health disparities (Thomas et al. 2011). Early childhood exposure to various factors ranging from exposure to toxins to family violence to poor nutrition and poverty has been associated with poor CAMH outcomes (Shonkoff et al. 2012). Results from the Great Smoky Mountain Study in the United States has supported the association between socioeconomic constraints on parents and behavioral disorders (Costello et al. 2003). As a result, many interventions have been targeted at mitigating inequities in early childhood (Table 13–5) by expanding access to early childhood education, improving prenatal and infant nutrition, using wealth/cash transfer programs that support vulnerable populations by distributing transfers to low-income households or helping low-income parents deal with the stress and challenge of having young children (Mistry et al. 2012).

Geopolitical Situation

Although war and conflict zones affect both HICs and LAMICs, the majority of the affected population belongs to the latter region (Brundtland 2000). Children growing up in LAMICs already lack resources for proper nurturing, especially in early life. The situation is worse for children and adolescents who reside in areas affected by armed conflict as a part of the war against terrorism and those who are displaced from their homes by natural and human-made disasters. During the past few years, there has been an increase in the numbers of refugees in HICs, and about half of the people seeking refuge from the uninhabitable conditions in their countries are younger than 18 years. Literature suggests that refugees who face restrictive policies such as temporary visa status, detention, and limited access to welfare are less likely to use health care services and are at higher risk of compromised mental health compared with the native-born population, adding to the public health crises in the host country (Lu 2008). Vulnerable countries direct a significant portion of capital resources toward defense to maintain regional stability, taking resources away from areas of health, education, and the fight against poverty. This significantly affects the well-being of its at-risk child and adolescent population, which is already vulnerable to developing mental health disorders.

However, the situation in HICs has evolved during the COVID-19 pandemic. As of this writing, a number of HICs are experiencing significant upheaval due to limited capacity of health care systems to accommodate communities' needs; the resurfacing of preexisting structural inequities, health disparities, and racism; and the inability of systems to accommodate the ever-rising mental health needs triggered by social isolation, school disruption, anxiety over sick or lost family and friends, and loss of livelihoods.

Evidence-Based Practice and Culturally Informed Care

Evidence-based practice is a three-legged stool that encompasses research evidence, clinician expertise, and patient preference (Spring 2007). However, given that diverse populations are remarkably underrepresented in clinical trials, the evidence-based practice approach often faces critique in LAMICs. Such practice often overlooks culturally informed care, which takes into account health care beliefs of religious, spiritual, and local faith healing practices (Patel 2011). As shown in Table 13–6, culturally informed care can be described by six levels along a continuum.

Economic Burden in CAMH

Mental health disorders in the general population are a major contributor to the economic burden of diseases (Table 13–7). The indirect costs of early-onset psychiatric disorders are high and are primarily hidden (Knapp et al. 1999). Consequences of untreated CAMH disorders include suicide, school failure, limited or nonexistent employment opportunities, poverty in adulthood, and juvenile and criminal justice involvement (Kessler et al. 1995). Lu et al. (2018) published a report on the level of financial aid and developmental assistance for child and adolescent mental health in 132 developing countries from 2007 to 2015. The top 10 cumulative recipients are shown in Figure 13–4. Although mental health disorders are the leading causes of disability and mortality among this population, only 0.1% of total developmental assistance has been spent on CAMH. Of these funds, most of the short-term humanitarian assistance has been directed to trauma-related mental health disorders through nongovernmental organizations (Table 13–8).

Multiple sectors intersect in providing CAMH-based services, including primary health care, education, child welfare, early childhood intervention, substance abuse treatment, and juvenile justice. Given the lack of financial commitment and fluctuations in the distribution of aid and funding, overreliance on external funding is not a sustainable solution to the CAMH crisis (see Table 13–8).

Inadequate Systems

The burden of disease is assessed by calculating DALYs (Murray and Lopez 1994), which requires the estimation of three parameters: prevalence, disability weight, and average duration of the case until remission or death. This information is gathered by epidemiological and opinion surveys, polls, and expert knowledge. In LAMICs, many health-related events take place outside health facilities, limiting the acquisition of information in centralized data sources. For example, parents often seek care for their children's illnesses from pharmacy shops or street vendors. Most births and neonatal deaths occur at home and often are unrecorded. These factors

TABLE 13-6. **Cultural competence continuum**

Level	Description
Cultural proficiency	• This is the most advanced type of cultural competence.
	• Culture and cultural differences are valued and seen as strengths.
	• Providers make continual efforts to augment their knowledge and improve practices.
	• Advocacy for cultural competence and for improved relations among diverse groups occur throughout the system.
Cultural competence	• This level represents a form of advanced competence.
	• Providers exhibit acceptance and respect for differences.
	• There is a commitment to incorporating new knowledge and service models to better meet changing needs of minority populations.
Cultural precompetence	• There is recognition of the limitations of services and staffing and an effort to improve.
	• At this level, there may be a false sense of accomplishment from partial improvement.
	• An example is tokenism with regard to establishing a diverse workforce.
Cultural blindness	• Providers attempt to be unbiased and embrace the idea that "we are all the same."
	• Such an approach disregards the relevance of color, race, and culture in provision of service.
	• This philosophy undermines the ability to provide an individualized approach to treatment and treatment planning.
Cultural incapacity	• Providers lack the capacity to help children, families of color, and their communities.
	• There is no conscious intention to be destructive, but some assumptions and practices are discriminatory and/or paternalistic.
Cultural destructiveness	• This is the most negative level.
	• Providers' attitudes and practices are destructive to cultures and therefore to individuals in these cultures.
	• The most extreme examples include cultural genocide.

Source. Adapted from American Academy of Child and Adolescent Psychiatry 2019; Cross et al. 1989.

result in a wide margin of uncertainty with regard to statistics from LAMICs, with limited availability of diagnostics for precise determination of causes of illness and death, which may pose challenges to and contribute to the uncertainty of the DALY estimates (Murray et al. 2000).

Call for Action

The complex needs of CAMH services require a comprehensive approach to service coordination, joint care pathways, integrated psychosocial care, and embedding of CAMH services within the general medical services. The unique needs of the child and adolescent population and caregivers or parents must play a central role in shaping service planning, development, re-

TABLE 13–7. **Overall economic burden of mental health disorders**

	Care costs	Productivity costs	Other costs
Patients	Payment for treatment and service fees	Work disability and lost earnings	Anguish and suffering, treatment side effects, suicide
Family and friends	Informal caregiving	Time off work	Anguish, isolation, stigma
Employers	Contributions to treatment and care	Reduced productivity from employee	Not applicable
Society	Provision of mental health care and general medical care (taxation and insurance)	Reduced productivity	Loss of lives, untreated illness (unmet needs), social exclusion

Source.   Adapted from World Health Organization 2003.

search, and evaluation. In this section, we present potential opportunities based on actions taken at system, group, and individual levels.

System-Based Actions

A system of care is a coordinated network that builds significant partnerships with families and the child and adolescent population. It addresses each individual's cultural and linguistic needs to enhance his or her functioning at home, in school, in the community, and throughout the person's life span (Stroul and Friedman 1986). The implementation of a well-researched and well-designed system of care is one effective way to address the tension between evidence-based practice and culturally informed care. It is a spectrum of effective, community-based services and provides support for the child and adolescent population with or at risk for mental health problems. One example of a system of care is the Child and Adolescent Service System Program (CASSP), initiated by the United States and implemented in 1984. This program follows six core principles that are important caveats to consider while developing CAMH-based services: CAMH care should be child centered, family focused, community based, multisystem, culturally competent, and least intrusive (Table 13–9) (American Academy of Child and Adolescent Psychiatry 2019). A similar approach can be adapted for use in LMICs to develop community CAMH services. This ethnoculturally contextualized approach provides insight into the public system, where limited funds, poverty, lack of attention to overall health needs, and bureaucracy add to the daily challenges.

Group-Based Actions

The key to addressing the increasing burden of CAMH disorders is early prevention (Little and Mount 2018). Particular focus needs to be delivered to strengthen and build capacity in LAMICs. Two efficient strategies used to improve access to CAMH services are telepsychiatry and pri-

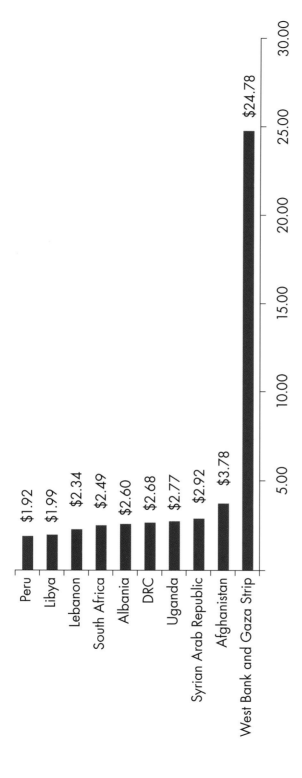

FIGURE 13–4. **Recipients of developmental assistance for child and adolescent mental health, 2007–2014.**

Note. Values are in millions in 2013 U.S. dollars.
Abbreviation. DRC=Democratic Republic of the Congo.
Source. Adapted from Lu et al. 2018.

TABLE 13–8.   Trends in developmental assistance provided for child and adolescent mental health (CAMH) from 2007 to 2014

Disorder	Percent of total developmental assistance
Trauma-related mental disorders	1.13
Substance abuse	0.76
Autism	0.19
Suicide	0.02
Depression	0.02
Anxiety	0.01

Source.   Adapted from Lu et al. 2018.

mary care integration. The former provides a solution to the geographic barriers to health care access and reduces inefficiencies related to clinical services; the latter further leverages child and adolescent psychiatrists' time and expertise through collaboration with primary care providers. Use of the Internet, videoconferencing, and mobile phones to deliver psychoeducation, self-help. and life skill teachings has been well established as a way to improve CAMH services (Kleintjes et al. 2010; Rocha et al. 2015; Sharifi et al. 2016). Belkin and Fricchione (2005) recommended establishing regional centers of excellence that include resource libraries, access to psychiatric consultants, support, training, and clinical diagnostic functions. This can lead to an increased number of adequately trained and culturally competent CAMH professionals within the region as well as training of everyone who comes in contact with the child, including teachers, nurses, and community health workers (Mian et al. 2015).

Individual-Based Actions

Bridging the Gap

CAMH professionals from UMICs and HICs (see Figure 13–1) can play a significant role in providing a bridge between the demand for care and available services globally. In the next subsections, we describe three approaches for practitioners that can have global impact.

Global Collaboration

International consultations can make an essential contribution to policy development, especially when the experts have experience in several other countries that are similar in terms of level of economic development, health system organization, and governmental arrangements. Similarly, more developed countries can be actively encouraged to share resources with less developed countries (World Health Organization 2018).

International Associations

CAMH professionals from UMICs and HICs should actively support the creation and strengthening of associations and organizations for CAMH professionals. Fricchione et al. (2012) proposed a strategy of development of global health institutes and global mental health divisions

TABLE 13–9.   Core principles of the Child and Adolescent Service System Program (CASSP)

Guiding principle for care	Description
Child centered	Services meet the individual needs of the child; consider the child's family and community contexts; and are developmentally appropriate, strengths based, and child-specific
Family focused	Service providers recognize that the family is the primary support system for the child and participates as a full partner in all stages of the decision-making and treatment planning process
Community based	Whenever possible, services are delivered in the child's home community, drawing on formal and informal resources to promote the child's successful participation in the community
Multisystem	Services are planned in collaboration with all the child-serving systems involved in the child's life
Culturally competent	Service providers recognize and respect the behavior, ideas, attitudes, values, beliefs, customs, language, rituals, ceremonies, and practices characteristic of the child and family's ethnic group
Least restrictive/least intrusive	Services take place in settings that are the most appropriate and natural for the child and family and are the least restrictive

Source.   Adapted from American Academy of Child and Adolescent Psychiatry 2019.

within academic medical centers and medical schools that will promote interprofessional and transprofessional education to break down professional silos and enhance collaboration.

Prevention and Psychoeducation

In conceptualizing the unique CAMH challenges, CAMH professionals in LAMICs must focus on preventive aspects of CAMH such as community-, school-, and parenting-based programs. According to Revet et al. (2018), CAMH professionals in LAMICs have a dual role of clinician-scientists and clinician-educators who engage in clinical, training, and research activities, including biomedical, epidemiological, educational, or clinical research. Kieling et al. (2011) proposed interventions to prevent CAMH problems in LICs and middle-income countries (see Table 13–10).

Conclusion

The current geopolitical situation and resulting refugee crisis, as well as prevailing migration patterns, make it imperative that CAMH service providers be familiar with the needs of the population they serve and systems of care from a global health perspective. There is a risk of a significant knowledge gap in understanding challenges and vulnerability, service delivery options, and treatment effectiveness when encounters are seen through more limited frames. LAMICs have historically faced significant constraints in resources in multiple areas, including training, fiscal needs, and research. Given these limitations, there are several examples in which LAMICs have been able to

TABLE 13–10.   Important considerations when devising a strategic plan for CAMH services development

There is the danger that systems of care will be fragmented, ineffective, expensive, and inaccessible if there is a lack of cultural and local guidance for developing child and adolescent mental health policies and plans

Several different systems of care (e.g., education, welfare, health) may need to be involved to ensure that services for youth are effective

A developmental perspective is needed for an understanding of all mental disorders and for designing an appropriate mental health policy

The strategic plan should focus on health promotion, not assistance, and provide an integrated framework, not a list of competencies or skills underpinned by a particular value and view of health

use creative and enterprising avenues to develop effective, impactful, and ethnoculturally informed services. Given the realities of globalization and transnational, cross-border traffic, these models may be shared with HICs as an effective means for developing adapted services in low-resource and challenging settings of marginalized communities such as rural populations, immigrants, and refugees. Global child and adolescent mental health offers CAMH service providers, educators, and researchers an informed lens for developing culturally contextual programs at an organizational level as well as for delivering individualized, ethnically sensitive service in clinical settings.

Clinical Pearls

- The pathway to care is often long and arduous in CAMH. By the time patients present to a CAMH specialist, a significant amount of money, time, and resources may have already been used. It is important to use the time with the patient wisely. Listen, listen, and listen. Then offer your assessment and recommendation.

- Collaboration with pediatricians and schools is part of good care. It includes creating new abbreviated pathways for multidisciplinary CAMH training that is well equipped with considerable ethnocultural sensitivity to help trainees master competencies in the changing landscape of G-CAMH.

- CAMH professionals have responsibility beyond direct clinical care. On the basis of their work setting, they may choose to advocate for raising awareness and improved mental health services at the community level; seek engagement with national and international mental health organizations, including nongovernmental organizations; engage in increasing child mental health literacy of general physicians, nurses, obstetricians, and schoolteachers; or advocate for robust CAMH training in medical school curricula, general psychiatry, pediatrics, and primary care residency training programs.

Self-Assessment Questions

1. There is the danger that systems of care will be fragmented, ineffective, expensive, and inaccessible if

    A. The approach focuses on health promotion.
    B. The approach is culturally contextualized.
    C. The approach is developmentally appropriate.
    D. Local guidance is not sought for policies.
    E. The approach is multisectoral.

2. In the task-shifting approach, tasks are shifted from specialists to which of the following?

    A. Policy makers.
    B. Health ministry.
    C. General physicians.
    D. Peer specialists.
    E. Public health officials.

3. According to the WHO World Mental Health Survey Consortium (Kessler et al. 2007), what is the median age of onset distribution of ADHD?

    A. 7–15 years.
    B. 7–9 years.
    C. 4–8 years.
    D. 9–14 years.
    E. 13–21 years.

4. On a cultural competence continuum, the ability of a health care provider to accept and respect the relevance of color, race, and culture to service provision and to make a commitment to incorporating new knowledge and best practices to better meet changing needs of their clinical population represents which of the following?

    A. Cultural proficiency.
    B. Cultural competence.
    C. Cultural precompetence.
    D. Cultural blindness.
    E. Cultural incapacity.

5. List five of the World Health Organization (WHO) Report 2001 proposed solutions to the growing concerns of global mental health.

Answers

1. D
2. C
3. B
4. B
5. Possible answers: integration and provision of treatment in primary care; ensuring the availability of psychotropic medications; community-based care; public awareness and psychoeducation; a holistic approach involving communities, families, and patients; national policies and legislation; capacity building and human resources; multisectoral approach; promotion of community mental health.

References

American Academy of Child and Adolescent Psychiatry: Systems-based practice overview. Revised August 2019. Washington, DC, American Academy of Child and Adolescent Psychiatry, 2019. Available at: www.aacap.org/App_Themes/AACAP/docs/resources_for_primary_care/training_toolkit_for_systems_based_practice/Overview-Module-August-2019-(8.19.19).pdf. Accessed October 1, 2020.

Barrett E, Jacobs B, Klasen H, et al: The Child and Adolescent Psychiatry: Study of Training in Europe (CAP-STATE). Eur Child Adolesc Psychiatry 29(1):11–27, 2020

Belkin GS, Fricchione GL: Internationalism and the future of academic psychiatry. Acad Psychiatry 29(3):240–243, 2005

Brundtland GH: Mental health in the 21st century. Bull World Health Organ 78(4):411, 2000

Clausen CE, Bazaid K, Azeem MW, et al: Child and adolescent psychiatry training and services in the Middle East region: a current status assessment. Eur Child Adolesc Psychiatry 29(1):51–61, 2020

Coleman WL, Dobbins MI, Garner AS, et al: Policy statement—the future of pediatrics: mental health competencies for pediatric primary care. Pediatrics 124(1):410–421, 2009

Costello EJ, Compton SN, Keeler G, et al: Relationship between poverty and psychopathology: a natural experiment. JAMA 290(15):2023–2029, 2003

Cross TL, Bazron BJ, Dennis KW, et al: Towards a Culturally Competent System of Care: A Monograph on Effective Services for Minority Children Who Are Severely Emotionally Disturbed, Vol I. Washington, DC, National Technical Assistance Center for Children's Mental Health, Georgetown University Child Development Center, 1989. Available at: www.ncjrs.gov/App/publications/abstract.aspx?ID=124939. Accessed August 12, 2020.

Cullins LM, Mian AI: Global child and adolescent mental health: a culturally informed focus. Child Adolesc Psychiatr Clin 24(4):823–830, 2015

Degenhardt L, Charlson F, Ferrari A, et al: The global burden of disease attributable to alcohol and drug use in 195 countries and territories, 1990–2016: a systematic analysis for the Global Burden of Disease Study 2016. Lancet Psychiatry 5(12):987–1012, 2018

Dubicka B, Bullock T: Mental health services for children fail to meet soaring demand. BMJ 358:j4254, 2017

Engle PL, Fernald LCH, Alderman H, et al: Strategies for reducing inequalities and improving developmental outcomes for young children in low-income and middle-income countries. Lancet 378(9799):1339–1353, 2011

Erskine HE, Baxter AJ, Patton G, et al: The global coverage of prevalence data for mental disorders in children and adolescents. Epidemiol Psychiatr Sci 26(4):395–402, 2017

Fegert JM, Vitiello B, Plener PL, Clemens V: Challenges and burden of the coronavirus 2019 (COVID-19) pandemic for child and adolescent mental health: a narrative review to highlight clinical and research needs in the acute phase and the long return to normality. Child Adolesc Psychiatry Ment Health 14:1–11, 2020

Findling RL, Stepanova E: The workforce shortage of child and adolescent psychiatrists: is it time for a different approach? J Am Acad Child Adolesc Psychiatry 57(5):300–301, 2018

Ford T: Practitioner review: how can epidemiology help us plan and deliver effective child and adolescent mental health services? J Child Psychol Psychiatry 49(9):900–914, 2008

Fricchione GL, Borba CP, Alem A, et al: Capacity building in global mental health: professional training. Harv Rev Psychiatry 20(1):47–57, 2012

Griesinger W: Mental Pathology and Therapeutics, 2nd Edition (1845). Translated by Lockhart Robinson C, Rutherford J. London, New Sydenham Society, 1867

Hirota T, Guerrero A, Sartorius N, et al: Child and adolescent psychiatry in the Far East. Psychiatry Clin Neurosci 69(3):171–177, 2015

Houtrow AJ, Larson K, Olson LM, et al: Changing trends of childhood disability, 2001–2011. Pediatrics 134(3):530–538, 2014

Karp DA, Tanarugsachock V: Mental illness, caregiving, and emotion management. Qual Health Res 10(1):6–25, 2000

Kessler RC, Foster CL, Saunders WB, et al: Social consequences of psychiatric disorders, I: educational attainment. Am J Psychiatry 152(7):1026–1032, 1995

Kessler RC, Amminger GP, Aguilar-Gaxiola S, et al: Age of onset of mental disorders: a review of recent literature. Curr Opin Psychiatry 20(4):359–364, 2007

Key E: The Century of the Child. New York, GP Putnam's Sons, 1909

Kieling C, Baker-Henningham H, Belfer M, et al: Child and adolescent mental health worldwide: evidence for action. Lancet 378(9801):1515–1525, 2011

Kleintjes S, Lund C, Flisher A, et al: A situational analysis of child and adolescent mental health services in Ghana, Uganda, South Africa and Zambia. Afr J Psychiatry (Johannesbg) 13(2):132–139, 2010

Knapp MRJ, Almond S, Percudani M: Costs of schizophrenia, a review, in Schizophrenia. Edited by Maj M, Sartorius N. Chichester, UK, Wiley, 1999, pp 407–454

Kohn R, Ali AA, Puac-Polanco V, et al: Mental health in the Americas: an overview of the treatment gap. Rev Panam Salud Publica 42:e1655, 2018

Koplan JP, Bond TC, Merson MH, et al: Towards a common definition of global health. Lancet 373(9679):1993–1995, 2009

Kyu HH, Stein CE, Boschi Pinto C, et al: Causes of death among children aged 5–14 years in the WHO European region: a systematic analysis for the Global Burden of Disease Study 2016. Lancet Child Adolesc Health 2(5):321–337, 2018

Lapouse R, Monk MA: An epidemiologic study of behavior characteristics in children. Am J Public Health Nations Health 48(9):1134–1144, 1958

Levy DM: Beginnings of the child guidance movement. Am J Orthopsychiatry 38(5):799–804, 1968

Little M, Mount K: Prevention and Early Intervention with Children in Need. New York, Routledge, 2018

Lu C, Li Z, Patel V: Global child and adolescent mental health: the orphan of development assistance for health. PLoS Med 15(3):e1002524, 2018

Lu Y: Test of the 'healthy migrant hypothesis': a longitudinal analysis of health selectivity of internal migration in Indonesia. Soc Sci Med 67(8):1331–1339, 2008

MacDonald K, Fainman-Adelman N, Anderson KK, et al: Pathways to mental health services for young people: a systematic review. Soc Psychiatry Psychiatr Epidemiol 53(10):1005–1038, 2018

Maudsley H: The Pathology of Mind: A Study of Its Distempers, Deformities, and Disorders. London, Macmillan, 1895

Mian AI, Milavić G, Skokauskas N: Child and adolescent psychiatry training: a global perspective. Child Adolesc Psychiatr Clin N Am 24(4):699–714, 2015

Mistry KB, Minkovitz CS, Riley AW, et al: A new framework for childhood health promotion: the role of policies and programs in building capacity and foundations of early childhood health. Am J Public Health 102(9):1688–1696, 2012

Morris J, Belfer M, Daniels A, et al: Treated prevalence of and mental health services received by children and adolescents in 42 low-and-middle-income countries. J Child Psychol Psychiatry 52(12):1239–1246, 2011

Murray CJ, Lopez AD: Quantifying disability: data, methods and results. Bull World Health Organ 72(3):481–494, 1994

Murray CJ, Salomon JA, Mathers C: A critical examination of summary measures of population health. Bull World Health Organ 78(8):981–994, 2000

Parry-Jones WL: The history of child and adolescent psychiatry: its present day relevance. J Child Psychol Psychiatry 30(1):3–11, 1989

Patel V: Traditional healers for mental health care in Africa. Glob Health Action 4:doi: 10.3402/gha.v4i0.7956, 2011

Patel V, Kieling C, Maulik PK, et al: Improving access to care for children with mental disorders: a global perspective. Arch Dis Child 98(5):323–327, 2013

Polanczyk GV, Salum GA, Sugaya LS, et al: Annual research review: a meta-analysis of the worldwide prevalence of mental disorders in children and adolescents. J Child Psychol Psychiatry 56(3):345–365, 2015

Revet A, Hebebrand J, Bhide S, et al: Dual training as clinician-scientist in child and adolescent psychiatry: are we there yet? Eur Child Adolesc Psychiatry 27(3):263–265, 2018

Rey JM, Assumpção FB Jr, Bernad CA, et al: History of child psychiatry, in IACAPAP Textbook of Child and Adolescent Mental Health. Edited by Rey JM. Geneva, Switzerland, International Association for Child and Adolescent Psychiatry and Allied Professions, 2015, pp 1–72

Rocha TBM, Graeff-Martins AS, Kieling C, et al: Provision of mental healthcare for children and adolescents: a worldwide view. Curr Opin Psychiatry 28(4):330–335, 2015

Rogler LH, Cortes DE: Help-seeking pathways: a unifying concept in mental health care. Am J Psychiatry 150(4):554–561, 1993

Rutter M, Tizard J, Whitmore K (eds): Education, Health, and Behaviour. London, Longman, 1970

Rutter M, Tizard J, Yule W, et al: Research report: Isle of Wight Studies, 1964–1974. Psychol Med 6(2):313–332, 1976

Schowalter JE: A history of child and adolescent psychiatry in the United States. Psychiatric Times 20(3), 2003

Sharifi V, Mojtabai R, Shahrivar Z, et al: Child and adolescent mental health care in Iran: current status and future directions. Arch Iran Med 19(11):797–804, 2016

Sheikh S, Furnham A: A cross-cultural study of mental health beliefs and attitudes towards seeking professional help. Soc Psychiatry Psychiatr Epidemiol 35(7):326–334, 2000

Shonkoff JP, Garner AS; Committee on Psychosocial Aspects of Child and Family Health, Committee on Early Childhood, Adoption, and Dependent Care, Section on Developmental and Behavioral Pediatrics: The lifelong effects of early childhood adversity and toxic stress. Pediatrics 129(1):e232–e246, 2012

Spring B: Evidence-based practice in clinical psychology: what it is, why it matters; what you need to know. J Clin Psychol 63(7):611–631, 2007

Stroul BA, Friedman RM: A System of Care for Severely Emotionally Disturbed Children and Youth. Washington, DC, CASSP Technical Assistance Center, Georgetown University Child Development Center, 1986. Available at: www.ncjrs.gov/pdffiles1/Digitization/125081NCJRS.pdf. Accessed January 29, 2020.

Thomas SB, Quinn SC, Butler J, et al: Toward a fourth generation of disparities research to achieve health equity. Annu Rev Public Health 32:399–416, 2011

Thomsen PH: Schizophrenia with childhood and adolescent onset—a nationwide register-based study. Acta Psychiatr Scand 94(3):187–193, 1996

Trivedi JK, Jilani AQ: Pathway of psychiatric care. Indian J Psychiatry 53(2):97–98, 2011

Vikram P, Flisher AJ, Nikapota A, et al: Promoting child and adolescent mental health in low and middle income countries. J Child Psychol Psychiatry 49(3):313–334, 2008

Vostanis P: Editorial: Global child mental health—emerging challenges and opportunities. Child and Adolescent Mental Health 22(4):177–178, 2017

Walker SP, Wachs TD, Grantham-McGregor S, et al: Inequality in early childhood: risk and protective factors for early child development. Lancet 378(9799):1325–1338, 2011

World Bank: World development indicators 2016. Washington, DC, World Bank, 2016. Available at: http://databank.worldbank.org/data/download/site-content/OGHIST.xls. Accessed October 14, 2019.

World Health Organization: The World Health Report 2001: Mental health: New Understanding, New Hope. Geneva, Switzerland, World Health Organization, 2001. Available at: www.who.int/whr/2001/en/whr01_en.pdf?ua=1. Accessed March 10, 2020.

World Health Organization: Investing in mental health. Geneva, Switzerland, World Health Organization, 2003. Available at: https://apps.who.int/iris/bitstream/handle/10665/42823/9241562579.pdf. Accessed October 27, 2019.

World Health Organization: Mental Health Atlas 2017. Geneva, Switzerland, World Health Organization, 2018. Available at: https://apps.who.int/iris/handle/10665/272735. Accessed April 30, 2020.

Yoder HN, Tol WA, Reis R, et al: Child mental health in Sierra Leone: a survey and exploratory qualitative study. Int J Ment Health Syst 10:48, 2016

CHAPTER 14

Digital Media, Culture, and Child and Adolescent Mental Health

Brittnie Fowler, M.D.
Sarah Y. Vinson, M.D.

IN *Bowling Alone*, Robert D. Putnam (2000) examined American society's decline in social capital, which he defined as "connections among individuals, social networks and the norms of reciprocity and trustworthiness that arise from them." (p. 19). Four social characteristics of American society that were contributing to this drop were identified: pressures of time and money, mobility and sprawl, television, and generational differences. Putnam argued that social capital is important because it facilitates the resolution of problems, results in improved social environments, renders business transactions easier because of mutual trust, widens awareness of mutual connectivity, helps to increase the flow of information, and improves health and happiness because humans are social creatures primed for contact with one another.

Bowling Alone was published in 2000. Four years later came Facebook, the first social media platform to gain widespread adoption. YouTube, Instagram, and Snapchat, the social media platforms most commonly used by youth, arrived in 2005, 2010, and 2011, respectively. Although older adult populations often prefer printed material, television, and desktop computers as means to access information, younger generations prefer portable forms of online streaming and online information via such devices as smartphones and tablets (Rideout 2015). These portable forms lend themselves to increased ubiquity of access, are more readily tailored to youth's interests, and can be harder to monitor.

Online culture is a critical influence on youth who are trying to understand their society and find their place in it. In order to master these tasks, they must develop emotional regulation, prac-

TABLE 14–1. **Media definitions**

Term	Definition
Media	Channel or system of communication, information, or entertainment
Digital media	Media in which the information is transmitted via the Internet through devices such as computers, tablets, gaming systems, and smartphones
Social media	Subset of digital media through which users engage in online communities to share content such as information, ideas, images, videos, and personal messages

Source. Merriam-Webster, 2020. Available at: www.merriam-webster.com/dictionary/media. Accessed June 30, 2019.

tice adaptive coping mechanisms, and fine-tune social skills. Emotionally salient and cognitively engaging content can be stressful, calming, encouraging, or demoralizing. The online environment can be a place of ridicule and exclusion or belonging and purpose. It can model and normalize risk behaviors or provide opportunities for growth and learning. Additionally, peer influence can now take place around the clock as exposure to peers reaches beyond school cafeterias and playgrounds to car rides, dinner tables, and bedrooms because of virtually ubiquitous smartphones.

The four drivers of the drop in social capital—time and money, mobility and sprawl, media, and generational differences—continue to be characteristics of our society. More importantly, media, which was represented by "television" in Putnam's book, appears to have stepped into the void, especially as it relates to youth. Currently, tweens spend an average of nearly 6 hours per day on entertainment media. For teenagers, it is nearly 9 hours per day (Rideout 2015). The quantity and quality of content consumed on media platforms not only can shape adolescents' worldview but also can impact their thoughts, feelings, and behaviors. In this chapter, we discuss media and children's mental health, with an emphasis on social media.

Background Information
History of Media

From the beginning of human history, people have found ways to pass along pertinent information about feelings, guidelines, laws, expectations, and experiences. Although the medium (from cave walls to silk paper to cell phones and the Internet) by which these ideas have been exchanged has changed, the desire to be social beings, obtain knowledge, and express ourselves has not. Table 14–1 includes information about various forms of media. Although this chapter will have an emphasis on social media, with the prominence and widespread use of sites such as YouTube, digital and broadcast media can and often do converge on these platforms.

Current Considerations for Culture Media and Youth

In the United States, with its cultural emphasis on individual responsibility and the free market, society currently relies largely on social media companies to regulate themselves (Raval 2019).

Although much attention is given to the sheer volume of media currently consumed by youth, an important consideration is the origin and desired effect of that media. The digital era has broadened the reach of individuals and companies that generate content. Consider the fact that youth can experience others' pain, joy, and fear in real time, even sometimes unsolicited, at the click of a button or the tap of an app. Anyone with a social media account or smartphone capable of taking pictures or video can go "viral." Ideas can be spread to developmentally vulnerable populations en masse and can range from positive to negative, such as being affirming of sexual minority youth or being used to out them—sometimes with tragic consequence. For better or for worse, this broad reach does not go through the historical media gatekeepers such as government agencies and family members. This has contributed to the emergence of the MeToo and Black Lives Matter messages but also has been a factor in the horror of mass shootings and trends such as the blue whale online suicide challenge.

In July 2020, President Donald Trump issued an executive order aimed at preventing social media companies from moderating content on their platforms. A result of this policy would be that vulnerable youth populations would have access to content that is not regulated or fact-checked, and the burden of filtering and education would fall on caregivers and clinicians who may not feel comfortable or may not have the resources (e.g., access, time) to do so. Youth tend to go to peers for answers because they have less fear of being judged and believe that peers are easier to talk to and understand them better. More pressure should be placed on media platforms to take responsibility, engage with agencies and organizations that desire to promote social capital, and keep the best interest of youth in mind.

Of particular concern is that the messaging most frequently reaching children and adolescents is not consistently filtered through a family or local community member who is invested in the youth's healthy emotional and social development. When media consisted of print and broadcast and households had just one or two screens in the form of bulky televisions, it was easier for caregiver rules and government regulations to limit exposure to potentially harmful content. Now, corporate interests can target youth more directly and in less obvious ways. As the case of electronic cigarettes demonstrates, they can do so quite effectively, to the point that even after the ads stop, the message continues to be perpetuated organically, reaching users with up to four degrees of separation from the original ad (Chu et al. 2018). Teenagers commonly retweet or reuse content (e.g., by recreating it in a TikTok video), and because youth trust each other, the information continues to be shared and passed on without further push or influence from the creator of the content. Popularity and views feed the desire for others to use the original in hopes of getting likes and views themselves. Additionally, there are fears about individual bad actors reaching youth through these platforms. Further complicating matters, in current society, *digital natives*, who have never experienced life without instantaneous access to information and images from around the world, may in fact be more savvy than the adults who are trying to monitor or guide their use.

Digital Culture and Youth Mental Health

Media, particularly social and digital media, is designed to capture the attention of its consumers, and it does so by using the brain's existing pathways and structures related to attention and salience. Similar to drugs of abuse, digital stimuli can hijack the brain's endogenous reward system by providing highs that outpace those of natural stimuli. The human brain continues to grow and create new neural connections known as synapses to a large extent into a person's 20s, but the biggest period of brain development is completed within the first 3 years of life. This period is associated with rapid development of language, cognition, social, emotional, and motor skills. As a result, media content—in terms of both quality and duration of exposure—can have significant impacts on a child's development. As the saying goes, practice makes perfect. For developing brains, this can be translated as referring to the use and strengthening of neural circuitry—or the lack thereof—during a critical window.

Of note, certain characteristics of young children may have an impact on their amount of media exposure. Excessive television viewing is more likely among infants and toddlers with self-regulation problems or a difficult temperament (Sugawara et al. 2015; Thompson et al. 2013). Additionally, mobile devices are more likely to be deployed by parents as calming mechanisms for toddlers with socioemotional delays (Radesky et al. 2016).

As in the case with substance use, which is more likely to become problematic or excessive when early brain exposure to the chemical occurs, it appears that early exposure to digital media can predispose youth to attentional problems and shape brain connectivity. In a longitudinal study of a nationally representative sample, a higher number of hours of television per day at both ages 1 and 3 was associated with attentional problems at age 7. It is notable that this finding was present even while controlling for a number of potential confounding factors such as prenatal substance use and gestational age, measures of maternal psychopathology, and socioeconomic status (Christakis et al. 2004). This result could be due, at least in part, to the influence of early media exposure on key areas of the brain dealing with cognitive processing and regulation (Gao et al. 2013). These processes aid in emotional regulation, behaviors, shaping of preferences, and internalization of social norms. This is important to consider when thinking about the media content being presented to a child and its implications on the developing mind, be it for better or worse. Recommendations regarding media and screen use are presented in Table 14–2.

A study of 19 healthy 8- to 12-year-old American children examined the functional connectivity of their reading-related brain regions and their exposure to screen-based media (Horowitz-Kraus and Hutton 2018). Youth with more screen time had lower connectivity between the visual word form area and the language, visual, and cognitive control regions of the brain. In contrast, brain connectivity in these areas was enhanced by reading books.

The adolescence period is notable for maturation of the frontoparietal systems, which are related to developing and fine-tuning executive functioning as well as other social, behavioral, and emotional skills (Paus 2005). During this time, adolescents are moving from a caregiver-child relationship to more peer-peer interactions. Youth at this age are suggestible, and therefore the duration and quality of media content can have significant impact on development and quality of life.

An important consideration in early childhood development is that these same attention grabs can impact caregivers as well. Distracted caregivers cannot actively, consistently engage their children. Although the evidence base regarding parent social media use has yet to catch up to societal realities, studies have concluded that associations between excessive media consumption by infants and toddlers in the form of television and cognitive, language, and socioemotional delays was likely secondary to decreases in parent-child interaction (Christakis et al. 2009).

TABLE 14–2.   Recommendations for children's screen and media use

Age	Recommendations	Notes
Younger than 18 months	Avoid use of screen media	Video chatting is OK
18–24 months	Watch content with children and help them understand what they are watching	Children should watch only high-quality programming
2–5 years	Limit use to 1 hour per day	Children should watch only high-quality programming, and parents should view programs with the child and explain content and relevance
6 years and older	Place consistent limits on time spent and types of media	Time spent should not replace essentials such as adequate sleep, hygiene, grooming, and physical activity

Source.   American Academy of Pediatrics: "American Academy of Pediatrics Announces Recommendations for Children's Media Use." January 21, 2020. Available at: www.pathwaypeds.com/american-academy-of-pediatrics-announces-new-recommendations-for-childrens-media-use. Accessed May 1, 2020.

The developmental impact of media is not uniformly negative; the type of content does make a difference. Although most media has not been demonstrated to be effective at promoting healthy development, there is some experimental evidence that switching from violent content to educational or prosocial content improves behavioral problems, particularly for boys from low-income families (Christakis et al. 2013). Well-designed television programs, such as *Sesame Street*, and applications have been demonstrated to have positive cognitive effects and to teach literary skills effectively to preschoolers (Chiong and Shuler 2016). That said, in order for toddlers to learn from educational commercial media, it is necessary for caregivers not only to watch it with them but also to reteach the content (Roseberry et al. 2014).

Psychological Impact

It is noteworthy that moderate social media use can have benefits, such as advanced social support and connection. The reality is that digital interactions are now a key part of peer engagement, and complete restriction may come with its own problems of alienation or fear of missing out. In fact, research has suggested a U-shaped relationship between Internet use and depression. In other words, the risk goes up at both the high and low ends of Internet use (Bélanger et al. 2011). In addition to how often, *how* youth use social media matters, too. One study found that older adolescents who use social media passively (e.g., viewing others' photos) reported declines in life satisfaction, whereas those who use it more actively (interacting with others and sharing content) did not experience these declines (Kross et al. 2013).

The Youth Internet Safety Survey of 150 Internet-using youth ages 10–17 years found that talking with strangers online, using the Internet most frequently for e-mailing others, and more intense Internet use differentiated youth reporting depressive symptoms from asymptomatic peers. Additionally, personal disclosure (e.g., name, school, address and phone number, sexual orientation) was significantly more likely to be reported by youth who reported major depressive symptomatology versus mild or no symptomatology (Ybarra et al. 2005). A study of 467 Scottish adolescents found that adolescents who used social media more—both overall and at night—and those who were more emotionally invested in social media experienced poorer sleep quality, lower self-esteem, and higher levels of anxiety and depression (Woods and Scott 2016). Of note, even after controlling for anxiety, depression, and self-esteem, nighttime-specific social media use predicted poorer sleep quality. Although emotional arousal may be a contributor, the mere presence of light (particularly blue light) before bed and its resultant impact on melatonin levels can be detrimental (Wahnschaffe et al. 2013).

With the sheer volume of time youth spend consuming media, it stands to reason that part of the psychological impact of media use may be mediated by its crowding out adequate sleep as well as other protective factors. Excessive media consumption can mean decreased engagement with caregivers and inadequate physical activity. Many youth are using electronic media while doing homework (Rideout 2015). Not surprisingly, evidence suggests that this has negative consequences on learning and academic performance (Carrier et al. 2015). Overreliance on virtual interactions may also decrease exposure to anxiety-provoking situations in real life, creating an environment where cognitive distortions remain unchallenged. Finally, self-comparisons to the curated social media personas of peers and influencers may negatively impact self-esteem and contribute to depressive feelings and cognitions.

The *Diagnostic and Statistical Manual of Mental Disorders*, Fifth Edition (DSM-5; American Psychiatric Association 2013) does not characterize problematic Internet use as a diagnosis, although Internet gaming disorder is included as a condition in need of further research. However, a significant proportion of youth today are experiencing symptoms related to problematic Internet use similar to the DSM-5 symptoms for proposed Internet gaming disorder, including a preoccupation with the activity, decreased interest in offline or "real life" relationships, unsuccessful attempts to decrease use, and withdrawal symptoms. The prevalence of problematic Internet use among children and adolescents is estimated to be between 4% and 8% (Jelenchick et al. 2015), and up to 8.5% of U.S. youth ages 8–18 years meet criteria for Internet gaming disorder (Gentile 2009). Additionally, a review of 23 peer-reviewed papers related to problematic smartphone use found that depression severity was consistently related to problematic smartphone use, demonstrating at least medium effect sizes; that anxiety was consistently related to problem use, but with small effect sizes; that stress was somewhat consistently related, with small to medium effects; and that self-esteem was inconsistently related, with small to medium effects when found (Elhai et al. 2017).

Behavioral Impact

Functional Improvement

Just as peer pressure in the traditional sense can promote adaptive behaviors, so too can socialization that occurs online. For youth who are isolated or are minority members of their local communities, digital communities can be a critical channel for connection and a place for belonging. Research indicates that social media can foster a sense of inclusion among users who may feel excluded (Krueger and Young 2015). Although a robust evidence base is lacking at this time, it stands to reason that this type of socialization could have potential benefit for minority groups such as immigrant populations, racial and ethnic minorities, sexual minorities, and individuals with chronic or debilitating illness or other physical impairments. Virtual communities can decrease feelings of isolation. Select social media threads may allow youth in marginalized groups to see themselves adequately and positively represented.

Additionally, social media can be used to inspire healthy behaviors, such as joining a support group to promote self-care or creating a GoFundMe page for a charitable cause (Chou et al. 2009). There is also potential for mitigating some of the functional limitations that arise because of mental illness. One example is the use of video modeling and video self-monitoring, which have been shown to be efficacious in helping children and adolescents with autism spectrum disorder improve behavioral, functional, and social skills. For older children and adolescents with executive function deficits, the use of apps can help with executive functioning tasks such as self-management, planning, and organization. Finally, for youth in rural areas or hypersegregated poverty-stricken communities, media may allow for exposure to content that helps youth to learn about the world as is and dream in a more expansive way about their place in it.

Sexuality

Youth share, emote, connect with peers, and meet new people online. Therefore, it is not surprising that adolescent sexual exploration would find a place there as well. *Sexting*, the electronic transmission of nude or seminude images or sexually explicit text messages, is common. It is estimated that approximately 12% of youth ages 10–19 years have sent a sexual photo to someone else (Temple and Choi 2014). Some studies have found that young people view sexting with indifference or even positively, as fun, natural behavior (Kerstens and Stol 2014; Lee and Crofts 2015; Nielson et al. 2015). This can cause a significant disconnect for youth when parent- or caregiver-led discussions about sexual online behaviors take on an alarmist tone.

Understandably, there are concerns, especially among people in generations that are less familiar with these platforms, of sexual exploitation and victimization (Mitchell et al. 2007) and/or posting of content that exposes youth to harassment or even criminal charges related to child pornography (Lorang et al. 2016). Additionally, sexting's relationship to other forms of media has been explored. One study of teenagers in the Netherlands found a bidirectional relationship between teen viewing of sexual reality television content and sexting but did not find the same relationship for Internet pornography (Vandenbosch et al. 2015). This impact may be mediated by an effect on youth perceptions of what is normative behavior, with reality television cast members being viewed as more relatable than pornography actors.

Suicidality

In March 2017, on-demand streaming service Netflix released *13 Reasons Why*, a series that followed the aftermath of a teenager's suicide. The professional mental health community raised concerns about the content, primarily the fact that it seemed to romanticize suicide instead of exposing its true harm and finality. Unfortunately, 2 years later, research data supported the validity of those concerns. Studies published by prominent medical journals found an association between the show and a significant increase in monthly suicide rates among U.S. youth ages 10–17 years (Bridge et al. 2020).

Assortativity, the propensity of similar people to be socially connected with one another more often than with dissimilar counterparts, has been found in suicidal behaviors. A recent study of suicide-related verbalizations coded 64 million posts from 17 million Twitter users. These verbalizations were significantly more assortative than chance, even through six degrees of separation. In other words, if a youth's friend's friend's friend's friend's friend posted about suicide online, that youth was more likely than chance to also post about suicide despite having never met the person who posted originally. Notably, in relationships with two degrees of separation, the assortativity was not attributable to the known assortativity of mood (Cero and Witte 2019).

Because youth are more suggestible, they are more vulnerable to imitation than are adults (De Veirman et al. 2019). Given what is known about salience, it is not surprising that stronger imitating effects are seen when there are similarities between the young person and the model (e.g., in age, gender, mood status, or background situation). This is also seen when the model is a celebrity or someone who is admired. The public response matters as well. When the behavior is condoned or regarded as positive or understandable, it is more likely to be imitated. Finally, media depictions, in both quantity and quality, impact the effect, with research showing a dose-effect relationship (O'Connor and Pirkis 2016). Although this knowledge has influenced approaches to coverage in some print and broadcast media, such policy has not been widely adopted in social media.

Risk Behaviors

The adolescent period is marked by risk-taking behaviors in a way that is distinct from childhood or adulthood. This phenomenon is not new; however, the current social implications are different because of the ease of documentation and dissemination of content related to the behaviors. Not surprisingly, studies indicate that some youth are more likely to engage in online risk behaviors. For example, boys are more likely to do so than girls (Morrongiello and Rennie 1998) and may have more benefit from a sheltered Internet environment (Segers and Verhoeven 2009). Compared with females, adolescent males tend to browse more and read less in open searches on the Internet; less risky behavior was seen in males when using media in environments with closed-search groups and delimited options (Segers and Verhoeven 2009).

Youth have shown vulnerability to peer influence as it relates to social media depictions of substance use (Winpenny et al. 2014). In addition, cyberbullying, which has the distinctions of potential anonymity and the ability to reach victims in spaces that would traditionally be safe from physical bullying, can be even more harmful for its victims than traditional bullying. Cyberbullying can lead to a myriad of negative short- and long-term social, academic, and health effects, not only for the victim but also for the perpetrator (Gini and Espelage 2014; Twyman et al. 2010).

Clinical Considerations in Serving Youth and Families

Supporting Parents

Caregivers live in the same society as their children, and they, too, are inundated with digital media intentionally designed to grab their attention. Not surprisingly, parent media use is a strong predictor of child media habits (Jago et al. 2012). Psychoeducation and support are needed for parents about the media use choices they make for themselves and for their children. Families of the children represented in specialty mental health clinical settings may be at particular risk of using media for distraction, calming, or even management.

It is noteworthy that just as online communities can provide meaningful connections and sources of inspiration and information for youth, they can provide the same for parents. Digital media can help caregivers navigate local systems and locate mental health and ancillary services. Additionally, validating interactions on social media may mitigate parents' feelings of being overwhelmed and/or isolated.

Family Media Plan and Intentionality Regarding Protective Factors

As the popular adage goes, "If you fail to plan, you plan to fail." Youth will use and be exposed to media. It is up to those who care for them to be intentional about *how*. Thus, the education and support of youth and caregivers in developing media plans are an essential part of promoting mental health. The American Academy of Pediatrics (2019) recommends that families work together to create a personalized family media use plan and provides an online tool to assist in the process. The tool is interactive and takes a developmental approach. Even though some families may opt to not use this tool, it can still provide a useful example for clinicians who are assisting families.

When new screens are gifted to or earned by youth, it is important that boundaries are set around use. Given the ample evidence of the detrimental effects of nighttime media use and the inherent challenges bedroom and late-night use pose for monitoring, a *media curfew* at bedtime is recommended. Taken in context, such a curfew makes perfect sense. Curfews in the traditional sense were imposed to keep youth from being exposed to higher-risk experiences before they were developmentally equipped to handle them. The Internet presents youth with a myriad of constant choices about what to say, share, and consume, and a youth's control over access should be increased over time with increasing maturity.

Ongoing Engagement and Open Dialogue

With tweens and teenagers spending most of their waking hours consuming media, their online life can hold just as much value to them, and may even hold more value, than what happens in real life. It can be tempting to dismiss events online as less important than those in real life or to just dispense advice; however, the issues raised by topics, trends, and stories in the news and on social media can provide opportunities for meaningful dialogue and critical thinking. Given the centrality of media in the lives of youth, patient-centered care demands an ongoing, open dialogue with youth about their online lives. Blanket, unilateral cautionary statements such as "Don't sext—you'll go to jail" or "You spend too much time on your phone" are woefully inadequate. This dialogue can extend beyond families in clinics to community leaders and organizations that work with youth.

When working with youth, clinicians should ask about their media use history. Some possible questions to ask include the following:

1. Do you have your own phone, tablet, or gaming system that you use to communicate with others?
2. What social media platforms are you on? Which one do you use most?
3. Do your parents know about your accounts? Are they friends with you or do they follow your accounts?
4. Do you engage with people online whom you have never met in real life?
5. Have you ever shared or received pictures of private body parts through social medial? What do you understand about the implications of sending or receiving those pictures?
6. What do you typically do on social media?
7. Where is your phone or tablet when you go to bed at night?

Some of the above questions may need to be modified on the basis of the age of the child or youth to make them more age appropriate. If clinicians do not feel that they have time to ask these questions during the session, they may want to consider having the teenager or family fill out a questionnaire before the visit.

Advocacy for Mental Health–Informed Media and Legal Policies

The skill set and knowledge base of children's mental health professionals can, and should, be deployed outside traditional treatment settings in order to shape a healthier media culture for children and families. Mental health professionals can play a key role in informing educators, school administrators, community leaders, and legislators about socioemotional development as well as research findings. In so doing, they can help systems serving children develop policies, procedures, and laws that are psychologically informed. For example, discussions with lawmakers about healthy development, the sexual maturation process, normative teenage behaviors, and the negative mental health outcomes associated with juvenile and/or criminal system involvement can help to inform school policies and laws related to sexting behaviors.

COVID-19 and the Syndemic

As 2020 rolled in with New Year resolutions to make it a better year than the previous one, the world began to face new realities and setbacks. Words such as quarantine, social distancing, distance learning, health, quality of life, safety, violence, brutality, rights, and justice began trending, entering our homes at what seemed like a faster pace than ever before. Although these ideas are not entirely new to humanity, having access to media has created an overabundance of information related to them. As discussed in this chapter, such information can have varying effects on youth and their caregivers, especially when considering that the vast amount of information gained through media and other sources may be frightening, exciting, upsetting, or a mixture.

Adding to the equation is the world's shift to operating from home during quarantine for the novel coronavirus SARS-CoV-2 (COVID-19). According to an article published by the *New York Times*, the United States has changed not just the frequency of use of the Internet but also the reasons for use (Koeze and Popper 2020). The *Times*'s research showed that there has been an increase in ways for people to connect with each other, learn, work, engage in pleasurable activities, and gain information. Also notable from the study was the fact that individuals have been branching out from use of smartphones to other devices as means to make connections and accomplish these activities. Access to the digital age, now considered a necessity for those wishing to shop online, socialize, engage in social learning, attend telemedicine visits, keep up with current events, or work remotely has become the new norm for many people. However, although some people are adapting to life online, others lack the resources needed to complete the transition. In addition to health disparities and economic difficulties, the COVID-19 pandemic has also resulted in an increase in digital inequalities (Beaunoyer et al. 2020).

As the world continues to grapple with COVID-19, political and social unrest, natural disasters, and isolation on a global level, clinicians are faced with new challenges to continue providing quality care. Creating a space for youth and their caregivers to talk about current concerns, experiences, and needs is a reasonable place to start. We do not yet know the full psychosocial impact of the syndemic, including the effects of increased use of media and technology during isolation, and we should continue to monitor for stress reactions, identify unhealthy or unsafe media usage, and work with families around healthy ways to incorporate media appropriately.

The Center for the Study of Traumatic Stress (2020) has provided guidelines for psychiatrists caring for patients during COVID-19 that include the following: "1) acknowledge concerns and uncertainty about emerging diseases, 2) share medical knowledge that is accurate and timely, and 3) identify steps the patient can take to reduce distress and sustain normal health behaviors, particularly sleep." These guidelines reach beyond the pandemic and the psychiatrist and can be used by clinicians, regardless of their specialty, to help guide conversations about many trending topics. Once the clinician has been able to discern the family's concerns, he or she can than work toward adapting the guidelines. For example, consider a case in which a clinician learns that family members have been feeling scared about spending time outside because of killer hornets and have spent hours on the Internet watching videos about hornet attacks, leading to poor sleep and increasing levels of anxiety. The clinician can follow the above steps by 1) acknowledging concerns ("Killer hornets sound scary"); 2) sharing knowledge that the provider may know about the hornets (e.g., medical risks if stung) or directing the family to reputable resources about the topic (e.g., an article from *National Geographic*); and then 3) promoting sleep hygiene and encouraging the family to reduce the amount of time spent on electronics researching hornets. For more sensitive topics such as police brutality and social injustice, clinicians should seek guidance from caregivers about the level of information desired to be shared with their child prior to giving an age-appropriate explanation where warranted.

On the macro level, we again want to encourage clinicians to consider using their platform for advocacy. Examples include speaking out regarding the need for reform in legal policies, addressing inequalities, and encouraging media platforms to take ownership and responsibility for the content made accessible to the public, specifically vulnerable populations. For further discussion, see Chapter 22, "Advocacy."

A final thought relates to the clinician. It is important that we as clinicians ensure our own well-being given the current health crisis. Increased work demands, risks to frontline workers, media coverage of the pandemic, and social injustices can be equally as distressing to clinicians as to the families we treat. It is imperative to recognize the signs of burnout, promote an appropriate work-life balance, and seek help when warranted. "The self-aware, balanced, energized, and resilient physician is one who is less susceptible to burnout and one who will become part of the solution by contributing to a positive work environment for his colleagues" (Lacy and Chan 2018, p. 316).

Conclusion

The pixelated cat is out of the bag. Media, particularly digital media, is a major force in child and adolescent mental health and is not going away. One could even argue that gathering a pertinent history and actively engaging patients and families about their media use are necessary components of cultural humility. Media use has clear implications for cognitive and emotional development in younger children. There are concrete steps that mental health professionals can, and should, take as clinicians and as members of the broader society to address the issue of digital media culture and youth mental health.

Clinical Pearls

- An understanding of a child's media use and online life is an essential part of patient-centered care for children and adolescents in the digital age.

- Psychoeducation and support for parents about the media use choices they make for themselves and for their children are needed.

- What happens online may be just as, if not more, important to youth as what happens in real life, and inquiring about it is a key component of a thorough social history.

- A curious, collaborative, open stance rather than a critical and prematurely directive one is likely to be more effective in gathering a social media history. Youth should be asked about their access to devices and the existence of social media accounts.

- Providers should familiarize themselves with state laws regarding sexting.

Self-Assessment Questions

1. What are the current recommendations regarding screen time?

2. During which phase of life is brain development most pertinent? What is the significance of brain development at this age when considering exposure to digital media?

3. What impact does media use have on the changes that occur during puberty?

4. What are some of the beneficial ways social media can be used?

5. What is a family media plan? How might it be helpful when talking with families?

6. What is the role of mental health providers regarding social media and the youth and their families?

Answers

1. No screen time for children younger than 18 months, screen time with parents for ages 18–24 months, 1 hour per day for children ages 2–5 years, and consistent limits for ages 6 years and older.

2. The biggest period of brain development occurs during the first 3 years of life, with rapid development of language, cognition, social, emotional, and motor skills. Therefore, the quality of media content and duration of use can have significant impacts on a child's development.

3. The frontoparietal systems, which are related to developing and fine-tuning executive functioning as well as other social, behavioral, and emotional skills, mature during adolescence. Youth are transitioning from a caregiver-child relationship to more peer-peer interactions, and they are suggestible. This is also a period of risk-taking behavior. Therefore, the duration and quality of media content can have significant impacts on adolescents' development and quality of life.

4. Advocacy, networking, education, decreasing disparities by increasing accessibility.

5. A family media plan consists of guidelines established by a family related to the use of media in their household. The plan should consider the health, education, and entertainment needs of each child and the family as a whole. Even if the family chooses not to create one, explaining use of a media plan can serve as an icebreaker for the clinician to initiate discussion on the risks and benefits of media and guidelines for media use in the home baed on the child's age.

6. The mental health provider's role can include advocacy on both the community and policy levels; open dialogue with families about use of social media in their homes; documentation of the patient's social media history; and provision of resources, guidance, and support for caregivers and their children regarding healthy use of media. Clinicians should be knowledgeable about the varied media platforms and the ways they impact youth.

References

American Academy of Pediatrics: How to make a family media use plan. Itasca, IL, HealthyChildren.org, American Academy of Pediatrics, November 2019. Available at: www.healthychildren.org/English/family life/Media/Pages/How-to-Make-a-Family Media-Use-Plan.aspx. Accessed December 15, 2019.

American Psychiatric Association: Diagnostic and Statistical Manual of Mental Disorders, Fifth Edition. Arlington, VA, American Psychiatric Association, 2013

Beaunoyer E, Dupéré S, Guitton MJ: COVID-19 and digital inequalities: reciprocal impacts and mitigation strategies. Comput Human Behav 111:106424, 2020

Bélanger RE, Akre C, Berchtold A, et al: A U-shaped association between intensity of Internet use and adolescent health. Pediatrics 127(2):e330–e335, 2011

Bridge JA, Greenhouse JB, Ruch D, et al: Association between the release of Netflix's 13 Reasons Why and suicide rates in the United States: an interrupted times series analysis. J Am Acad Child Adolesc Psychiatry 59(2):236–243, 2020

Carrier LM, Rosen LD, Cheever NA, et al: Causes, effects, and practicalities of everyday multitasking, in Living in the "Net" Generation: Multitasking, Learning, and Development. Developmental Review 35(special issue):64–78, 2015

Center for the Study of Traumatic Stress: Taking care of patients during the coronavirus outbreak: a guide for psychiatrists. Bethesda, MD, Center for the Study of Traumatic Stress, 2020. Available at: www.cstsonline.org/assets/media/documents/CSTS_FS_Taking_Care_of_Patients_During_Coronavirus_Outbreak_A_Guide_for_Psychiatrists_03_03_2020.pdf. Accessed: August 10, 2020.

Cero I, Witte TK: Assortativity of suicide-related posting on social media. Am Psychol doi.org/10.1037/amp0000477, 2019

Chiong C, Shuler C: Learning: is there an app for that? Investigations of young children's usage of learning with mobile devices and apps. New York, Joan Ganz Cooney Center at Sesame Workshop, 2016. Available at: http://dmlcentral.net/wp-content/uploads/files/learningapps_final_110410.pdf. Accessed May 5, 2020.

Chou WY, Hunt YM, Beckjord EB, et al: Social media use in the United States: implications for health communication. J Med Internet Res 11(4):e48, 2009

Christakis DA, Zimmerman FJ, DiGiuseppe DL, et al: Early television exposure and subsequent attentional problems in children. Pediatrics 113(4):708–713, 2004

Christakis DA, Gilkerson J, Richards JA, et al: Audible television and decreased adult words, infant vocalizations, and conversational turns: a population-based study. Arch Pediatr Adolesc Med 163(6):554–558, 2009

Christakis DA, Garrison MM, Herrenkohl T, et al: Modifying media content for preschool children: a randomized controlled trial. Pediatrics 131(3):431–438, 2013

Chu K-H, Colditz JA, Primack BA, et al: JUUL: spreading online and offline. J Adolesc Health 63(5):582–586, 2018

De Veirman M, Hudders L, Nelson MR: What is influencer marketing and how does it target children? A review and direction for future research. Front Psychol 10:2685, 2019

Elhai JD, Dvorak RD, Levine JC, et al: Problematic smartphone use: a conceptual overview and systematic review of relations with anxiety and depression psychopathology. J Affect Disord 207:251–259, 2017

Gao W, Gilmore JH, Shen D, et al: The synchronization within and interaction between the default and dorsal attention networks in early infancy. Cerebral Cortex 23(3):594–603, 2013

Gentile D: Pathological video-game use among youth ages 8 to 18: a national study. Psychol Sci 20(5):594–602, 2009

Gini G, Espelage DL: Peer victimization, cyberbullying, and suicide risk in children and adolescents. JAMA 312(5):545–546, 2014

Horowitz-Kraus T, Hutton JS: Brain connectivity in children is increased by the time they spend reading books and decreased by the length of exposure to screen-based media. Acta Paediatr 107(4):685–693, 2018

Jago R, Stamatakis E, Gama A: Parent and child screen-viewing time and home media environment. Am J Prev Med; 43(2):150–158, 2012

Jelenchick L, Eickhoff J, Zhang C, et al: Screening for adolescent problematic internet use: validation of the Problematic and Risky Internet Use Screening Scale (PRIUSS). Acad Pediatr 15(6):658–665, 2015

Kerstens J, Stol W: Receiving online sexual requests and producing online sexual images: the multifaceted and dialogic nature of adolescents' online sexual interactions. Cyberpsychology Journal of Psychosocial Research on Cyberspace 8(1):doi.org/10.5817/CP2014-1-8, 2014

Koeze E, Popper N: The virus changed the way we Internet. New York Times, April 7, 2020. Available at: www.nytimes.com/interactive/2020/04/07/technology/coronavirus-internet-use.html. Accessed August 10, 2020.

Kross E, Verduyn P, Demiralp E, et al: Facebook use predicts declines in subjective well-being in young adults. PLoS One 8(8):e69841, 2013

Krueger EA, Young SD: Twitter: a novel tool for studying the health and social needs of transgender communities. JMIR Ment Health 2(2):pii:e16, 2015

Lacy BE, Chan JL: Physician burnout: the hidden health care crisis. Clin Gastroenterol Hepatol 16(3):311–317, 2018

Lee M, Crofts T: Gender, pressure, coercion and pleasure: untangling motivations for sexting between people. Br J Criminol 55(3):454–473, 2015

Lorang MR, McNiel DE, Binder RL: Minors and sexting: legal implications. J Am Acad Psychiatry Law 44(1):73–81, 2016

Mitchell K, Finkelhor D, Wolak J: Youth internet users at risk for the most serious online sexual solicitations. Am J Prev Med 32(6):532–537, 2007

Morrongiello BA, Rennie H: Why do boys engage in more risk taking than girls? The role of attributions, beliefs, and risk appraisals. J Pediatr Psychol 23(1):33–43, 1998

Nielson S, Paasonen S, Spisak S: 'Pervy role-play and such': girls' experiences of sexual messaging online. Sex Education 15(5):472–485, 2015

O'Connor R, Pirkis J: Suicide clusters, in International Handbook of Suicide Prevention, 2nd Edition. Edited by O'Connor RC, Perkis J. Chichester, UK, Wiley, 2016, pp 758–774

Paus T: Mapping brain maturation and cognitive development during adolescence. Trends Cogn Sci 9(2):60–68, 2005

Putnam RD: Bowling Alone: The Collapse and Revival of American Community. New York, Simon & Schuster, 2000

Radesky JS, Peacock-Chambers E, Zuckerman B, et al: Use of mobile technology to calm upset children: associations with social-emotional development. JAMA Pediatr 170(4):397–399, 2016

Raval T: Regulating social media companies. Forbes, June 10, 2019. Available at: www.forbes.com/sites/forbestechcouncil/2019/06/10/regulating-social-media-companies/#112ea2e062b9. Accessed May 1, 2020.

Rideout V: The Common Sense Census: media use by tweens and teens. San Francisco, CA, Common Sense Media, 2015. Available at: www.commonsensemedia.org/sites/default/files/uploads/research/census_researchreport.pdf. Accessed May 1, 2020.

Roseberry S, Hirsh-Pasek K, Golinkoff RM: Skype me! Socially contingent interactions help toddlers learn language. Child Dev 85(3):956–970, 2014

Segers E, Verhoeven L: Learning in a sheltered internet environment: the use of WebQuests. Learning and Instruction 19(5):423–432, 2009

Sugawara M, Matsumoto S, Murohashi H, et al: Trajectories of early television contact in Japan: relationship with preschoolers' externalizing problems. Journal of Children and Media 9(4):453–471, 2015

Temple JR, Choi H: Longitudinal association between teen sexting and sexual behavior. Pediatrics 134(5):e1287–e1292, 2014

Thompson AL, Adair LS, Bentley ME: Maternal characteristics and perception of temperament associated with infant TV exposure. Pediatrics 131(2):e390–397, 2013

Twyman K, Saylor C, Taylor LA, et al: Comparing children and adolescents engaged in cyberbullying to matched peers. Cyberpsychol Behav Soc Netw 13(2):195–199, 2010

Vandenbosch L, van Oosten JM, Peter J: The relationship between sexual content on mass media and social media: a longitudinal study. Cyberpsychol Behav Soc Netw 18(12):697–703, 2015

Wahnschaffe A, Haedel S, Rodenbeck A, et al: Out of the lab and into the bathroom: evening short-term exposure to conventional light suppresses melatonin and increases alertness perception. Int J Mol Sci 14(2):2573–2589, 2013

Winpenny EM, Marteau TM, Nolte E: Exposure of children and adolescents to alcohol marketing on social media websites. Alcohol Alcohol 49(2):154–159, 2014

Woods HC, Scott H: #Sleepyteens: social media use in adolescence is associated with poor sleep quality, anxiety, depression and low self-esteem. J Adolesc 51:41–49, 2016

Ybarra ML, Alexander C, Mitchell KJ: Depressive symptomatology, youth Internet use, and online interactions: a national survey. J Adolesc Health 36(1):9–18, 2005

CHAPTER 15

Culture of Technology

Use of Telepsychiatry and Other Advances to Engage Children, Adolescents, and Transitional-Age Youth

R. Dakota Carter, M.D., Ed.D.

IN the current accelerated era of technology, cultural psychiatry is a vital component for mental health practitioners in providing competent care to patients and families, and as practitioners, we must understand the influence these advances have on the culture of psychiatry. Technological developments have altered the delivery of care and the practice of psychiatry, mediated by the generalized use of technology by patients and health care systems. Technology has changed the ways in which we learn and communicate and, for health care providers, diagnose and treat. As individuals who use technology more than any cohort in history, the youth population offers new, innovative, and revolutionary opportunities for diagnosis, treatment, and management of their mental health care through the devices they use every day.

As technology has progressed, so has its use, expanding extensively in the past two decades. Clinicians use telepsychiatry services to engage patients, including youth, in order to provide care and opportunities for health care intervention. This includes populations that might not otherwise be served, bridging gaps (e.g., health disparities; lack of access to quality, culturally competent care) commonly found in diverse populations seeking care. New technology is allowing better access to treatment despite shortages of child and adolescent psychiatrists. With the use of telepsychiatry and other video-monitoring solutions, geographic limitations no longer prevent families in rural areas from accessing psychiatric care. Numerous new programs ranging from schools and local clinics to local communities use technology to improve mental health. These advances allow communities that have historically faced discrimination, prejudice, and health care disparities access to culturally informed providers capable of not only treating psychiatric symptoms but also addressing the effects of stigmatization associated with mental illness, and doing so with humility and compassion. With the help of technology, psychiatrists work with collaborative teams to improve mental health outcomes and cultural competency by training local providers familiar with the community. Innovation has been a powerful influence on the practice of child and adolescent mental health care, and the very culture of psychiatry has been altered drastically through technology and advances in information and communication technologies.

Research in telepsychiatry has demonstrated positive effects in the child and adolescent population, including diverse populations of varying cultures. New smart technology and applications continue to emerge, helping youth engage in mindfulness-based practice, coping skills, and effective management of their diagnoses. New advances in artificial intelligence, mobile applications, wearable gadgets, and remote patient monitoring have been purposed for mental and behavioral health and show efficacy in younger populations, with high engagement and satisfaction.

However, with these changes in technology, numerous ethical, legal, and treatment challenges arise, offering a robust debate on the role of technology in the practice of psychiatry. Despite these debates, innovation continues to have effects on the culture of psychiatry itself, creating a culture of technology that impacts youth and their families.

Clinical Vignette

Martin, a 14-year-old eighth grader with a reported history of ADHD, was referred to an outpatient clinic because of mood dysregulation and recent suspensions from school due to increased aggression. Reports from the school indicated that Martin may be on the autism spectrum because he has difficulties during social interactions, has few friends, and is noted to have rigid thinking much of the time. He is being raised by his maternal grandmother, the only relative involved in his care, who has lived in the community most of her life. The small community has a majority population below the poverty level, and resources are scarce. The clinic where Martin was referred recently contracted with a rural school district two counties away in order to provide support via telepsychiatry sessions to local counselors referring patients with behavioral or mood disorders or who exhibit disruptive behaviors.

The psychiatrist immediately noticed that Martin has a connection with the local clinician, a nurse who serves all the students in the district. They seem to have good rapport, talking in the clinical room despite Martin's poor eye contact and tendency to change the subject back to a car magazine he is holding. The psychiatrist noted that Martin's grandmother is present but appears to be somewhat uncomfortable. On evaluation, Martin was cooperative but had difficulties remaining calm and still within the scope of the session and at one point left the room entirely. With Martin gone, his grandmother shared with the psychiatrist that this experience is strange for her because she only recently got a smartphone and Wi-Fi at home. She noted that she likes to meet her doctors and "look them in the eye" but said she knows that Martin really needs help to be successful in school. She asked the psychiatrist where she is from, where she went to school, and whether she has ever been to "this neck of the woods." After the psychiatrist made her recommendations, Martin's grandmother asked how to contact her between visits, how medications will be sent, and what to do if there is a need or question outside scheduled appointments.

Telepsychiatry and Mental Health Care Via Telehealth Services

Over the past two decades, the culture of psychiatry has seen a dramatic shift in the use of technology and videoconferencing in the delivery of care to patients. With flexibility and a few adaptations as needed, telepsychiatry is an effective means to connect care to patients and demonstrates continued ability to capture verbal, nonverbal, and clinical observations as compared with in-person care (American Academy of Child and Adolescent Psychiatry 2017; Gloff et al. 2015). Telepsychiatry has been helpful in bridging gaps and bringing psychiatrists and specialists to help youth in need. Importantly, telepsychiatry moves psychiatric care from clinic to community, engaging families, local providers and resources, and the cultural influences that impact patient care (Gloff et al. 2015).

Access to care has been impacted significantly by this cultural shift. As noted in Chapter 1, "Introduction to Cultural Psychiatry," 20% of youth in the United States have a psychiatric diagnosis, and with increasing legislation expanding care and parity, more individuals and families are seeking mental health care. Unfortunately, a majority of children and adolescents are unable to find psychiatric care, and clinicians have needed to be inventive in the provision of care for this expanding care-seeking population (American Academy of Child and Adolescent Psychiatry 2017, 2019; Gloff et al. 2015).

Telepsychiatry has been one avenue to increase the access to mental health care despite a continued and increasing national shortage of child psychiatrists, higher levels of retirees than new practitioners, and geographic maldistribution of providers (American Academy of Child and Adolescent Psychiatry 2017, 2019; Flaum 2013; Gloff et al. 2015). Importantly, the expansion of services has offered youth populations opportunities to receive evidence-based services from specialists, especially for young people living in rural and underserved communities facing declining economies; poor access to care, insurance, and transportation; and possible stigmatization in traditional mental health clinics (Gloff et al. 2015). The cultural impact of telepsychiatry is broad, with several ethical, financial, clinical, and legal implications (see section "Legal, Ethical, and Practical Considerations in Technology"). Additionally, technology impacts culture through its geographic reach and by its ability to provide diverse clinical sites that include day care centers, schools, detention centers, pediatricians' offices, and even patients' homes.

Notably, telepsychiatry studies in youth are sparse but promising. Several technology-based mental health studies have been completed in diverse adult populations, with findings that equal or surpass clinical outcomes of office-based, in-person patients. Studies on children and adolescents have shown similar, comparable results; the American Academy of Child and Adolescent Psychiatry "Practice Parameter for Telepsychiatry With Children and Adolescents" (American Academy of Child and Adolescent Psychiatry 2017) offers a robust meta-analysis of studies that have been completed in youth and adult populations. Randomized control trials in youth have demonstrated equal efficacy between in-person and online treatment of major depression, Tourette's disorder and tic disorders, behavioral therapy and interventions for ADHD, oppositional defiant disorder (ODD), other disruptive behavior disorders, and parent management training (American Academy of Child and Adolescent Psychiatry 2017). Other trials have even demonstrated increased efficacy of telepsychiatry compared with in-person visits in obsessive-compulsive disorder, anxiety, and insomnia (Aboujaoude et al. 2015; American Academy of Child and Adolescent Psychiatry 2017; American Telemedicine Association 2017; Siemer et al. 2011).

Other studies have shown improvements in family relationships, symptom severity, treatment compliance, and psychoeducation. In customer satisfaction studies, youth, parents, and consulting providers all reported high levels of satisfaction in the remote delivery of care when compared with in-person management; in fact, some studies showed higher satisfaction than with face-to-face encounters (Myers et al. 2008). Diagnostic validity was comparable to in-person visits, and telepsychiatry was a reasonable alternative for treatment of psychosomatic complaints in youth (Aboujaoude et al. 2015; American Academy of Child and Adolescent Psychiatry 2017; American Telemedicine Association 2017; Siemer et al. 2011). Although few studies have tracked the use of teletherapy in the child and adolescent population, this mode of therapy, especially in manualized modalities, is feasible and comparable to in-person therapy, acceptable and satisfying for patients in varying settings, and appropriate for a myriad of diverse patient populations (Aboujaoude et al. 2015; American Academy of Child and Adolescent Psychiatry 2017; American Telemedicine Association 2017; Borders 2017; Siemer et al. 2011).

Additionally, these findings have been replicated in culturally diverse populations, indicating that telepsychiatry is helpful in providing support to youth and families from various backgrounds (American Academy of Child and Adolescent Psychiatry 2017; American Telemedicine Association 2017). Studies have also extrapolated cultural aspects of care in telepsychiatry with adult patients to youth populations facing similar psychiatric and behavioral needs (Aboujaoude et al. 2015; American Academy of Child and Adolescent Psychiatry 2017; American Telemedicine Association 2017; Borders 2017; Siemer et al. 2011). Many clinicians note that the youth population, which is more adept with technology, may benefit from the use of these modalities, even without robust evidence of efficacy demonstrated in specific youth populations. Those studies that have captured diverse youth have supported findings in similar adult populations. Additionally, studies and systematic literature reviews have shown efficacy in telepsychiatry and teletherapy use within rural, underserved urban communities; immigrant, ethnic, and racial minority populations; incarcerated youth; and other diverse populations, many of which currently lack access to quality mental health care outside this delivery mode.

Mobile Technology, Teletherapy, Remote Patient Monitoring, and E-Health Solutions

With smartphones, tablets, and the advent of applications and broad mobile service, technology has begun to expand beyond telepsychiatry to services that patients can access from their own home, using their own devices. These services range from synchronous to asynchronous care, mood and symptom tracking, therapy, and a myriad of others. According to data from the Pew Research Center (Anderson and Jiang 2018), the reach of these technologies may be broad: 95% of teens, as young as 13 years, have access to a smartphone, and 88% have access to a computer; additionally, technology use and access are nearly universal among teens of different genders, races, ethnicities, and socioeconomic backgrounds. Another study (Torous et al. 2014) noted that 97% of individuals with a mental health diagnosis own a smartphone, with a vast majority of these patients being supportive of using mobile applications to monitor their condition. The advent of technology and its widespread use has created a unique opportunity for the free market to create mental health–related applications, services, and tools that expand or extend existing care to patients.

Ongoing advances are constant and create new trends for youth to engage in technology for auxiliary and direct care services to improve mental health outcomes, even in challenging areas such as compliance, adherence, education, and engagement. New evidence continues to show that children and adolescents are ever more engaged with mobile technology and e-health, using technology and texting for appointment and medication reminders, engaging in mobile therapy, and using remote patient monitoring and mobile symptom reports to relay real-time data to their providers (Carter 2018). There is a paucity of literature regarding newer technologies such as virtual reality exposure therapy, but existing studies have indicated positive results for patients (Aboujaoude et al. 2015). All child mental health technicians should be aware of these new advances, screen for their use, and be familiar with potential strengths and risks associated with the use of these tools (Torous and Roberts 2017). Use of unvetted applications can lead to patients being exposed to information that is not evidence based and is potentially even harmful to their health, whereas other apps may be a helpful adjunct to their provider-based care. Because not all providers are tech-savvy, understanding these advances may require some research on the provider's end, which will prove necessary when it comes to educating and supporting the youth population and their families. New tools are being developed to help providers navigate these applications. One such tool that can be used by multiple disciplines is an online resource that allows providers to review applications and online services that impact mental health (American Psychiatric Association 2019). Understanding these services being used by patients, psychiatrists, or other mental health professionals can help providers evaluate these technology-based mental health platforms in order to make an informed decision regarding their use (Table 15–1).

Other solutions outside of traditional telepsychiatry have also been evaluated. One meta-analysis revealed efficacy in the use of computerized cognitive-behavioral therapy models, both standalone and therapist-guided, specifically among pediatric populations as compared with psychoeducation and traditional therapy (Aboujaoude et al. 2015; American Academy of Child and Adolescent Psychiatry 2017; American Telemedicine Association 2017; Borders 2017; Siemer et al. 2011). Studies also showed positive outcomes in online therapy use, regardless of whether therapy was conducted in real time with videoconferencing or in asynchrony (Aboujaoude et al. 2015; Yellowlees et al. 2008). Teletherapy continues to be highly utilized and has the potential to reach the youth population. Although synchronous and asynchronous therapy have been provided via teleconferencing systems, newer and more readily available application-based therapy has proven efficacious, increasing access to care and helping to train clinicians on the various therapy modalities, thus expanding patient care (American Academy of Child and Adolescent Psychia-

TABLE 15–1.   **Model for evaluating applications**

Step	Description
Access and background	Decide whether to proceed with further evaluation of the app by reviewing basic features such as conflicts of interest, costs, accessibility, and updates
Security	Evaluate risks, including data costs, social profiling, loss of insurance benefits or insurability, and privacy
Clinical foundation and effectiveness	Download the app to verify the content for correctness, relevance, and evidence of benefit
Usability	Review the engagement styles, features, and functional scope; determine if the app is customizable and easy to use
Interoperability	Determine whether the data can be integrated toward therapeutic goals

Source.   American Psychiatric Association: App evaluation model. 2020. Available at: www.psychiatry.org/psychiatrists/practice/mental-health-apps/app-evaluation-model. Accessed May 5, 2020.

try 2017; American Telemedicine Association 2017). However, teletherapy often is provided anonymously, creating unique ethical dilemmas and unclear long-term efficacy or outcomes.

Remote patient monitoring (RPM), a technology that has been used in chronic health conditions, has recently begun to embrace care for patients with mental health diagnoses. RPM, provided via mobile applications (usually using a patient's own smartphone) or devices provided by the treating clinician, can be an effective tool for patient engagement and symptom monitoring in the patient's home setting. The technology can deliver interactive and educational content, collect self-report and biometric data, provide insights based on collected data, and support users in receiving assistance during crises. Many RPM applications also incorporate telepsychiatry and videoconferencing, allowing patients to interact with psychiatrists and their health care team outside outpatient or hospital settings. Studies have shown efficacy in increased medication compliance due to medication reminders, better symptom reporting and tracking, resolution of clinical issues and improvements in health (e.g., medication side effects, medication titration, symptom control) before appointments, higher satisfaction and engagement from patients, and prevention of self-harm and suicide attempts (Adams et al. 2017; Carter 2018; Dhulipala et al. 2016; Faurholt-Jepsen et al. 2014; Naslund et al. 2015). Use of this technology also allows for physician resources and time to be utilized judiciously by triaging and engaging with patients who may need more acute, in-person care while collecting needed self-report and biometric data to track and treat any clinical needs for future encounters.

Legal, Ethical, and Practical Considerations in Technology

There is a vital need for psychiatrists to be active and knowledgeable about the legal and ethical components of telepsychiatry. Along with competency in the practice of psychiatry, practitioners should be abreast of federal and state regulations overseeing technology and telepsychiatry. Issues related to these regulations include, but are not limited to, billing and coding for

TABLE 15-2.   Goals of the Interstate Medical Licensure Compact

Expand reach of child psychiatrists (and other subspecialists) to facilitate access to care in communities
located in rural, underserved areas

Increase collaboration and communication between primary or pediatric care and psychiatrists

Streamline emergency and disaster responses by addressing licensing concerns

Support the clinical leadership of psychiatrists in special communities (e.g., schools, juvenile justice,
reservations, rural areas)

Enhance care coordination for patients and families relocating to underserved areas

Source.   Interstate Medical Licensure Compact, https://imlcc.org. Accessed November 9, 2019.

these services, licensure and the provision of care in multiple states, malpractice insurance requirements, and prescribing of controlled substances. The Ryan Haight Online Pharmacy Con-
sumer Protection Act of 2008 increased restrictions on the practice of psychiatry and
telemedicine, offering confusing and conflicting regulations on the use of technology in the delivery of care for patients. Increased precaution and diligence must provide for confidentiality
to comply with federal regulations that include the Health Insurance Portability and Accountability Act of 1996 and the Family Educational Rights and Privacy Act, and clear informed consent procedures are vital for the safe practice of telepsychiatry (American Academy of Child
and Adolescent Psychiatry 2017; American Telemedicine Association 2017).

Medical licensure is also an important consideration in the delivery of remote mental health
care. Initiatives such as the Interstate Medical Licensure Compact (IMLC) have sought to expand
care via telemedicine to underserved areas through expediting licensure in multiple states by using
physician licensing information from the primary state in which they practice. This compact ex-
pands needed care while increasing patient rights and public protection by enhancing the ability
of states to share licensing, investigative, and disciplinary information (Interstate Medical Licensure Compact 2019). As noted by the American Academy of Pediatrics (2020), the use of this
compact via telemedicine delivers subspecialty consultation, including psychiatry, to children
and families residing in underserved communities. Telemedicine can impact the youth population goals of the IMLC noted in Table 15–2.

Another area of concern is the need to understand the development of rapport and therapeutic alliance through teletherapy. Other issues that must be addressed are confidentiality and privacy concerns. High dropout rates and the need to increase continuity of care are reported in
some studies (Aboujaoude et al. 2015; American Academy of Child and Adolescent Psychiatry
2017; American Telemedicine Association 2017). Financial concerns related to health insurance coverage, malpractice coverage, and ongoing licensing issues are also an area of concern.
Additionally, in application-based and Web-based therapy, anonymous or asynchronous counseling may not adequately respond to patients in immediate crisis, preventing these individuals
from receiving emergency care from the same practitioner who has been providing their treatment. Online security and confidentiality breaches remain prevalent concerns, especially with
privacy scandals recently reported among several major technological corporations.

Practitioners will also need to be proactive in defining the scope of their practice. The use
of technology within the field of child and adolescent psychiatry may include consultative services to pediatricians, therapists, or school counselors who are involved in direct patient care.

Mental health workers coordinate administrative tasks and safety and emergency planning while determining what type of patients are appropriate to participate in telepsychiatry and distant care. It is also important for practitioners to discuss with patients specifics of care delivery, including therapy, prescriptions, and escalation of care.

More research is needed to understand safety around telepsychiatry use, despite the efficacious outcomes seen in studies. As noted by several researchers, the mindset that "if it does not help, it does not hurt" cannot be accepted regarding the use of these modalities (Aboujaoude et al. 2015). The role of a mental health provider should be to provide quality, evidence-based care to patients, especially with newer mediums that can present new challenges. Patient security and safety are needed, along with more understanding of when and how the technology should be used. In ongoing debates, some mental health professionals see telepsychiatry as a supplement or alternative to the gold standard of face-to-face treatment, whereas others highlight the positive outcomes seen in research and clinical practice as an indication that a standalone practice of telepsychiatry can be efficacious in any setting. There is also a need for further research in working with diverse populations, from demographics to diagnosis, to understand how this technology can best be further used (Aboujaoude et al. 2015; American Academy of Child and Adolescent Psychiatry 2017; American Telemedicine Association 2017).

Additionally, with more free market engagement in providing services for patients outside the scope of traditional physician-led care, there is a need for caution and careful evaluation of unregulated mental health applications and technology. Several national organizations have begun to review and rate various applications available to patients to determine their safety, efficacy, and relevance to patient care. Especially when treating the youth population, providers should be abreast of the latest applications, devices, and technology used by patients and should also screen for use, educating patients of the risks or how the technology may supplement their care.

Clinical Vignette *(Continued)*

Martin continued monthly remote sessions with his therapist, and a therapeutic relationship was built with both Martin and his grandmother. They were happy to meet the psychiatrist when she came to the clinic a few months ago. Following the psychiatrist's recommendations, Martin's grandmother sought applied behavioral analysis therapy near her home but without success. She asks if there is a way for Martin "to use the computer to do his therapy" or if there is an app she can download to help with his progress.

Martin's grandmother recently saw a news report regarding health information and technology, and she asks about privacy and confidentiality concerns. They live in a small town, and she is worried about Martin being judged for being "different" because he is seeing a mental health provider. She has multiple questions regarding who has access to his records, whether the videos are recorded, how information is communicated between the clinic and the doctor, and how Martin's privacy is protected. She also asks about communicating directly with the psychiatrist between visits via e-mail or phone calls for any issues or questions that arise.

Technology, Culture, and the Impact on Psychiatric Care for Youth

Rarely has the discussion of culture included the multidimensional, reflexive dynamic it has within health care and advances in technology. It is widely known that cultural beliefs regarding the nature of illness and the effectiveness of conventional, traditional, and alternative therapies impact health care delivery and outcomes; these beliefs impact behavior and how families interact with health systems, comply with medications, and engage in treatment (Savin et al. 2011). Culture also impacts the time, money, and resources that a family will spend in seeking health and wellness commensurate with their beliefs and means. Meanwhile, the prevalent health care culture determines what resources and clinical services will be offered to various populations on the basis of available resources, current needs, and practical allocation opportunities in communities—that is, finding partnerships and networking opportunities to expand care. Therefore, clinicians must recognize the interplay between culture, politics, and health care in order to provide leadership in navigating the complex, nuanced issues that may arise in providing quality, technology-based care to patients in need.

It is important for practitioners who work with youth populations to recognize the cultural influences that must be addressed in any provision of care; these issues are central to practicing culturally competent care and must be at the forefront when providing care remotely through technology. There is a significant need for providers to be aware of local child-rearing practices in communities that they are serving, observe the child's behavior to determine deviations from a cultural standard, and understand their role in diagnosing and treating as perceived by the patient and family (Savin et al. 2011). Research highlights the need for the psychiatrist to be an ethnographer, seeking to understand and incorporate the local culture into treatment, while also understanding how the provider's own culture, as well as beliefs around medication use, will influence the delivery of care, especially in telepsychiatry (Kleinman and Benson 2006). As with in-person care, practitioners providing distant care must be more diligent about understanding patients' culture, their own personal culture and biases, and the interplay between these sometimes differing views.

Collaboration to Expand Access to Care

In order to address the needs of culturally diverse youth populations and to expand access to care, the practice of psychiatry in areas lacking mental health resources has gone through a cultural shift that includes working within current systems while including colleagues from other specialties. It is important to seek consultation with local practitioners and psychiatric colleagues familiar with the needs of the community being treated, especially when the person providing care is not a member of the patient's cultural group or lacks understanding of local cultural influences (Savin et al. 2011). Integrated care models or patient-centered medical homes have also been developed in several areas, using existing providers, such as local pediatricians, who have been trained by psychiatrists to treat mental health disorders (American Academy of Child and Adolescent Psychiatry 2017; Margolis et al. 2018). This shift in practice has focused on psychiatrists becoming trainers, educators, and consultants in addition to clinicians, adapting to a role that can serve communities seeking care. Various models exist in rural or low-access areas, with psychiatrists providing direct care, serving only as a consultant, or practicing a mixture of these two modalities (Gloff et al. 2015; Margolis et al. 2018).

Telepsychiatry has been used effectively in diverse child and adolescent populations; findings have shown that this medium is useful for diverse patient populations with varying races, ethnicities, socioeconomic levels, geographical locations, and practice settings (Savin et al. 2011). Research has provided numerous examples of telepsychiatry supporting culturally sensitive collaborative treatment (CSCT) and helping practitioners recognize symptoms in patients from populations that stigmatize mental illness (Yeung et al. 2010). CSCT is focused on 1) training primary care providers on mental health and cultural competency and use of appropriate screening measures to identify particular cultural identities within a population, using an appropriate clinical interview that incorporates the patient's culture into the discussion and collaboration and consultation between the psychiatrist and community physicians and 2) care management (Kleinman and Benson 2006; Yeung et al. 2010). The CSCT model has been applied to telepsychiatry with significantly positive results for patients with poor access to mental health care needing providers versed in cultural competency and psychiatry.

Cultural Competency and Technology

When interacting with and treating diverse populations, culturally competent care is vital in order to achieve positive health outcomes. Telepsychiatry can create opportunities for communities to access specialists who are trained in mental health and common cultural manifestations of mental illness. Technology-based care can also create connections via culture. It can expand access to care and build powerful connections via a provider who shares the patient's cultural background or speaks the patient's primary language (Yeung et al. 2010). Psychiatrists must also recognize their position of privilege when providing care for diverse populations. Minority groups that have historically or traditionally experienced ostracism, persecution, or discrimination by the majority population may view the provider as a member of that oppressing group. The literature expounds on examples such as rural versus urban, indigenous peoples versus government, race relations, and class and socioeconomic systems (Savin et al. 2011; Shore et al. 2006). It is important for psychiatrists to understand these unique power dynamics in the provision of mental health care while also understanding the role telepsychiatry, technology, and lack of face-to-face contact might play in influencing this gradation.

The Cultural Formulation Interview from the 5th Edition of the *Diagnostic and Statistical Manual of Mental Disorders* (American Psychiatric Association 2013) provides a cultural framework for delivery of culturally competent care that is relevant to telepsychiatry and the use of technology in the practice of psychiatry. Research and clinical experience with cultural formulation and telepsychiatry are limited but promising. Clinicians have used the four core components in the delivery of care distantly through telepsychiatry (see Chapter 21, "DSM-5 Outline for Cultural Formulation and Cultural Formulation Interview"), and use of the CFI has improved patient experiences, satisfaction, and outcomes (Brooks et al. 2013; Hilty et al. 2018).

Telepsychiatry can help address health disparities that commonly are seen in minority communities and increase access to care for vulnerable populations. Health care disparities are especially substantial within mental health, and technology and telepsychiatry have the potential to shorten such disparities by facilitating care delivery to rural, remote, and underserved populations (Savin et al. 2006; Shore et al. 2006). Interestingly, traditional racial disparities in access are reversed for smartphones: regardless of household income, 85% of non-Hispanic Black teens have access to a smartphone, compared with 71% of non-Hispanic white teenagers and 71% of Hispanic teenagers (Powell et al. 2017). Recent findings note that these numbers are even higher in all demographic groups, with little impact of gender, race, ethnicity, and socioeconomic status (Anderson and Jiang 2018). These findings highlight that technology, when used strategically and appropriately, can be used more easily than more traditional, in-person approaches to reach underserved communities.

Telepsychiatry studies related to psychiatry and cultural and identity in children remain limited; however, it can be extrapolated from adult studies that effective, competent care can be provided to children and adolescent populations of ethnic and racial minorities. Adult studies have shown positive health outcomes in distance, technology-based care in underserved Hispanic, Asian, immigrant, and lower socioeconomic populations; in fact, telepsychiatry has high rates of use in these populations, which lack access to child psychiatrists in their community (Pumariega and Rothe 2003; Savin et al. 2006, 2011). Additionally, families living in remote rural areas have worse mental health outcomes that have been linked to poor access to care and lack of mental health services and support. Several studies have indicated that the use of telepsychiatry can improve outcomes for families living in remote areas and alleviate some costs and protect resources (Savin et al. 2011). Although research continues to highlight health disparities for many of these populations, access issues can be alleviated with the appropriate use of technology-based remote interventions.

Technology, Culture, and Practical Application

Via technology, providers with expertise in mental health and cultural competency can expand their personal reach to educate patients and other providers to better understand and alleviate culturally based disparities and barriers. When determining the appropriate patient population for technology-based care, providers must not only evaluate clinical diagnosis and treatment considerations but also appreciate the roles race, ethnicity, geography, socioeconomic status, and other cultural factors play in the delivery of care. Often, psychiatrists providing care via telepsychiatry do not live in the community they are treating, an important cultural consideration that may influence the efficacy of telepsychiatric care. Providers raised, trained, or practicing in an urban area must be aware of the nuances of living in a rural environment and the impact this may have on patients' communication, culture, and world view (Savin et al. 2011; Shore et al.

2006). Although technology may increase access to care, providers must account for cultural considerations in order to ensure effective care. When considering culture and technology related to patient care, there is a heightened need to evaluate the patient and his or her specific needs when using telepsychiatry. Before addressing common features of a patient's cultural identity, the clinician must first understand the patient's experience with technology and the use of video-conferencing devices (Pumariega and Rothe 2003; Savin et al. 2006).

A patient's experience with technology is affected by age and education; younger patients and those with higher levels of education tend to be the most adept at using technology in health care (Shore et al. 2006). This bodes well for the child and adolescent psychiatrist treating youth and transitional-age populations distantly. Often, the cultural challenges in telepsychiatry are related to the interactions with parents and guardians who may be less familiar with the use of certain technologies. For those patients and families who are uncomfortable or unfamiliar with telepsychiatry, a significant portion of the initial visit should be dedicated to querying this comfort level and determining if adjustments can or should be made; in addition, throughout treatment, patient feedback should be elicited regarding the continued use of the technology for their care (Shore et al. 2006).

Poor access to care seems to be a major cultural factor in the advent and sustained use of telepsychiatry and technology. Cultural barriers to care that may be mediated by the use of technology include geography and access to care from a remote location. Technology can address patients' lack of transportation and alleviate specific issues such as lack of language proficiency or cultural stigma regarding mental health and health seeking (Borders 2017). Several studies have indicated that specific adult populations, such as the elderly and veterans, may benefit from telepsychiatry and access to care, but the technology may also be applicable to diverse youth populations such as recent immigrants, rural families, refugee and asylum seekers, and families with low proficiency in the language of the majority culture (Borders 2017). Findings have shown that patients are able to build strong therapeutic alliances and have high satisfaction scores and that technology may alleviate potential barriers in such domains as culture, age, language, geography, cognition, and income inequality (Borders 2017; Kopel et al. 2001). Providers and patients have noted some apprehension and concerns about the lessening of humanity when using technology to deliver care, despite growing literature on the satisfaction and high level of engagement from patients. However, current research indicates that over time, technology fades to the background, sometimes after an initial awkwardness, to create a natural, therapeutic relationship between doctor and patient (Savin et al. 2011).

Psychiatrists need to recognize and address fears of a confidentiality breach using this medium and address the positive and negative clinical impacts that distance care may have on the therapeutic relationship. Providers might find that some patients, especially those coming from rural or remote communities, may prefer the level of confidentiality technology provides (Shore et al. 2006). Clinical anecdotes support the use of teletherapy in patients who struggle with establishing close interpersonal relationships, such as in patients with PTSD and autism spectrum disorders, who may prefer distance from the psychiatrist providing care (Shore et al. 2006).

It is also important to understand verbal and nonverbal cues relevant to culture as well as communication styles influenced by culture and/or technology that may impact treatment decisions. Examples include culturally accepted lack of eye contact or the need for the psychiatrist to be more assertive and direct than is necessary during in-person evaluations (Shore et al. 2006). Some patients are hesitant to interact with a provider they cannot meet in person, wanting to have a concrete, physical interaction with their psychiatrist (e.g., a handshake, eye contact); other patients may have issues with physical interaction that are rectified via telepsychiatry, alleviating potential negative experiences that can occur between providers and patients of different cultures.

Other aspects of nonverbal communication that should be considered in telepsychiatry pertain to the mental status examination, behavioral observations and assessments, developmental milestones, and play. Appropriate staffing (i.e., consistent facilitators at the clinical site) may alleviate any cultural and observational gaps that might be present. These facilitators may be able to provide needed in-person experiences, such as offering play opportunities, collecting and sharing data and information (e.g., patient drawings), and discussing observations not conveyable via technology (e.g., odor, parent-child interactions before the session) (Gloff et al. 2015; Margolis et al. 2018; Savin et al. 2011; Shore et al. 2006). Interestingly, telepsychiatry may also allow for newer, more innovative ways to engage with technologically inclined cohorts, such as watching YouTube videos or listening to songs on Spotify to build rapport (Savin et al. 2011). These experiences can also provide the clinician cultural insight into the child, adolescent, or family that may otherwise not happen in a traditional, in-person format. Appropriate staffing and a strong relationship with facilitators from the treatment community present an avenue for information about local history, geography, and culture. These local liaisons can also help the telepsychiatrist keep up with local news and events (Savin et al. 2011; Shore et al. 2006).

Providers may be able to alleviate cultural and communication barriers by visiting the clinical location to understand the community's values and resources and introduce themselves in person (Gloff et al. 2015; Margolis et al. 2018; Savin et al. 2011; Shore et al. 2006). This alleviation of cultural differences can also be achieved by becoming acquainted with the nuances and values exhibited in clinical locations such as schools, reservations, rural areas, and detention centers (Gloff et al. 2015; Margolis et al. 2018; Myers et al. 2006; Pumariega and Rothe 2003; Savin et al. 2006, 2011; Shore et al. 2006). Examples in the literature range from provider visits to gain an experiential understanding of local remoteness and poverty to rapport-building measures such as learning about local foods and the geographic layout of the area where patients live (Savin et al. 2011). Shared experiences, regardless of patient and provider location, are pivotal for the development of a therapeutic relationship, and a local visit may help develop these connections in distance mental health care (Savin et al. 2006; Shore et al. 2006).

In addition, telepsychiatry can provide several clinical benefits to the psychiatrist. Telepsychiatry can open educational opportunities for providers to learn about new cultures and expand their clinical expertise in diverse patient populations (Savin et al. 2011). From a practical sense, distance care can also cut down on commute times, allowing providers to see more patients, thus increasing time and financial resources. Telepsychiatry reports have shown higher utilization of services, with positive outcomes and improvement in patients; decreased costs for patients due to lower travel expenses; and an increase in market competition, with decreased operation costs and potential for higher earnings for psychiatrists (Powell et al. 2017).

Educational and Systems-Based Shifts in Psychiatry

There has been a cultural shift in the education of future psychiatrists toward understanding culture and the use of innovative technology in the practice of psychiatry. Programs across the country are embracing new educational modalities that increase education on culturally sensitive use of technology in the delivery of mental health care. Telepsychiatry education is being associated with training competencies and milestones with support from the American Psychiatric Association, American Academy of Child and Adolescent Psychiatry, and American Telemedicine Association. These organizations seek to ensure standardized frameworks and evidence-based metrics based on current research via proven models such as the one used by the U.S. Department of Veteran Affairs (American Academy of Child and Adolescent Psychiatry 2017). Research and emerging literature highlight the need to train clinicians in both cultural competency and changing technologies impacting the practice of psychiatry (Khan and Ramtekkar 2019; Shore et al. 2006).

In the changing practice of psychiatry and technology, there is a need to understand that common terms may also be evolving. Providers must recognize that *system transference* may be an important phenomenon in the use of telepsychiatry. These positive and negative feelings or experiences may influence patients' perspectives on the use of technology in their care; negative emotions must be met with inquiry, empathy, and support to help patients work within systems that utilize telehealth (Shore et al. 2006).

Understandably, the use of telepsychiatry commonly includes interactions between bureaucratic systems, various electronic medical records, other providers, and support staff; these dynamics must be met with the understanding that care and organizational culture must be focused on the patient, not the organizations coordinating delivery (Shore et al. 2006). Psychiatrists must also recognize that with increasing use of technology, they may have to spend considerable time navigating multiple institutional and administrative cultures. This can often impede, rather than support, ease of care. These competing operational and clinical cultures usually exist through differing clinical procedures, goals of service, and bureaucratic policy. Strategies to address administrative and clinical issues impacting telehealth delivery and utilization should be an integral part of an organization's structure and should include specific processes to address any problems that are bound to arise. Telepsychiatry requires a team-based approach between the home and clinical sites to create a united approach to patient care that is analogous to the therapeutic alliance pursued between provider and patient (Savin et al. 2011).

Conclusion

The culture of psychiatry and mental health care has been highly impacted by the expansion of technology, including telepsychiatry and other services, in the delivery of services to youth patients and their families. This shift has allowed for traditionally underserved patients to have access to care and to expand culturally humble care to these populations. The use of these mediums presents unique legal, ethical, and practical considerations while also increasing the knowledge requirements needed by child psychiatrists regarding new applications, services, and tools used by their patients.

The use of telepsychiatry, specifically, creates new opportunities for collaboration with other providers, expanding the role of the psychiatrist from clinician to include educator, trainer, and consultant. With the expansion of care, more patient populations have access to treatment, which is especially important for patients coming from underserved communities with no previous access to mental health care. Often, the telepsychiatrist must also be a cultural psychiatrist, recognizing the challenges associated with long-distance care while considering the cultural factors that may influence such care. This requires cultural humility and consideration of the practical application of psychiatry via teleconferencing, understanding the dynamics between patient, family, and provider, and taking into account larger influences such as the local community, the patient's culture, and systems-based challenges that may interplay when providing care for culturally diverse children, adolescents, and families.

Self-Assessment Questions

1. Which of the following describes system transference in mental health telecare?

    A. Positive or negative emotions that *patients* may experience regarding the use of telecare as they navigate bureaucratic or organizational systems of care, teledelivery experiences, technology use, and distance care.
    B. Positive or negative emotions that *providers* may experience regarding the use of telecare as they navigate bureaucratic or organizational systems of care, teledelivery experiences, technology use, and distance care.
    C. Positive or negative emotions that patients experience regarding bureaucratic delivery of care in large health systems.
    D. The way in which patients navigate systems of care that provide mental health care via telehealth services.

2. What is the primary goal of the Interstate Medical Licensure Compact?

    A. To create partnerships between multiple states to increase support for physicians and to expand physician geographical reach.
    B. To expand care to underserved areas via licensure in the physician's primary practice state, thereby increasing patient rights and public protection by enhancing the ability of states to share licensing, investigative, and disciplinary information.
    C. To alleviate costs for state licensure boards and expand licensure to physicians in multiple states.
    D. To help urban areas meet the demand for providers for their large patient populations.

3. Research on the efficacy of mental health care via telehealth services, even with diverse patient populations, has shown which of the following?

A. Varying outcomes compared with in-person delivery.
B. Equivalent or better outcomes compared with in-person delivery.
C. Worse outcomes compared with in-person delivery.
D. Telehealth services are limited and cannot be compared with in-person delivery.

Answers

1. A
2. B
3. B

References

Aboujaoude E, Salame W, Naim L: Telemental health: a status update. World Psychiatry 14(2):223–230, 2015

Adams ZW, McClure EA, Gray KM, et al: Mobile devices for the remote acquisition of physiological and behavioral biomarkers in psychiatric clinical research. J Psychiatr Res 85:1–14, 2017

American Academy of Child and Adolescent Psychiatry: Workforce maps by state. Washington, DC, American Academy of Child and Adolescent Psychiatry, 2019. Available at: www.aacap.org/aacap/Advocacy/Federal_and_State_Initiatives/Workforce_Maps/Home.aspx. Accessed November 9, 2019.

American Academy of Child and Adolescent Psychiatry (AACAP) Committee on Telepsychiatry and AACAP Committee of Quality Issues: Clinical update: telepsychiatry with children and adolescents. J Am Acad Child Adolesc Psychiatry 56(10):875–893, 2017

American Academy of Pediatrics: Interstate Medical Licensure Compact: advocacy action guide for AAP chapters. Itasca, IL, American Academy of Pediatrics, 2020. Available at: www.aap.org/en-us/advocacy-and-policy/state-advocacy/Documents/Interstate%20Medical%20Licensure%20Compact-Advocacy%20Action%20Guide%20for%20AAP%20Chapters.pdf. Accessed May 5, 2020.

American Psychiatric Association: Diagnostic and Statistical Manual of Mental Disorders, 5th Edition. Arlington, VA, American Psychiatric Association, 2013

American Psychiatric Association: Mental health apps. Washington, DC, American Psychiatric Association, 2019. Available at: www.psychiatry.org/psychiatrists/practice/mental-health-apps. Accessed November 9, 2019.

American Telemedicine Association Telemental Health with Children and Adolescents Work Group: Practice guidelines for telemental health with children and adolescents. March 2017. Available at: https://higherlogicdownload.s3.amazonaws.com/AMERICANTELEMED/618da447-dee1-4ee1-b941-c5bf3db5669a/UploadedImages/Practice%20Guideline%20Covers/NEW_ATA%20Children%20and%20Adolescents%20Guidelines.pdf. Accessed November 9, 2019.

Anderson M, Jiang J: Teens, social media & technology. Washington, DC, Pew Research Center, 2018. Available at: http://publicservicesalliance.org/wp-content/uploads/2018/06/Teens-Social-Media-Technology-2018-Pew-Research-Center.pdf. Accessed September 4, 2020.

Borders CB: Realizing the promises of telepsychiatry in special populations. Ment Illn 9(1):7135, 2017

Brooks E, Spargo G, Yellowlees PM, et al: Integrating culturally appropriate care into telemental health practice, in Telemental Health: Clinical, Technical, and Administrative Foundations for Evidence-Based Practice. Edited by Myers K, Turvey CL, Waltham, MA. Saint Louis, MO, Elsevier Science, 2013, pp 63–80

Carter RD: Case study: improving behavioral health outcomes: utilizing enterprise virtual care technology. Parsippany, NJ, Medocity, 2018. Available at: https://medocity.com/wp-content/uploads/2018/12/Carter CaseStudy.pdf. Accessed May 5, 2020.

Dhulipala VRS, Devadas P, Murthy PHST: Mobile phone sensing mechanism for stress relaxation using sensor networks: a survey. Wireless Personal Communications 86(2):1013–1022, 2016

Faurholt-Jepsen M, Frost M, Vinberg M, et al: Smartphone data as objective measures of bipolar disorder symptoms. Psychiatry Res 217(1):124–127, 2014

Flaum M: Telemental health as a solution to the widening gap between supply and demand for mental health services, in Telemental Health: Clinical, Technical, and Administrative Foundations for Evidence-Based Practice. Edited by Myers K, Turvey CL. Waltham, MA, Elsevier, 2013, pp 11–25

Gloff NE, LeNoue SR, Novins DD, et al: Telemental health for children and adolescents. Int Rev Psychiatry 27(6):513–524, 2015

Hilty DM, Evangelatos G, Valasquez GA, et al: Telehealth for rural diverse populations: cultural and telebehavioral competencies and practical approaches for clinical services. J Technol Behav Sci 3:206–220, 2018

Interstate Medical Licensure Compact: The IMLC. Denver, CO, Interstate Medical Licensure Compact, 2019. Available at: https://imlcc.org. Accessed November 9, 2019.

Khan S, Ramtekkar U: Child and adolescent telepsychiatry education and training. Psychiatr Clin North Am 42(4):555–562, 2019

Kleinman A, Benson P: Anthropology in the clinic: the problem of cultural competency and how to fix it. PLoS Med 3(10):e294, 2006

Kopel H, Nunn K, Dossetor D: Evaluating satisfaction with a child and adolescent psychological telemedicine outreach service. J Telemed Telecare 7 (suppl 2):35–40, 2001

Margolis K, Kelsay K, Talmi A, et al: A multidisciplinary, team-based teleconsultation approach to enhance child mental health services in rural pediatrics. J Educ Psychol Consult 28(3):342–367, 2018

Myers K, Valentine J, Morganthaler R, et al: Telepsychiatry with incarcerated youth. J Adolesc Health 38(6):643–648, 2006

Myers KM, Valentine JM, Melzer SM: Child and adolescent telepsychiatry: utilization and satisfaction. Telemed J E Health 14(2):131–137, 2008

Naslund JA, Marsch LA, McHugo GJ, et al: Emerging mHealth and eHealth interventions for serious mental illness: a review of the literature. J Ment Health 24(5):321–332, 2015

Powell AC, Chen M, Thammachart C: The economic benefits of mobile apps for mental health and telepsychiatry services when used by adolescents. Child Adolesc Psychiatr Clin N Am 26(1):125–133, 2017

Pumariega AJ, Rothe E: Cultural considerations in child and adolescent psychiatric emergencies and crises. Child Adolesc Psychiatr Clin N Am 12(4):723–744, vii, 2003

Savin D, Garry MT, Zuccaro P, et al: Telepsychiatry for treating rural American Indian youth. J Am Acad Child Adolesc Psychiatry 45(4):484–488, 2006

Savin D, Glueck DA, Chardavoyne J, et al: Bridging cultures: child psychiatry via videoconferencing. Child Adolesc Psychiatr Clin N Am 20(1):125–134, 2011

Shore JH, Savin DM, Novins D, et al: Cultural aspects of telepsychiatry. J Telemed Telecare 12(3):116–121, 2006

Siemer CP, Fogel J, Van Voorhees BW: Telemental health and Web-based applications in children and adolescents. Child Adolesc Psychiatr Clin N Am 20(1):135–153, 2011

Torous J, Roberts LW: Needed innovation in digital health and smartphone applications for mental health: transparency and trust. JAMA Psychiatry 74(5):437–438, 2017

Torous J, Friedman R, Keshavan M: Smartphone ownership and interest in mobile applications to monitor symptoms of mental health conditions. JMIR Mhealth Uhealth 2(1):e2, 2014

Yellowlees PM, Hilty DM, Marks SL, et al: A retrospective analysis of a child and adolescent emental health program. J Am Acad Child Adolesc Psychiatry 47(1):103–107, 2008

Yeung A, Shyu I, Fisher L, et al: Culturally sensitive collaborative treatment for depressed Chinese Americans in primary care. Am J Public Health 100(12):2397–2402, 2010

CHAPTER 16

Rural Psychiatry

L. Lee Carlisle, M.D., DFAACAP

THE challenges of rural psychiatry are widely known. Poverty, low rates of insurance, increased stigma of mental illness, higher levels of substance use disorders, ready access to guns, geographical isolation, a shortage of providers, and difficulties with confidentiality in small rural communities pose significant challenges within the field of rural psychiatry (New Freedom Commission on Mental Health 2004). In this chapter, I explore the context of these concerns and how mental health providers can best provide evidence-based and culturally competent care in rural communities. Because of the strong and varied cultural makeup of many rural communities (in general, they now more multicultural than are urban areas), utilization of cultural competence principles (Pumariega et al. 2013) is highly recommended when evaluating youth in these communities (Table 16–1).

Background: Psychiatric Care for Youth in Rural Communities

There are 13.4 million children younger than 18 years living in rural communities in the United States (U.S. Census Bureau 2016). Of these, 6.1 million are between ages 10 and 18, compared with 18.3 million urban youth and 11 million suburban youth of the same age. Between 2000 and 2010, minority populations comprised three-quarters of the population growth in rural communities (Housing Assistance Council 2012). Although still nearly 80% of the rural population are white non-Hispanics, rates of culturally diverse rural communities have significantly increased. The largest rate of increase (46%) was in the Latinx communities, followed by the Asian and Pacific Islander/Native Hawaiian populations, American Indian, and African American populations (Housing Assistance Council 2012). The white non-Hispanic rural population grew at a rate of only 1.8%, the slowest among all groups (Housing Assistance Council 2012).

TABLE 16–1. **Risk and protective factors for youth in rural communities**

Risk factors	Protective factors
Exposure to higher levels of violence	Positive ethnic/racial identity
Greater access to guns	Familial involvement
Greater access to substances	Teacher support
Less access to school or community mental health services	Positive peer support
Lower educational levels	
Mental health stigma	
Discrimination	
Low self-esteem	

Diversity in rural America is not a new phenomenon. In the past, rural minorities' locations were often not by choice: African American populations lived in "Black Belt" areas that were an outgrowth of slavery (Lichter et al. 2007; Wimberley and Morris 2002), and American Indian reservations were the product of involuntary resettlements meant to break the Indian Nations in what most people see as attempted genocide (Bombay et al. 2014). Many cities, including Atlanta, Baltimore, and San Antonio, became minority majority as whites drifted to the suburbs. In contrast, rural communities have a pattern of isolation and segregation of minority populations that has gone relatively unnoticed (Lichter et al. 2007, 2010). Latinx immigrants and urban minorities are migrating to rural communities for meat-packing and large agrobusiness employment. This influx is happening so rapidly that it has been disruptive to longstanding and fragile social pacts of rural communities, leading to concerns that intolerance and social segregation may be on the rise (Lichter 2012).

Suicide rates for youth ages 10–24, both male and female, are twice as high in rural versus urban communities (Fontanella et al. 2015). Suicide rates for male youth in urban areas are trending downward, but in rural communities they have remained the same (Fontanella et al. 2015). Suicide rates for females are increasing significantly in both rural and urban communities (Fontanella et al. 2015). Suicide completion rates by firearm are lowering in both rural and urban communities but remain higher for both sexes in rural communities than in urban ones (Fontanella et al. 2015). This has been attributed to youth descriptions of social and geographic isolation in rural communities and to having less access to basic mental health services, increased access to firearms, and fewer economic opportunities (Fontanella et al. 2015).

Firearms are the leading method of suicide in adolescents (Simonetti et al. 2015); therefore, firearm access is a major mental health concern for all youth. Rural youth have significantly higher access to firearms (28.1%) compared with urban youth (22.6%), and non-Hispanic white youth have higher access to firearms in rural areas than in urban ones. Simonetti et al. (2015) noted no difference in access to firearms for either rural or urban youth with risk factors for suicide.

Evidence of suicide risk among offspring of individuals who have attempted suicide compounds the problem in rural communities. A prospective study of 701 offspring of 334 parents with mood disorders, of whom 191 (57.2%) had attempted suicide, was conducted to assess this problem (Brent et al. 2015). During the study, 4.1% of the parents made an additional attempt.

Parental suicide attempt was the strongest predictor of offspring attempts, with an odds ratio of 4. In rural communities, where the risk of suicide is already higher, this connection only magnifies the risk (Brent et al. 2015).

Visits to the emergency department are 1.6 times higher in rural children ages 3–17 with autism spectrum disorder when compared with their urban counterparts (Zhang et al. 2017). These patients have significant comorbidities requiring occupational therapy, speech therapy, and behavioral interventions. When these services are not provided, children with autism spectrum disorder are in crisis more often, requiring more frequent visits to the emergency department (Zhang et al. 2017).

Role of Primary Care Providers in Mental Health Care for Rural Youth

When additional care is needed, primary care providers (PCPs) act as gatekeepers, referring patients to appropriate specialists. In large urban settings, this gatekeeper function is often bypassed or unnecessary. In the rural setting, this role is vital.

Access

In both Canada and the United States, rural communities have less access to mental health services (Gill et al. 2017). Data from a population-based study of 118,851 Canadian youth found that increased contacts with PCPs regarding mental health concerns appear to improve outcomes for youth from rural, immigrant, refugee, and low-income families (Gill et al. 2017).

Detection

Primary care is a critical place to detect early signs of mental health issues. The youth, family, and community can be assessed holistically, and the patient's physical, behavioral, emotional, developmental, and mental well-being can be evaluated in order to detect indications of problems in these areas (Holden et al. 2014).

Collaborative Care

Innovations to reduce suicide rates include integrative care with PCPs and mental health providers, school-based mental health service providers, and telemental health providers (Fontanella et al. 2015). In Texas, Myers et al. (2010) conducted a 14-month study of collaborative care in treating rural versus urban Latinx youth ages 6–12 years with a model that included a case manager who acted as a go-between for the pediatrician and the psychiatrist. The collaborative care model was effective in both settings in reducing ADHD symptoms, but differences were noticed. Clinicians in the urban setting provided more visits in the first 2 months, collected more rating scales to guide dosing, adjusted ADHD medications more often, and provided more psychoeducation when compared with rural practitioners. Urban youth received higher dosages of medications, and their stabilization period was achieved faster. Resources in the rural clinic were less robust. Widespread utilization of collocated mental health providers with PCPs for children would most likely have brought the rural clinic to similar evidence-based practices as the urban clinic (Myers et al. 2010).

PCPs in rural communities appear to be more experienced in psychiatric medication management than those in urban communities. The telemental health provider can stabilize patients the PCP finds most challenging and after about six sessions refer them back to the PCP. This type of close collaboration between PCP and telemental provider makes more openings available for patients in the future. In rural communities where telemental health is the only option available for consulting with a mental health provider, collaboration between practitioners is critical in order for the telemental health provider to be able to focus on those patients most in need of services (Carlisle 2019).

Support for Rural PCPs

Because PCPs provide significant mental health treatment for rural youth, it is important to provide them with support through programs such as the Partnership Access Line (PAL) in Washington State so that additional help is available when more psychiatric consultation is needed. Programs such as PAL are present in several other states, but PAL is the first to cover a large rural population; it also provides a Medicaid second opinion service to community mental health providers (Barclay et al. 2017). One positive result of the PAL program is that it has cut second-generation antipsychotic medication prescribing in half (Barclay et al. 2017). These medications are commonly used for externalizing disorders, which are seen at higher rates in rural and minority youth (Barclay et al. 2017).

Challenges for Youth With Psychiatric Illness in Rural Communities

Poor health outcomes in rural communities such as chronic obstructive pulmonary disease, suicide, unintentional injuries, and obesity (Eberhardt and Pamuk 2004) have been attributed to increased stressors and limited resources. However, although the challenges of caring for mentally ill rural youth are significant, there are also protective factors at play.

Risk Factors

In general, rural youth have increased risk factors for poor health as compared with their urban peers (Office of Population Affairs 2018). They are less likely to have access to community and recreation activities, spend more time on media, and have fewer means of transportation. Rural youth are more likely to have shortages of health providers, especially mental health providers. They have higher rates of obesity and are more likely to live with someone who smokes (Office of Population Affairs 2018). They also have more access to illicit substances (Mink et al. 2005) and experience greater geographic isolation (Hook et al. 2005).

Education

Educational challenges such as higher school dropout rates in rural communities compared with urban or city communities of low socioeconomic income levels are evidence of the increased vulnerability of rural youth (Provasnik et al. 2007). Evidence supports that these issues begin in middle school, when rural youth are more likely to develop feelings of "not belonging" to the school environment (Witherspoon and Ennett 2011). Youth who leave school early are less likely to pull out of poverty or have access to basic health and mental health care (Witherspoon and Ennett 2011).

Stigma

A creative study using qualitative interviews and data collection with 163 rural African American caregivers looked at barriers to mental health care for rural African American adolescents in the southeastern United States (Murry et al. 2011). The surveys and interviews focused on understanding the views of caregivers around barriers to finding help for their adolescents in the mental health system. Stigma was the most common barrier to seeking mental health care. Caregivers feared that people in their small communities would blame and ostracize them as parents and think poorly of their families. Caregivers overwhelmingly thought that professionals could help but preferred support from "friends, family members, clergy or church members" (Murry et al. 2011, p. 1125). The study concluded that identifying ways to support faith-based mental health services for African American families is needed. As is often seen among other minority families, African American caregivers are more likely to have children with severe mental health issues, especially externalizing behaviors. Caregivers reported that the bulk of their support came from PCPs and schools (Murry et al. 2011).

Discrimination

In a study comparing social discrimination in Latinx high school students in Los Angeles and urban and rural North Carolina, rural youth reported a greater level of social discrimination than youth in Los Angeles or urban North Carolina (Potochnick et al. 2012). Being male, Latinx, and from a rural community have been correlated with externalizing disorders (Forster et al. 2015; Kessler et al. 2005). Ponting et al. (2018) explored more directly the effects of discrimination on externalizing behaviors in rural Latinx adolescents. Both male and female adolescents reported that *familismo* (a Latinx cultural concept in which a family's values are held in higher esteem than the values of the individual) lowered discrimination stress; however, there were differences between genders. For females, *familismo* was more likely to protect against discrimination stress, with family conflict increasing the likelihood of externalizing behaviors. For males, *familismo* was not as likely to mitigate the effects of discrimination, and family conflict was not as often identified as being likely to increase externalizing behaviors (Ponting et al. 2018).

The Ponting et al. (2018) study is instructional for the development of interventions for Latinx youth living in rural environments who struggle with discrimination stress. Programs that focus on family are likely to have a robust response in young Latinas. This study supports that interventions to reduce family conflict and increase *familismo* can reduce externalizing symptoms in all Latinx youth but will have a more robust response in female Latinx youth.

Low Self-Esteem and Depression

More than 4,000 middle-schoolers from the rural South were sampled in a study by Smokowski et al. (2014a). The participants were from two counties with robust participation, which increased the power of the study. This research revealed that low income, poor parenting, and being female were factors associated with elevated levels of depression and low self-esteem.

Protective Factors

Ethnic Identity

Depression and self-esteem were studied in 4,431 ethnically diverse sixth to eighth graders in two southern rural communities (Smokowski et al. 2014a). Ethnic identity, along with supportive relationships with parents and friends, positive views of academic life, and positive identification with a religion, predicted lower levels of depression and higher levels of self-esteem (Smokowski et al. 2014a).

In a 5-year study of a large, diverse rural adolescent community (28.5% Lumbee American Indian, of whom 51.4% were female), positive ethnic identity improved mental health functioning, especially in American Indian youth (Smokowski et al. 2014b). The researchers explored two pathways for ethnic identity to mediate improved mental health: self-esteem and future optimism (Smokowski et al. 2014b, p. 343). For all ethnic groups, self-esteem in relation to ethnic identity mediated improvement across all symptoms. Future optimism that was mediated through ethnic identity decreased externalizing behaviors for all groups in the sample; future optimism among American Indians significantly mediated the relationship between ethnic identity and depression. For the Lumbee adolescents in the study, incorporating evidence-based programs to promote ethnic identity in a culturally competent manner significantly lowered depression. Because American Indians are at much higher risk for depression and suicidality, these results provide further support for specific interventions for this rural ethnic group (Smokowski et al. 2014b).

Familial Involvement and Teacher Support

In an investigation into what they referred to as promotive factors, Cotter and Smokowski (2017, p. 754) found familial involvement helpful in battling an increase in adolescent female aggression in two rural communities. Teacher support was also a significant factor in lowering aggression among female adolescents; peer support was also found to be critical. Conflicts with parents, delinquent peers, peer pressure, and internalizing symptoms were associated with increased aggression in rural females. A need to focus more on peer relationships while at the same time continuing to promote support from the adults in a teenage girl's life was found to be necessary in this study (Cotter and Smokowski 2017).

Best Mental Health Practices

A 1-year longitudinal study among 2,617 diverse rural sixth to eighth graders focused on the parent-child relationship and youth mental health (Smokowski et al. 2015). This disadvantaged, diverse population was from a conservative southeastern community with authoritarian parenting styles and high levels of corporal punishment. Parental support associated with authoritative parenting correlated with higher mental well-being (lower rates of depression, anxiety, and aggression) and lower parent-child conflict. Practical recommendations stemming from this study include the use of more evidence-based treatment to promote positive parenting programs (Smokowski et al. 2015). Two recommended programs are Entres Dos Mundos (Between Two Worlds), which was developed to address acculturation in Latinx families (Bacallao and Smokowski 2005), and Active Parenting of Teens, which has been favorably evaluated in rural communities and is used to promote positive parenting (Pilgrim et al. 1998).

Puskar et al. (2015) reported the effects of Teaching Kids to Cope with Anger, a randomized controlled trial using a school-based program focusing on anger reduction interventions for high school–age youth in rural southwest Pennsylvania (86% white). The study revealed a significant difference at the 1-year postintervention point between the control group and the group receiving the intervention. The authors recommended further research on this school-based program because lowering anger has the potential to reduce injuries, homicides, and suicides, which are all great concerns for rural youth.

Investigators in rural Appalachia looked at caregivers of children ages 3–12 (95% white) and found that children of parents with higher rates of trauma also reported higher rates of trauma (Sprang et al. 2013). Higher rates of trauma were associated with greater parenting stress, perceptions of their child as difficult, and parent-child conflict. Investigators suggested focusing mental health interventions on parents who have experienced trauma as a prevention intervention.

Chavira et al. (2017) explored cognitive-behavioral therapy (CBT), an underutilized evidence-based treatment for youth diagnosed with anxiety disorders—particularly effective among white youth with anxiety disorders—with parents of rural Latinx children ages 8–13 who met criteria for anxiety disorder. In this "telephone-based, therapist-supported bibliotherapy" intervention for anxiety disorders, parents were more open to treatment because, as compared with traditional therapy in an office setting, it addressed many of the barriers to CBT. Providers, however, expressed more reservations. Other supports and adaptations are being considered to meet the needs of Latinx families, such as providing recorded materials on DVD or audio recordings to serve as adjuncts to telephone-based treatment or providing tablets and teletherapy support if the family has access to Wi-Fi. Parents found telephone or video therapy support with a mental health provider in the evenings and on weekends to be helpful. Parents and therapists agreed that at least one face-to-face meeting was needed because Latinx family cultural values such as *personalismo* emphasize warm interpersonal relationships to develop trust.

Clinical Vignette 1

Susan, a 13-year-old white female with a history of social anxiety and longstanding dysthymia, presented to the local clinic for evaluation. An only child to parents who allow her to make decisions about all health issues alone, she prides herself on taking high school classes while in the eighth grade. Her father, Mr. Pearce, recently lost the family farm—which had been in the family for generations—to bankruptcy and is now gathering fruit as a seasonal worker. He had a farming accident 5 years ago and has been in and out of drug rehabilitation because of opioid addiction. Susan's mother works as a bank teller and is the sole breadwinner for most of the year. Susan's parents argue frequently, mostly about financial insecurities. They live in a one-bedroom apartment, and Susan sleeps in the living room. She has been receiving CBT for 6 months and has developed a good therapeutic relationship with her therapist, but her symptoms have improved only slightly. Susan is quite close to her father, and they enjoy outdoor activities such as fishing and camping; her mother does not engage in these activities. Mr. Pearce has a history of social anxiety and depression and is more understanding of Susan's difficulties in these areas. He and Susan are against antidepressants and believe Ms. Pearce is pushing Susan to take them in order to rush her recovery. Susan and her father tend to isolate and have few friends. Her mother's family is from a large city, and Ms. Pearce desires to move there, but Susan and her father prefer rural life.

The treatment team reviewed different medication options and the research around the use of CBT and selective serotonin reuptake inhibitors for treatment of anxiety and depression. Susan listened but chose to continue CBT only. Her symptoms did not improve, and she returned a few months later after reconsidering her treatment options. Because Susan's psychosocial issues were clearly impacting her recovery, the therapist attempted family therapy. However, Mr. Pearce does not believe in therapy or psychiatry, and Ms. Pearce felt too overworked to attend.

Susan was open to a series of psychoeducational sessions with the psychiatrist and continued CBT with the therapist. Both providers closely coordinated care throughout the process. Because of her keen intellect, after learning about the treatment modalities, Susan made the decision to take medication. She also explored more about how large farms were forcing family farmers out of business and the effect this can have on people like her father who knew no other life. She also developed a better appreciation of her mother for remaining in the rural community to support her husband even though she could likely be more prosperous in the city. Susan's family remains poor, but she and her father continue to fish and camp, and her father has been clean and sober for a year now. Susan is in Advanced Placement classes, and her symptoms are improving.

Clinical Vignette 2

Rosa, a 14-year-old Latina, was seen in the community mental health center after an overnight medical stay for her third suicide attempt. She had been sexually abused by her mother's former boyfriend. After sneaking out and drinking with an older white boy, she was bullied by white girls at her school. The girls also cyberbully Rosa, sending her social network messages telling her to try again to "kill yourself." Rosa has panic attacks when attempting to attend school and was ultimately suspended for hitting one of the bullies. Using the DSM-5 Cultural Formulation Interview (American Psychiatric Association 2013), a clinician reviews Rosa's history (Table 16–2).

Rosa's family felt disrespected when called to school to meet with the white principal to discuss the suspension. During the meeting, Rosa's mother, who speaks only Spanish, was not provided an interpreter, and instead, school staff insisted on having Rosa interpret for her mother.

At home, intergenerational conflicts over Rosa's increasing level of acculturation are prominent. Rosa and her single mother live with Rosa's maternal grandparents, who have a significant impact on decision-making in the household. Rosa makes a special effort to continue the cultural activities she has always found comforting, such as painting and needlepoint with her grandmother. The extended family includes Rosa's former day care provider, Marie, who assists Rosa's grandparents and mother in decision-making. As fictive kin, Marie is respected for her ability to incorporate the best qualities of the host community while retaining the best of her culture of origin. She bridges the gap between the elders in the family and Rosa's mother, who feels caught between her parents' beliefs and the needs of her daughter.

Rosa's grandparents are resistant to Rosa's receiving psychiatric treatment and to her relationship with a white high school senior. Marie has been helpful negotiating the intergenerational conflict within the family. However, although Rosa's grandparents eventually accepted CBT, they balked when antidepressants were recommended, and another intergenerational acculturation conflict ensued.

TABLE 16–2.   DSM-5 Cultural Formulation Interview (CFI) for Rosa

CFI	Rosa's case
Cultural definition of the problem	
Core problems	Discrimination and bullying by white females
	Harassment on social media
Cultural perceptions of cause, context, and support	
Cause	Bullying for crossing cultural color lines
Stressors	Acculturation conflict
	Romantic relationship forbidden by grandparents
	Peer discrimination
Supports	Fictive kin
	Church
Role of cultural identity	Desired friendships and romantic relationships both outside and inside her native culture
	Cultural activities
	Religion
Cultural factors affecting self-coping and past help seeking	
Self-coping	Suicide attempts
	Painting and needlepoint projects with grandmother
Barriers	Grandparents strongly opposed to medication
Cultural factors affecting current help seeking	
Preferences	Desire to have friendships with both white and Latinx peers in school
Clinician-patient relationship	Certified interpreter at every school meeting

As one would expect, the acculturation conflict predicted worsening depression and less positive ethnic regard by Rosa. When Latinx adolescents experience peer discrimination as well as acculturation conflicts at home and in their community of origin, ethnic identity is adversely affected. Youth have described this psychosocial situation as not being Latinx enough for their family but not American enough for their peers (Huq et al. 2016). Discrimination is significantly associated with negative Latinx ethnic identity, and negative ethnic identity is associated with depression in unauthorized immigrants (Cobb et al. 2017).

Rosa's treatment team recognized these conflicts and worked with the family to create a treatment plan that included in-home visits from the center's Latinx community peer support person and family support person along with treatment with the therapist and a telemental health provider. Insisting on a certified interpreter at every school meeting was essential to the successful transition back to school so that Rosa's Spanish-speaking mother is a full partner in developing a plan for safe return to school.

In the case of Rosa, use of the cultural competence principles for intergenerational acculturation conflict and involvement of the entire family, including extended family (Table 16–3), were vital. Using the child as an interpreter for the parent in disciplinary school situations is inappropriate, per principle 2 of the American Academy of Child and Adolescent Psychiatry (AACAP)

TABLE 16–3. Principles in the American Academy of Child and Adolescent Psychiatry Practice Parameter for Cultural Competence in Child and Adolescent Psychiatric Practice

	Description
Principle 1	Identify and address barriers that may prevent children from obtaining mental health services
Principle 2	Conduct the evaluation in the language in which the child and family are proficient
Principle 3	Understand the impact of dual-language competence on the child's adaptation and functioning
Principle 4	Be cognizant of your own cultural biases and address them
Principle 5	Apply knowledge of cultural differences in development, idioms of distress, and symptomatic presentation to clinical formulation and diagnosis
Principle 6	Assess for history of immigration-related loss or trauma and community trauma and address them in treatment
Principle 7	Evaluate and address acculturation stress and intergenerational acculturation family conflict
Principle 8	Make special effort to include family members and key members of traditional extended families in assessment, treatment planning, and treatment
Principle 9	Evaluate and use the child and family's cultural strengths in treatment interventions
Principle 10	Treat the child and family in familiar settings within their community when possible
Principle 11	Support parents in developing appropriate behavioral management skills compatible with their cultural values and beliefs
Principle 12	Use evidence-based psychological and pharmacological interventions specific for the child and family's ethnic/racial population
Principle 13	Identify ethnopharmacological factors that may influence the child's response to medications, including side effects

Source.   Adapted from Pumariega et al. 2013.

Practice Parameter for Cultural Competence in Child and Adolescent Psychiatric Practice: "Clinicians should conduct the evaluation in which the child and family are proficient" (Pumariega et al. 2013, p. 1104). Use of the child in language brokering (instead of an interpreter) is associated with higher levels of family stress and poorer academic functioning. It goes against AACAP and the American Psychiatric Association's principles and practices. Principles 7, 8, and 9, are also relevant (see Table 16–3).

Conclusion

The demographics of rural America have changed significantly to the extent that, in general, rural communities are now more multicultural than are urban areas. Youth of indigenous heritage; youth from ethnic minorities; youth with recent immigrant heritage; and youth with white immigrant heritage whose parents, grandparents, and great-grandparents came to their communities generations ago are now all walking through the same doors of rural mental health centers.

They have many common needs and are influenced by many of the same stressors—poverty, higher suicide rates, fewer educational opportunities, higher rates of substance use disorders, geographic isolation, shortages of mental health professionals, foster care shortages, and stigma associated with mental illness. Although these issues are not unique to rural youth, they are magnified in comparison with the experiences of urban youth. And although rural youth of varied ethnicities face similar stressors, research is showing that a culturally competent approach to diagnosis and treatment planning is key to improving outcomes. In the future, all mental health providers will be serving more diverse populations and will need to develop the culturally competent skills to do so. For mental health providers currently serving rural communities, the future is now.

Rural Psychiatry in the Time of COVID-19

The novel coronavirus SARS-CoV-2 (COVID-19) pandemic has adversely impacted children with mental illness (Fegert et al. 2020) through increasing social isolation (Hossain et al. 2020), loss of family income (Parker et al. 2020), loss of child care, limited free and reduced breakfast and lunch, limited access to Individual Education Programs in remote learning programs, and reduced access to mental health services. Although these impacts are not unique to children with mental illness, these children are more reliant on school and community mental health services and acutely feel the changes and loss of access. For children of rural communities—already affected by social isolation and poverty at a higher rate than suburban and urban youth—the COVID-19 crisis has intensified these issues. The families who live close to the parents' place of employment, such as those harvesting fruits and vegetables or employed at meat-packing facilities, are required to go to town to pick up groceries at school at a time of day when both parents are working. While these parents work to keep the food chain intact for our nation, their children experience food insecurity.

During this pandemic, parents everywhere are stressed by being the financial, childcare, and education providers for their children. In rural communities, these stressors may be amplified because many parents are unable to be home when their children are attempting to connect with remote learning and therapy, often on tablets and Internet hot spots provided by the schools. School-based therapists are quite popular with families of color (Pumariega et al. 2013), especially in rural communities that are some distance from the mental health center. The switch to remote therapy is acutely felt.

For families with adequate bandwidth to support telehealth and children old enough and cognitively capable of managing the demands of the technology, telepsychiatry can be an adequate replacement for in-person therapy. Telepsychiatry is an effective treatment modality that has been a common form of treatment delivery in rural communities where these services would otherwise be unavailable. Some rural families are accustomed to telepsychiatry through point-to-point technology in the many rural mental health centers (Carlisle 2019). Many rural school districts provide tablets and hot spots for remote learning, and some do not require them to be turned in over the summer, which is fortuitous for continued summer education and telehealth.

However, families who live in remote, especially mountainous, areas where telehealth is unreliable do not have this option. Telephone landlines are the most reliable backup plan for these families. However, because of financial issues, many families have chosen smartphones, which are unreliable because of connectivity problems.

Developmental disabilities services, applied behavioral therapy, and wraparound services are school- and home-based supports for many children. Typically less available in rural communities in the best of times, these services are quite limited during the pandemic because of the need for decreased close interpersonal contact.

Parents of color are overrepresented in employment that carries a high risk of developing COVID-19 (disproportionately working in essential workforce service jobs that do not provide options of sick leave or ability to telework). Similarly, African American and Latinx families are less likely to have emergency funds to cover their expenses (Parker et al. 2020). Early in the epidemic, urban areas had higher numbers of cases, hospitalizations, and deaths, but at the time of this writing, rural areas were seeing rising numbers. If rural parents are hospitalized, they are commonly sent to urban areas because ICU beds are quickly being overrun in rural communities because of closures of rural hospitals over recent years. Children of color are more likely to be dealing with COVID-19 in the family (Wood 2020), and rural children will be physically far away from hospitalized parents, which is an added burden.

Clinical Pearls

- In rural communities, coordination between the mental health provider and the primary care provider is critical to ensure that treatment is available for those youth most in need.

- For depressed rural American Indian youth, promotion of ethnic identity, which significantly enhances future optimism, greatly improves treatment outcomes.

- For depressed male white youth, assessment of access to firearms is of the highest importance.

- Rural Latinx high school students were found to have higher levels of social discrimination than urban Latinx youth of comparable age.

- Looking at ways to support faith-based services for rural African American and Latinx youth is indicated.

- Use tools such as the Cultural Formulation Interview and the Practice Parameter for Cultural Competence in Child and Adolescent Psychiatric Practice to help recognize cultural aspects in working with patients.

Self-Assessment Questions

1. Which of the following is *not* true regarding mental health issues in rural communities?

    A. Suicide rates are twice those of urban communities.
    B. Rural primary care providers are more experienced with mental health medications.
    C. Discrimination against Latinx youth is lower in rural areas.
    D. Emergency department visits for youth with autism spectrum disorder are 1.6 times higher for rural than for urban youth.

2. Which of the following needs to be supported to improve the mental health outcomes of rural youth?

    A. Colocate mental health providers and primary care physicians.
    B. Address access to firearms, especially by white males.
    C. Decrease stigma of mental health services.
    D. All of the above.

3. The American Academy of Child and Adolescent Psychiatry practice parameter principles support all but which of the following?

    A. Fictive kin participation in the treatment team.
    B. Extended family involvement in the treatment team.
    C. Youth providing interpretation for parents when time is short.
    D. Assessment of acculturation stress is essential.

4. Describe why it is particularly important to think about culture and diversity in rural mental health.

5. List and explain three areas that you currently include in your cultural assessment of patients and discuss ways to improve these areas.

6. Discuss three specific aspects you can add to your cultural formulation and treatment of rural patients.

Answers

1. C
2. D
3. C

References

American Psychiatric Association: Cultural Formulation Interview, in Diagnostic and Statistical Manual of Mental Disorders, Fifth Edition. Arlington, VA, American Psychiatric Association, 2013, pp 750–757

Bacallao M, Smokowski PR: "Entre dos mundos" (between two worlds): bicultural skills training and Latino immigrant families. J Prim Prev 26(6):485–509, 2005

Barclay RP, Penfold RB, Sullivan D, et al: Decrease in statewide antipsychotic prescribing after implementation of child and adolescent psychiatry consultation services. Health Serv Res 52(2):561–578, 2017

Bombay A, Matheson K, Anisman H: The intergenerational effects of Indian residential schools: implications for the concept of historical trauma. Transcult Psychiatry 51(3):320–338, 2014

Brent DA, Melham NM, Oquendo M, et al: Familial pathways to early onset suicide attempt: a 5.6-year prospective study. JAMA Psychiatry 72(2):160–168, 2015

Carlisle LL: Child and adolescent telemental health, in Telemental Health: Clinical, Technical and Administrative Foundations for Evidence-Based Practice. Edited by Myers MK, Turley C. Kidlington, UK, Elsevier, 2013, pp 197–221

Carlisle LL: Child and adolescent telepsychiatry toolkit. Washington, DC, American Psychiatric Association and American Academy of Child and Adolescent Psychiatry, 2019. Available at: www.psychiatry.org/psychiatrists/practice/telepsychiatry/toolkit/child-adolescent. Accessed May 14, 2019.

Chavira DA, Bustos CE, Garcia MS, et al: Delivering CBT to rural Latino children with anxiety disorders: a qualitative study. Community Ment Health J 53(1):53–61, 2017

Cobb CL, Xie D, Meca A, et al: Acculturation, discrimination, and depression among unauthorized Latinos/as in the United States. Cultur Divers Ethnic Minor Psychol 23(2):258–268, 2017

Cotter KL, Smokowski PR: An investigation of relational risk and promotive factors associated with adolescent female aggression. Child Psychiatry Hum Dev 48(5):754–767, 2017

Eberhardt MS, Pamuk ER: The importance of place of residence: examining health in rural and nonrural areas. Am J Public Health 94(10):1682–1686, 2004

Fegert JM, Vitiello B, Plener PL, Clemens V: Challenges and burden of the Coronavirus 2019 (COVID-19) pandemic for child and adolescent mental health: a narrative review to highlight clinical and research needs in the acute phase and the long return to normality. Child Adolesc Psychiatry Ment Health 14(20):1–11, 2020

Fontanella CA, Hiance-Steelesmith DL, Phillips GS, et al: Widening rural-urban disparities in youth suicides, United States, 1996–2010. JAMA Pediatr 169(5):466–473, 2015

Forster M, Grigsby T, Soto DW, et al: The role of bicultural stress and perceived context of reception in the expression of aggression and rule breaking behaviors among recent-immigrant Hispanic youth. J Interpers Violence 30(11):1807–1827, 2015

Gill PJ, Saunders N, Gandhi S, et al: Emergency department as a first contact for mental health problems in children and youth. J Am Acad Child Adolesc Psychiatry 56(6):475.e4–482.e4, 2017

Holden K, McGregor B, Thandi P, et al: Toward culturally centered integrative care for addressing mental health disparities among ethnic minorities. Psychol Serv 11(4):357–368, 2014

Hook M, Murray M, Seymour A: Meeting the needs of underserved victims video discussion guide. Washington, DC, Office for Victims of Crime, U.S. Department of Justice, Office of Justice Programs, August 2005. Available at: www.ovc.gov/pdftxt/underserved_victims_vdguide.pdf. Accessed January 30, 2020.

Hossain MM, Sultana A, Purohot N: Mental health outcomes of quarantine and isolation for infection prevention: a systematic umbrella review of the global evidence. Epidemiol Health 42:e2020038, 2020

Housing Assistance Council: Race and ethnicity in rural America. Rural Research Brief, April 2012. Available at: www.ruralhome.org/storage/research_notes/rrn-race-and-ethnicity-web.pdf. Accessed June 29, 2019.

Huq H, Stein GL, Gonzales LM: Acculturation conflict among Latino youth: discrimination, ethnic identity, and depressive symptoms. Cultur Divers Ethnic Minor Psychol 22(3):377–385, 2016

Kessler RC, Berglund P, Demler O, et al: Lifetime prevalence and age-of-onset distributions of DSM-IV disorders in the National Comorbidity Survey Replication. Arch Gen Psychiatry 62(6):593–602, 2005

Lichter DT: Immigration and the new racial diversity in rural America. Rural Sociol 77(1):3–35, 2012

Lichter DT, Parisi D, Grice SM, et al: National estimates of racial segregation in rural and small-town America. Demography 44(3):563–581, 2007

Lichter DT, Parisi D, Taquino M, et al: Residential segregation in new Hispanic destinations: cities, suburbs, and rural communities compared. Social Science Research 39(2):215–230, 2010

Mink MD, Moore CG, Johnson A, et al: Violence and rural teens: teen violence, drug use, and school-based prevention services in rural America. Columbia, South Carolina Rural Health Research, 2005. Available at: www.ruralhealthresearch.org/publications/125. Accessed January 23, 2019.

Murry VM, Heflinger CA, Suiter SV, et al: Examining perceptions about mental health care and help-seeking among rural African American families of adolescents. J Youth Adolesc 40(9):1118–1131, 2011

Myers K, Vander Stoep A, Thompson K, et al: Collaborative care for the treatment of Hispanic children diagnosed with attention-deficit hyperactivity disorder. Gen Hosp Psychiatry 32(6):612–614, 2010

New Freedom Commission on Mental Health: Subcommittee on Rural Issues: Background paper (DHHS Publ No SMA-04-3890). New Freedom Commission on Mental Health, Rockville, MD, U.S. Department of Health and Human Services, June 2004. Available at: http://annapoliscoalition.org/wp-content/uploads/2014/03/presidents-new-freedom-commission-background-paper.pdf. Accessed January 22, 2019.

Office of Population Affairs: The changing face of America's adolescents. Washington, DC, Office of Population Affairs, U.S. Department of Health and Human Services, 2018. Available at: www.hhs.gov/ash/oah/facts-and-stats/changing-face-of-americas-adolescents/index.html. Accessed June 27, 2019.

Parker K, Horowitz JM, Brown A: About half of lower-income Americans report household job or wage loss due to COVID-19. Washington, DC, Pew Research Center, April 21, 2020. Available at: www.pewsocialtrends.org/2020/04/21/about-half-of-lower-income-americans-report-household-job-or-wage-loss-due-to-covid-19. Accessed July 5, 2020

Pilgrim C, Abbey A, Hendrickson P, et al: Implementation and impact of family based substance abuse prevention program in rural communities. J Prim Prev 18(3):341–361, 1998

Ponting C, Lee SS, Escovar EL, et al: Family factors mediate discrimination related stress and externalizing symptoms in rural Latino adolescents. J Adolesc 69:11–21, 2018

Potochnick S, Perreira KM, Fuligni A: Fitting in: the roles of social acceptance and discrimination in shaping the daily psychological well-being of Latino youth. Soc Sci Q 93(1):173–190, 2012

Provasnik S, KewalRamani A, Coleman MM, et al: Status of education in rural America (NCES 2007-040). Washington DC, National Center for Education Statistics, U.S. Department of Education, July 2007. Available at: https://nces.ed.gov/pubs2007/2007040.pdf. Accessed March 3, 2019.

Pumariega AJ, Rothe E, Mian A, et al: Practice parameter for cultural competence in child and adolescent psychiatric practice. J Am Acad Child Adolesc Psychiatry 52(10):1101–1115, 2013

Puskar KR, Ren K, McFadden T: Testing the 'Teaching Kids to Cope with Anger' youth anger intervention program in a rural school-based sample. Issues Ment Health Nurs 36(3):200–208, 2015

Simonetti JA, Mackelprang JL, Rowhani-Rahbar A, et al: Psychiatric comorbidity, suicidality, and in-home firearm access among a nationally representative sample of adolescents. JAMA Psychiatry 72(2):152–159, 2015

Smokowski PR, Evans CBR, Cotter KL, et al: Ecological correlates of depression and self-esteem in rural youth. Child Psychiatry Hum Dev 45(5):500–518, 2014a

Smokowski PR, Evans CBR, Cotter KL, et al: Ethnic identity and mental health in American Indian youth: examining mediated pathways through self-esteem, and future optimism. J Youth Adolesc 43(3):343–355, 2014b

Smokowski PR, Bacallao ML, Cotter KL, et al: The effects of positive and negative parenting on adolescent mental health outcomes in a multicultural sample in rural youth. Child Psychiatry Hum Dev 46(3):333–345, 2015

Sprang G, Staton-Tindall M, Gustman B, et al: The impact of trauma exposure on parenting stress in rural America. Journal of Child and Adolescent Trauma 6:287–300, 2013

U.S. Census Bureau: New Census Data Show Differences Between Urban and Rural Populations, December 2016. Available at: www.census.gov/newsroom/press-releases/2016/cb16-210.html. Accessed June 29, 2019.

Wimberley RC, Morris LV: The regionalization of poverty: assistance for the Black Belt South? Southern Rural Sociology 18(1):294–306, 2002

Wood G: What's behind the COVID-19 racial disparity? The Atlantic, May 27, 2020. Available at: www.theatlantic.com/ideas/archive/2020/05/we-dont-know-whats-behind-covid-19-racial-disparity/612106. Accessed July 5, 2020

Witherspoon D, Ennett S: Stability and change in rural youths' educational outcomes through the middle school and high school years. J Youth Adolesc 40(9):1077–1090, 2011

Zhang W, Mason AE, Boyd B, et al: A rural-urban comparison in emergency department visits for U.S. children with autism spectrum disorder. J Autism Dev Disord 47(3):590–598, 2017

PART IV
Developmental Stages, Family, and Clinical Implications

CHAPTER 17
Infant Psychiatry
Culture and Early Childhood

Wanjikũ F.M. Njoroge, M.D.
Amalia Londoño Tobón, M.D.

THE 2018 U.S. Census data reflect the country's changing demographics, with children younger than age 15 from diverse racial/ethnic backgrounds outnumbering non-Latinx/Hispanic white children (Colby and Ortman 2015). With these changes, cultural attunement, sensitivity, and humility are necessary in order to provide quality empathic psychiatric care, particularly in early childhood, when cultural environments are inextricably linked to development. The first 5 years of life are critical as rapid brain development and formation of millions of synaptic connections occur in the context of a child's environment (Londono Tobon et al. 2016). The Harvard Center on the Developing Child describes this period as a time when "the interactions of genes and experience shape the developing brain" (Center on the Developing Child 2009; Shonkoff and Phillips 2000). With this greater scientific knowledge, increasing attention is being paid to how the earliest environments influence development.

The impact of race/ethnicity on children's development can be seen beginning in pregnancy. African American women have two to three times higher rates of perinatal complications and pregnancy-related mortality compared with non-Latinx/Hispanic white women (Petersen et al. 2019). Postpartum challenges include disparate access to services and treatment. Research also reflects that children from diverse racial/ethnic backgrounds receive differential access to prevention and quality treatments relative to their non-Latinx/Hispanic white counterparts, which impacts child health outcomes (Flores and Committee on Pediatric Research 2010). Gilliam and colleagues also note disparities in early education settings, with young children of underserved backgrounds having limited access to quality preschools (Gilliam and Shahar 2006). In particular, African American boys have higher rates of preschool expulsions and suspensions (Gilliam et al. 2016).

The growing literature on health and educational disparities underscores how diverse families are not able to garner the services they need. Even if diverse families are able to overcome the myriad of systemic barriers preventing access to care, they still may not receive the same level and/or quality of care as non-Latinx/Hispanic white families do (Hall et al. 2015).

To meet the needs of diverse families and alleviate childhood health care disparities, clinicians must better understand the multiple frameworks and contexts that diverse families negotiate to accurately assess, formulate, and treat young children from diverse backgrounds. Beginning this nuanced cultural approach in early childhood is a wonderful opportunity for clinicians to optimally shape the trajectories of children and their families. In this chapter, we aim to provide a practical reference for including culture into clinical work with very young children and their families.

Earliest Efforts to Incorporate Culture in Infant Mental Health

Early researchers, including Anna Freud (1965), Erik Erikson (1950), John Bowlby (1958), and Mary Ainsworth (Ainsworth and Bell 1970), underscored the importance of parenting styles and the broader environmental context on the developing infant. Likewise, Frantz Fanon (1952/1967) discussed the impact of culture, racism, and the environment on the adult psyche, beginning an investigation of the effect of larger systems on emotional and psychological well-being. Despite this body of knowledge and understanding of how culture, race, and the environment affect the developing child, greater understanding of these factors and more consistent application of that knowledge to child psychiatry is needed, specifically with regard to infant mental health (IMH) clinical practice.

Mental health in the first 5 years of life requires healthy social and emotional development in the context of the environment (Fraiberg et al. 1975; Zeanah 2018). Infant and early childhood mental health focuses on young children's social-emotional development, caregiver-child interactions, contextual and cultural influences on child and family development, and all conditions that place young children and/or their families at risk for less than optimal development (Clinton et al. 2016; https://waimh.org/page/about_waimh). The psychological balance of the entire infant-family system is involved, requiring full consideration.

Understanding families and the broader environmental context remains a core tenet of IMH, and significant disparities remain in working with diverse families of young children (Ghosh Ippen 2009). The Harris Professional Development Network work group aimed to address this problem by drafting tenets focusing on justice and equity to address diversity and cultural aspects of IMH (Thomas et al. 2019). The tenets purport to add a richer understanding of how structural racism, stigma, and bias disproportionately impact the way families of color receive early childhood services and how diverse families and cultures are understood by teams with whom they interact. Along with greater appreciation of the importance of this earliest developmental period, having a nuanced understanding of the impact of culture and young children's environments is paramount (Thomas et al. 1997).

Assessments

Using a cultural framework ensures that diverse families with very young children experience high-quality, appropriate assessments. As clearly demonstrated in decades of research, infants and very young children are inextricably linked to the beliefs of their parents (Greenfield et al. 2006). Cultural researchers found significant differences in belief systems around a variety of parental caregiving tasks, including sleeping, feeding, speaking, and other developmental milestones occurring in the first 5 years of life (Bornstein et al. 2004; Harkness and Super 1992; Ogbu 1981). Therefore, explicitly asking parents about cultural beliefs around everyday parenting practices and the role that culture plays in their life and their young child's life is of utmost importance. The assessment should gather as much information as possible from the caregivers so that the clinician can accurately understand the child, family, and broader environmental context in order to provide culturally appropriate recommendations and interventions.

Standardized Assessments

Before the initial visit, primary caregivers often are asked to complete standardized assessment measurements and rating scales (Godoy et al. 2019). Although these measures are available in multiple languages, they have typically been standardized on an English-speaking population and/or specific racial/ethnic group. Therefore, as articulated in the literature on the use of such tools in diverse populations, these assessments may not capture particular cultural nuances and must be used thoughtfully (Lyman et al. 2007). It remains essential to use these tools in assessments, but the information obtained should be understood within a cultural context (Nikapota 2009). Because clinics may use instruments that have not been standardized for a particular population, reviewing the instrument and assessing its validity is essential. The tool may have items that are either not applicable or confusing, and asking the child's caregivers if they have any questions regarding the instrument may be helpful. Time permitting, reviewing these items with the caregiver and asking for more information can be fruitful. At the very least, discussing the questions about which the family had concerns is important. Standardized assessment results should be cautiously interpreted in the context of the child, family, environment, and instrument validity.

General Assessment Context

Briefly, the evaluation of young children involves engaging caregivers and assessing the child in various settings over multiple sessions (Thomas et al. 1997). Initial preparation includes ensuring that there is enough room to accommodate all participants and access to language services when needed (Misch et al. 2019). Allowing individuals to speak in their preferred language has been shown to facilitate their expression and concerns; therefore, medically trained interpreters are the gold standard for families who speak a primary language different from that of the clinician (Earner 2007). The Office of Minority Health (2001) National Standards for Culturally and Linguistically Appropriate Services in Health Care states that

> care organizations must offer and provide language assistance services, including bilingual staff and interpreter services, at no cost to each patient/consumer with limited English proficiency at all points of contact, in a timely manner during all hours of operation…. Family and friends should not be used to provide interpretation services (except on request by the patient/consumer). (p. 28)

If nonprofessional interpreters, such as office staff who speak the family's primary language, are used, careful consideration should be given to how the lack of training will impact the assessment and how the caregivers and/or young child may feel about these informal interpreters.

IMH assessments occur in a variety of settings, including but not limited to medical offices, hospitals, patient homes, schools, and child care centers. Preparing for assessments in various locations and thinking about how the child may react in multiple contexts is important when formulating the case. When there is flexibility in the appointment location, discussing with families how they feel about the various locations, including their perceptions of advantages and/or disadvantages for each, is important in ensuring that caregivers are on board and part of the decision-making process. However, the majority of mental health IMH assessments will most likely occur in a clinic-based setting. In recognizing the diverse needs of families, it is important to respect the family's wishes regarding who should be included in the assessment. If the primary caregivers would like to include multiple family members and/or other participants, it is essential to ensure that the evaluation occurs in a space that is a comfortable size, with enough appropriate seating for each participant.

An important note when conducting home-based assessment is that the clinician must understand the family's cultural view on having visitors in their home. Care should be taken to assess the family's comfort with the assessment and observation in more personal settings. It is essential to be respectful of the family's cultural practices (e.g., taking shoes off, entering only certain portions of the home, acknowledging fasting for religious purposes) and cultural expectations around having guests in their home (e.g., accepting offers of something to eat and/or drink). Having a more nuanced understanding of the family's cultural expectations will prevent misunderstanding and miscommunication.

Reason for Evaluation

Ideally, the initial session is completed with the caregivers alone, typically in an office setting or in the caregivers' home (Misch et al. 2019). However, caregiver interviews can pose challenges to some families with regard to child care, access to the clinic, and appointment times. Preferably, the clinician should discuss session structure with a caregiver via telephone prior to the first session so that caregivers can ask questions and discuss arrangements. Alternatively, the same detailed information can be sent in a form letter through the mail or electronically.

In order to engage caregivers, the evaluation should include a welcoming environment and openness to hearing their story and concerns. This includes ensuring that the meeting space reflects an appreciation of diversity and multiculturalism through books, handouts, art, and availability of interpreter services as described earlier. Before beginning a thorough exploration of the presenting problem, it is helpful to introduce yourself and your role as well as confirming the caregivers' understanding of the assessment structure and then inquiring what brings them in and/or asking about their understanding of the reason for the assessment. It is important to understand the referral source: some families may have been referred by another agency and may not understand the referral; some assessments may be court mandated; and some families may be self-referred. Including more extensive family and community systems in this line of questioning allows for a better understanding of the presenting problem in a broader familial or cultural context. For recommended questions to ask, see Table 17–1.

Assessment Participants

After thoroughly unpacking the initial concern, understanding everyone of importance in the child's life who might be included in future appointments is essential. Asking the primary caregivers who is involved in the care of the child and if they would like to involve those individuals in the assessment immediately lets them know that you understand the importance of these additional caregivers' perspectives (Villarreal et al. 2005). Cultural beliefs are not static and indeed may differ across and within different ethnic groups (Garcia Coll 1990). Because of heterogeneity, ensuring that families are queried and not making assumptions are a crucial part of a culturally informed assessment. For example, in some cultures, grandparents, uncles, aunts, neighbors, other extended family members, and church members may participate in providing care for the young child, whereas in others, only immediate family members participate in providing care.

Knowing about all of the caregivers with whom the child spends time and whether said caregivers have similar cultural references (e.g., language, parenting practices, beliefs around interacting with media) is key. It is crucial that each caregiver present his or her views regarding the child's upbringing because generational differences may exist around cultural beliefs and parenting practices (Benasich and Brooks-Gunn 1996). Directly asking if such differences exist and how they are managed is useful because there may be significant heterogeneity *within* the family.

Caregiver Assessments: What Else to Assess and How to Keep Culture in Mind

In addition to asking about the presenting problem and conducting a psychiatric and medical review of systems, asking more nuanced questions about the environmental context (family and social history) is important. For instance, asking about support systems, intergenerational parenting practices, traumas and adversities, discipline strategies, television viewing habits, sleeping habits, feeding/nutritional beliefs, language(s) used with the child, and other views on parenting and being a parent provides invaluable information (Bornstein 2013). If caregivers appear ill at ease, openly asking if some of the questions make them uncomfortable and giving them a choice to not answer the question may help them feel respected and understood, strengthening the assessment relationship. If caregivers endorse finding a question insulting or intrusive,

TABLE 17-1.   Mental health assessment, formulation, and treatment considerations

Prior to assessment

Actions for the clinician

- Discuss with the family who will be present at the first meeting.
- Discuss location of first meeting (school, home, hospital, clinic, or telemedicine) with family.
- Discuss with the family the organization of the assessment. Will assessment include multiple sessions in various settings? How does the family feel about this? What are the family's expectations and feelings about the location(s)?
- Ensure that the assessment space is welcoming to people of diverse cultures and backgrounds.
- Discuss potential barriers to engaging in assessment, including transportation and child care.

Initial assessment[a]

Questions for caregivers

- How are you feeling about being here during this assessment?
- What is your understanding about the referral?
- What are your thoughts on mental health or seeing a mental health provider for your child?
- What concerns you or troubles you the most about your child?
- What do you think is happening with your child?
- Who else is involved in the care of this child?
- What do other caregivers believe is happening with your child? Do they think there is a problem?
- How involved are other community members in the care of your child? What do they think is happening?
- Does your community believe there is a problem?
- What have you and other caregivers tried to do to alleviate the problem?
- Have you found anything helpful?
- Are there things that make the challenges worse or better?

Specific caregiver assessment

Questions for caregivers

- Could you say a few things about your cultural background?
- How have your cultural background and upbringing influenced how you raise your children?
- Are there any differences in parenting practices and beliefs among your child's various caregivers?
- What are some of your current stressors?
- Could you talk about support systems for you and your child?
- What languages are spoken at home?
- What are your views on feeding? Sleeping? Discipline? Use of media? Play? Other parenting practices?

Child assessment

Questions for caregivers

- What is your child able to do with regard to motor skills, emotional regulation, social interactions, cognition, language, and play? (Clinician may need to explain some of these concepts to caregivers.)
- How do you think your child is developing compared with other children in your community?

TABLE 17-1.   Mental health assessment, formulation, and treatment considerations *(continued)*

Play and dyadic evaluation

Questions for caregivers

*   How do you view play and adults playing with children? What does play mean to you?
*   What types of toys does your child enjoy playing with? What toys do you have at home?

Actions for the clinician

*   Ensure you have culturally diverse toys and a variety of types of toys.
*   Introduce culturally relevant themes that may add additional nuance to the session. Allow the child to take the lead and introduce themes of play if appropriate.

Cultural case formulation

Actions for the clinician

*   With the family, create a joint formulation of the case.
*   Evaluate your own implicit and explicit biases and reactions to the family and child.
*   Evaluate all the collected observations and material in light of the child's culture, taking into consideration your own biases and reactions.
*   Discuss with a diverse team the formulation of the case and ask for diverse opinions of the formulation.
*   Discuss barriers to care with the family and ways to reduce those barriers.
*   Review the literature and ask colleagues if the intervention you are considering (medication or psychosocial treatment) has been tried in a particular culture/race/ethnicity.

Culturally relevant interventions and treatment

Actions for the clinician

*   Discuss with the family their views of the evaluation.
*   Discuss with the family their views on treatment and intervention in young children.
*   What does the diagnosis mean to the family?
*   What is the caregivers' understanding of whether or not their family dynamic is contributing to the child's challenges?
*   What is their belief around very young children and mental health disorders? Their views around the environment impacting child behavior?

[a]Consider adapting the DSM-5 Cultural Formulation Interview (American Psychiatric Association 2013).

explaining the reasons behind asking the question and framing it as an opportunity to better understand their child, family, and concerns is often worthwhile.

It is important to explore parenting practices in the broader cultural group with whom the caregivers identify to determine whether this is a source of support or conflict (Bornstein et al. 2004). The literature on differences in parenting practices and beliefs reflects the significance of understanding caregivers' belief systems because they have been shown to directly impact not only child development but also caregivers' views regarding their child's development (Benasich and Brooks-Gunn 1996; Miller 1988). Compelling research on immigrant parents' beliefs systems shows that regardless of the child-rearing beliefs of the culture and/or the country in which they are currently living, many immigrants still adhere to the rearing expectations of their home culture and/or country (LeVine 1988). Understanding these cultural expectations is essential when considering caregivers' adherence to recommendations. It is unsurprising that if the recommendations are counter to the family's beliefs and there was never a discussion about these differences, caregivers often do not follow recommendations made by a well-intended team (Bornstein et al. 2004).

Evaluation of the child's development is another integral part of the assessment process. Beyond asking about milestones, which may be particular and normalized to certain U.S. standards (Rogoff 2003), discussing more broadly the child's abilities with regard to motor skills, emotional regulation, social interactions, cognition, language, and play allows for inclusion of culture and better understanding of the impact of culture on the child's developing skills. Furthermore, surveys reflect significant cross-cultural variances in parental understanding of child development and expectations around what is developmentally appropriate to the caregivers in the context of their culture. Therefore, understanding the primary caregivers' beliefs about the child's abilities at particular ages and developmental stages is crucial (Stevens 1984).

Child Assessment

Child assessment involves observation of the child's play with both caregivers and the clinician, using an assortment of toys with which the child and the caregiver engage. It is important to include culturally diverse toys and dolls in the play materials (Heller et al. 2019). However, caregivers may be anxious about such directions as "play as you normally would play at home." Discussing with families what play means to them is helpful because it may have a different meaning in the caregivers' particular culture (Rogoff 2003). For example, caregivers may not use toys to engage with their child. They also may not have time to "play" with their child but may interact with the child in other ways that are playful, such as engaging the child while completing tasks around the house. Other families may feel that play is for children and not for adults. Some may not have access at home to the same toys available in a clinic. Having these conversations before assessing the child-caregiver interaction is valuable and constructive for understanding the assessment and for future recommendations.

When assessing how the child and the caregiver interact with one another during the caregiver-child play interaction, the clinician should consider the ways in which culture informs the exchanges. For example, is it culturally acceptable for the caregiver to allow the child to express certain emotions? Do the caregivers interact with the child in certain culturally acceptable ways that differ from the majority culture? Similarly, when playing with the child, the clinician should take note of differences and similarities between child-caregiver, child-clinician, and child-peer play. Additionally, the clinician should consider deliberately introducing culturally relevant themes (e.g., having characters with diverse names and speaking multiple languages) when appropriate to add additional nuance to the session. Discussing the play sessions with the family allows for an assessment of the caregivers' ability to reflect on themselves and their child and may highlight culturally relevant issues.

Culturally Relevant Intervention and Treatment

After completion of the assessment as outlined in the previous section and obtaining collateral information from the school or day care, pediatrician, and other relevant sources, it is essential to understand the child's presentation in different contexts and with peers. It is vital to take into consideration implicit and explicit biases that caregivers, teachers, and others working with the child may have and how these biases may influence their reporting of the child's behavior. Clinicians should consider their own biases in order to ensure awareness of potential blind spots. When creating a culturally relevant formulation, developing a nuanced and complete narrative is key to avoiding assumptions and generalizations. Having a diverse group of clinicians formulating the case helps to avoid bias in the assessment interpretation. Additionally, discussing with the family their own thoughts and impressions is essential in creating a collaborative formulation.

Additionally, it is imperative to consider how implicit and explicit biases may contribute to the diagnosis and treatment of young children. Historically, when young children of color were referred to treatment for behavioral health concerns, they were underdiagnosed or misdiagnosed (Cross et al. 1989). Underutilization of services by racially/ethnically diverse families has long been noted. To address these issues, clinicians and researchers have provided recommendations of ways to be inclusive and to increase the cultural relevance of interventions (Sue and Sue 1995). Additionally, racial disparities in pharmacological treatments have also been noted. Specifically, a study by Zito et al. (2005) showed factors such as Medicaid eligibility having a significant impact on racial disparities in the prevalence of psychotropic medication use.

Many treatments and interventions currently available have been tested in non-Latinx/Hispanic white individuals. Unsurprisingly, researchers have experienced difficulties in widely using interventions that are not inclusive of diverse communities (Harachi et al. 2001). Recently, there has been a push to create more culturally informed interventions that take into account diverse families and cross-cultural differences (Liu et al. 2018). As a result, many treatments and interventions currently available have been tested in non-Latinx/Hispanic white individuals. For example, Brotman et al. (2011) tested a culturally informed universal intervention that showed efficacy in diverse, historically underserved populations.

Although much remains to be done in the area of culturally relevant treatment, before starting a medication or recommending a psychological or behavioral intervention, it is wise to review the literature and assess the intervention's efficacy in individuals from the patient's culture, race, or ethnicity. It is also important to discuss with families their views on treatment options and how their culture views such treatments. Treatment team–based discussion must include the family in order to ensure understanding of and comfort with the recommendations. Additionally, once the child is engaged in treatment, ongoing discussion with the family about how they and other family members or community members think the treatment is going is crucial because the family may stop the treatment if it does not align with their cultural values and beliefs (Liu et al. 2018).

Clinical Vignette

Chief Complaint and Developmental History

Abena is a 30-month-old multiracial girl presenting with a history of challenging behaviors observed at her preschool day care.

History of presenting illness and developmental history. Abena was the product of a planned and wanted pregnancy. Her mother worked throughout the pregnancy as a paralegal while attending law school, and her father worked in his family's accounting firm. Initial concerns were solely around naming their baby because they wanted to satisfy both families' traditions: Mr. Nayra is Ghanaian American, and Mrs. Nayra is Ecuadorian American.

After a full-term, normal spontaneous vaginal delivery with 9, 9 Apgars, Abena was discharged home after a typical stay. Abena's mother remained home for 6 weeks and her father for 2 weeks, although after going back to work, he returned daily for lunch. Mr. and Mrs. Nayra endorsed significant support from extended family. Mrs. Nayra denied any postpartum mood or anxiety symptoms but endorsed stress because multiple family members had differing ideas about child care, leading her to call her eldest sister frequently for help with managing the disparate advice.

After 6 weeks, a complex caregiving arrangement was established, shared between Abena's paternal Nigerian grandmother, maternal Ecuadorian grandmother, maternal aunt, and mother. Abena's parents said that the baby did well with the arrangement, but they had concerns about differing "rules" across households. Mrs. Nayra said that they "figured it wasn't such a big deal because she was going to start school soon." Mr. and Mrs. Nayra denied having any concerns in the first year of life, stating that Abena met all of her milestones on time, although talking was delayed because she was learning multiple languages.

After turning 1, Abena attended day care with children from diverse backgrounds. The day care was run by a Russian immigrant and focused on structure and education—values Mr. and Mrs. Nayra strongly endorsed. Abena liked the day care; however, because of distance, she transitioned to an in-home day care by a Somali neighbor. Within 2 weeks, her parents began receiving complaints that Abena was biting, hitting, and kicking the other children. Mr. and Mrs. Nayra were shocked by these behaviors but thought they were secondary to the new environment and would self-correct. However, after 2 months, the behaviors had not improved, and Abena was removed from the day care and returned to family care.

Shortly after Abena turned 2, her parents placed her in a day care closer to home, with a similar philosophy to the first day care, although it was not diverse. Abena liked the new day care and had friends. However, each time her parents spoke to day care staff about her academic performance, which was of paramount importance to them, the staff focused instead on Abena's behaviors. Mr. and Mrs. Nayra became increasingly concerned about the "fit" of the day care after witnessing a couple of incidents during which the teachers placed Abena in timeout even though another child had been the aggressor. At a parent-requested meeting with the day care, Mr. and Mrs. Nayra were given a document listing many behavioral difficulties, with a recommendation that they see a specialist for "testing." They promptly removed Abena from the day care and placed her back in family care while they searched for another preschool, simultaneously making an appointment at the clinic concerned that "something's wrong."

Assessment

Initial session.   To better understand Abena and her family, the clinician spent time learning about their cultural backgrounds, parenting beliefs (particularly around discipline strategies), education, behavioral expectations, and extended family members because of their significant involvement. After gathering an extensive history, the clinician and family came up with a plan that included meeting with the extended family to better understand all of the caregivers' concerns.

Session 2.   Abena's parents, both sets of grandparents, two maternal aunts, and her maternal great-grandmother met with the clinician in a large conference room. After introductions, the first question asked was about everyone's concerns about Abena's behavior, which allowed the clinician to observe the family dynamics, alliances, and disagreements. Initially, the family seemed ill at ease. However, after framing the session as the clinician wanting to understand *their* parenting cultural traditions and learn from and *partner with* them, there was increased comfort.

Although there were many areas of similarity between the family members, including respect for elders, the importance of children learning their indigenous and/or tribal languages, and the importance of education, there were also significant areas of disagreement. Time was spent discussing their profound cultural and generational differences. Both sets of grandparents believed in corporal punishment and did not understand why their American-reared children did not believe in spanking. Furthermore, they were appalled that their preferred discipline strategy was seen as abusive. Neither set of grandparents understood the significance of timeouts and described Abena as singing songs and/or talking to herself in timeout before returning to the original challenging behaviors after being released. All of the extended family members admitted that Abena was challenging, but they also agreed she was bright, sweet, curious, sassy, loving, and a delight.

At the close of the second session, the family stated that the discussion had been helpful. They now saw their caregiving roles differently, realizing that Abena had received mixed messages about expectations from all of them, such as praising her for her independence while simultaneously berating her for being willful. They proposed that these mixed messages and family discord may have been what was driving Abena's behavioral difficulties. With support from the IMH team, the family decided to postpone the sessions with Abena, determining that spending more time discussing a unified parenting strategy, simplifying the caregiving schedule, and finding a diverse school that incorporated their values of structure and a strong educational component might help with Abena's behavioral challenges.

Conclusion

In an ever-diversifying world, knowledge of cross-cultural differences is of utmost importance in providing appropriate treatment and care for children and families. During a child's earliest years, understanding cultural differences is important in assessment and treatment planning. Appropriately incorporating culturally sensitive practice in early childhood includes, but is not limited to, understanding diverse families, parenting practices, and cultural beliefs while recognizing significant differences that may exist across and within cultures and families. Inevitably, given the complexity of culture and intersectionality, all clinicians will have blind spots and biases. Working in diverse teams, participating in reflective supervision, and partnering with families in a humble and respectful manner is important. At times, the clinician's traditional script may need to be changed to honor the family's traditions while still ensuring that the child and family are receiving the highest standard of care. Using these concepts and strategies, clinicians will be able to better serve diverse families and young children in a culturally thoughtful way.

As evidenced in this chapter, there is still much more to learn about how culture influences the developing child and family, as well as how culture influences mental health presentations, diagnosis, and treatment in IMH. Additionally, more studies are needed to understand how the clinician's and family's backgrounds intersect and influence young children's development. Future studies should focus on a more nuanced understanding of these questions not only in U.S. populations but also populations around the world.

A Note on Race, Racism, and the COVID-19 Pandemic

This book was in production during the novel coronavirus SARS-CoV-2 (COVID-19) pandemic, a period when many diverse families—particularly, Black, brown, and immigrant families—found themselves at a crossroads of facing a syndemic- or synergistic aggregation of two epidemics: that of COVID-19 and that of racism. In the United States, the COVID-19 pandemic has disproportionately affected communities of color, specifically Black and brown communities with higher infection and mortality rates (Webb Hooper et al. 2020). This disproportionality also includes Black and brown children, who have been increasingly found to be at greater risk than non-Latinx white children from COVID-19 (Kim et al. 2020). The disparities evidenced during this crisis should be considered in the context of systemic and individual racism.

As we have addressed in this chapter the critical importance of understanding family and community contexts in a culturally appropriate way, this pandemic also highlights that it is imperative to concretely ask families about their experiences of discrimination and racism at both the systemic and individual levels. Some of these experiences with racism and discrimination may be subtle, and some are overt. The important key factor is that clinicians directly address racism, allowing families to discuss their experience in a supportive environment. Furthermore, during the rapid development that occurs in the first 5 years of life, very young children are becoming more aware of differences in color of skin, gender, religion, and language between themselves and others. Thus, during play, clinicians should create opportunities for exploration of these topics in a safe therapeutic environment.

The COVID-19 pandemic has highlighted the need for carefully investigating delivery of care and resources in young children and their families as discussed in this chapter. Much research remains to be conducted to examine the efficacy and effectiveness of interventions utilizing different modalities of delivery in diverse communities. Despite these gaps in the literature, when engaging family in services, clinicians should respect, understand, and ask about the individual, family, community and larger socioenvironmental context in which the services are provided to ensure culturally sensitive delivery of services for diverse very young children and their families.

Clinical Pearls

- In spite of changing U.S. demographics, racial and ethnic health and educational disparities still persist, even among very young children.

- The first 5 years of life are critically important for child development, and culture impacts all aspects of this period.

- Culture and diversity should always be kept in mind throughout an infant mental health assessment. Families should be asked explicitly at every point of the assessment about their parenting practices, structural barriers to care, and cultural influences, including their beliefs regarding mental health assessment and treatment.

- Reflective supervision with a diverse team of colleagues helps to unpack unintended slights and to ensure that assessments are less biased.

Self-Assessment Questions

1. When assessing young children and caregivers with standardized assessments, which of the following should be considered?

    A. Ensure that the standardized assessment is in the language that the caregiver prefers.
    B. Ensure that the scale is validated in the population with which the child and caregiver identify.
    C. Discuss the assessment with the family and questions they may have.
    D. All of the above.

2. When providing treatment to young children and their families, which of the following is incorrect?

    A. The clinician should discuss how the child and family feel about treatment and mental health services.
    B. The clinician should review the literature to see if the treatment has been associated with improved outcomes or side effects in the population with which the child and caregiver identify and then discuss these outcomes and side effects with the family.
    C. The clinician should discuss with the family possible barriers and facilitators to treatment.
    D. The clinician should decide whether the family will be able to comply with treatment and provide recommendations to the family.

3. Describe why it is particularly important to think about culture and diversity in infant mental health.

4. List and explain three areas that you currently include in your cultural assessment of young children and include ways to improve these areas.

5. Discuss three specific aspects you could add to your assessment of infants and young children that would take culture into account.

6. List and explain three areas that you currently include in your cultural formulation and treatment of young children and include ways to improve these areas.

7. Discuss three specific aspects you could add to your cultural formulation and treatment of infants and young children.

Answers

1. D
2. D

References

Ainsworth MD, Bell SM: Attachment, exploration, and separation: illustrated by the behavior of one-year-olds in a strange situation. Child Dev 41(1):49–67, 1970

American Psychiatric Association: Cultural Formulation Interview, in Diagnostic and Statistical Manual of Mental Disorders, 5th Edition. Arlington, VA, American Psychiatric Association, 2013, pp 750–757

Benasich AA, Brooks-Gunn J: Maternal attitudes and knowledge of child-rearing: associations with family and child outcomes. Child Dev 67(3):1186–1205, 1996

Bornstein MH: Parenting and child mental health: a cross-cultural perspective. World Psychiatry 12(3):258–265, 2013

Bornstein MH, Cote LR, Maital S, et al: Cross-linguistic analysis of vocabulary in young children: Spanish, Dutch, French, Hebrew, Italian, Korean, and American English. Child Dev 75(4):1115–1139, 2004

Bowlby J: The nature of the child's tie to his mother. Int J Psychoanal 39(5):350–373, 1958

Brotman LM, Calzada E, Huang KY, et al: Promoting effective parenting practices and preventing child behavior problems in school among ethnically diverse families from underserved, urban communities. Child Dev 82(1):258–276, 2011

Center on the Developing Child: Brain architecture. Cambridge, MA, Harvard University, 2009. Available at: https://developingchild.harvard.edu/science/key-concepts/brain-architecture. Accessed June 2019.

Clinton J, Feller A, Williams R: The importance of infant mental health. Paediatr Child Health 21(5):239–241, 2016

Colby SL, Ortman JM: Projections of the size and composition of the U.S. population: 2014 to 2060, Current Population Reports, Population Estimates and Projections. Suitland, MD, U.S. Census Bureau, March 2015. Available at: https://www.census.gov/content/dam/Census/library/publications/2015/demo/p25-1143.pdf. Accessed August 12, 2020.

Cross TL, Bazron BJ, Dennis KW, et al: Towards a Culturally Competent System of Care: A Monograph on Effective Services for Minority Children Who Are Severely Emotionally Disturbed, Washington, DC, Georgetown University Child Development Center, 1989

Earner I: Immigrant families and public child welfare: barriers to services and approaches for change. Child Welfare 86(4):63–91, 2007

Erikson EH: Childhood and Society. New York, WW Norton, 1950

Fanon F: Black Skin, White Masks [in French] (1952). Translated by Markmann CL. New York, Grove Press, 1967

Flores G; Committee on Pediatric Research: Technical report—racial and ethnic disparities in the health and health care of children. Pediatrics 125(4):e979–e1020, 2010

Fraiberg S, Adelson E, Shapiro V: Ghosts in the nursery: a psychoanalytic approach to the problems of impaired infant-mother relationships. J Am Acad Child Psychiatry 14(3):387–421, 1975

Freud A: Normality and Pathology in Childhood: Assessments of Development. New York, International Universities Press, 1965

Garcia Coll CT: Developmental outcome of minority infants: a process-oriented look into our beginnings. Child Dev 61(2):270–289, 1990

Ghosh Ippen CM: The sociocultural context of infant mental health: towards contextually congruent interventions, in Handbook of Infant Mental Health, 3rd Edition. Edited by Zeanah Jr CH. New York, Guilford, 2009, pp 104–119

Gilliam WS, Shahar G: Preschool and child care expulsion and suspension: rates and predictors in one state. Infants and Young Children 19(3):228–245, 2006

Gilliam WS, Maupin AN, Reyes CR, et al: Do early educators' implicit biases regarding sex and race relate to behavior expectations and recommendations of preschool expulsions and suspensions? Research Study Brief, New Haven, CT, Yale Child Study Center, 2016

Godoy L, Chavez AE, Mack RA, et al: Rating scales for social-emotional behavior and development, in Clinical Guide to Psychiatric Assessment of Infants and Young Children. Edited by Frankel KA, Harrison JN, Njoroge WFM. Cham, Switzerland, Springer, 2019, pp 217–251

Greenfield PM, Suzuki LK, Rothstein-Fisch C: Cultural pathways through human development, in Handbook of Child Psychology, Vol IV, 6th Edition: Child Psychology in Practice. New York, Wiley, 2006, pp 655–699

Hall WJ, Chapman MV, Lee KM, et al: Implicit racial/ethnic bias among health care professionals and its influence on health care outcomes: a systematic review. Am J Public Health 105(12):e60–e76, 2015

Harachi TW, Catalano RF, Kim S, et al: Etiology and prevention of substance use among Asian American Youth. Prev Sci 2(1):57–65, 2001

Harkness S, Super CM: Parental ethnotheories in action, in Parental Belief Systems: The Psychological Consequences for Children, 2nd Edition. Edited by Sigel IE, McGillicuddy-DeLisi AV, Goodnow JJ. New York, Psychology Press, 1992, pp 373–392

Heller SS, Wasserman K, Kelley A, et al: Observational assessment of the dyad, in Clinical Guide to Psychiatric Assessment of Infants and Young Children. Edited by Frankel KA, Harrison JN, Njoroge WFM. Cham, Switzerland, Springer, 2019 pp 107–141

Kim L, Whitaker M, O'Halloran A, et al: Hospitalization rates and characteristics of children aged <18 years hospitalized with laboratory-confirmed COVID-19—COVID-NET, 14 states, March 1–July 25, 2020. MMWR Morb Mortal Wkly Rep 69:1081–1088, 2020

LeVine RA: Human parental care: universal goals, cultural strategies, individual behavior. New Dir Child Adolesc Dev 1988(40):3–12, 1988

Liu J-L, Cherng H-YS, Rex-Kiss B, et al: Parents beyond oceans: a social group work curriculum for Chinese immigrant parents. Social Work With Groups 41(4):291–305, 2018

Londono Tobon A, Diaz Stransky A, Ross DA, et al: Effects of maternal prenatal stress: mechanisms, implications, and novel therapeutic interventions. Biol Psychiatry 80(11):e85–e87, 2016

Lyman DR, Njoroge WF, Willis DW: Early childhood psychosocial screening in culturally diverse populations: a survey of clinical experience with the Ages and Stages Questionnaires: Social-Emotional (ASQ:SE). Zero to Three 27(5):46–54, 2007

Miller SA: Parents' beliefs about children's cognitive development. Child Dev 59(2):259–285, 1988

Misch D, Billings G, Hong J, et al: Observational assessment of the young child, in Clinical Guide to Psychiatric Assessment of Infants and Young Children. Edited by Frankel KA, Harrison JN, Njoroge WFM. Cham, Switzerland, Springer, 2019, pp 143–184

Nikapota A: Cultural issues in child assessment. Child Adolesc Mental Health 14(4):200–206, 2009

Office of Minority Health: National Standards for Culturally and Linguistically Appropriate Services in Health Care, Final Report. Rockville, MD, Office of Minority Health, U.S. Department of Health and Human Services, March 2001

Ogbu JU: Origins of human competence: a cultural-ecological perspective. Child Dev 52(2):413–429, 1981

Petersen EE, Davis NL, Goodman D, et al: Vital signs: pregnancy-related deaths, United States, 2011–2015, and strategies for prevention, 13 states, 2013–2017. MMWR Morbid Mortal Wkly Rep 68(18):423–429, 2019

Rogoff B: The Cultural Nature of Human Development. New York, Oxford University Press, 2003

Shonkoff JP, Phillips DA (eds): From Neurons to Neighborhoods: The Science of Early Childhood Development. Washington, DC, National Academies Press, 2000

Stevens JH: Black grandmothers' and black adolescent mothers' knowledge about parenting. Dev Psychol 20(6):1017–1025, 1984

Sue D, Sue DM: Asian-Americans, in Experiencing and Counseling Multicultural and Diverse Populations, 3rd Edition. Edited by Vacc NA, DeVaney SB, Wittner J. Philadelphia, PA, Accelerated Development, 1995, pp 63–89

Thomas JM, Benham AL, Gean M, et al: Practice parameters for the psychiatric assessment of infants and toddlers (0–36 months): American Academy of Child and Adolescent Psychiatry. J Am Acad Child Adolesc Psychiatry 36 (10 suppl):21S–36S, 1997

Thomas K, Noroña CR, St John MS: Cross-sector allies together in the struggle for social justice: diversity-informed tenets for work with infants, children, and families. Zero to Three 39(3):44–54, 2019

Villarreal R, Blozis SA, Widaman KF: Factorial invariance of a pan-Hispanic familism scale. Hisp J Behav Sci 27(4):409–425, 2005

Webb Hooper M, Nápoles AM, Pérez-Stable EJ: COVID-19 and racial/ethnic disparities. JAMA 323:2466–2467, 2020

Zeanah CH Jr: Handbook of Infant Mental Health, 4th Edition. New York, Guilford, 2018

Zito JM, Safer DJ, Zuckerman IH, et al: Effect of Medicaid eligibility category on racial disparities in the use of psychotropic medications among youths. Psychiatr Serv 56(2):157–163, 2005

CHAPTER 18

Adoption and Foster Care Systems

Courtney L. McMickens, M.D., M.P.H., M.H.S.

THE adoption and foster care systems involve a complex network of public and private agencies, institutions, and individuals working to ensure that children live in a safe, supportive environment. Circumstances surrounding adoption and foster care vary greatly. Generally, research has shown that adoptees not involved with the child welfare system are well adjusted; however, they are more likely than nonadoptees to engage with mental health providers (Nickman et al. 2005). Within the child welfare system, it is estimated that up to 80% of children have at least one psychiatric diagnosis, and it has been well documented that psychotropic medications are prescribed at significantly higher rates to these youth than to the general population (McCue et al. 2012). In this chapter, I provide an overview of the adoption and child welfare systems as well as health care needs among children and adolescents within these systems. This includes factors that increase vulnerability to mental illness, long-term outcomes for children and adolescents within the foster care system, and the impact that involvement in the child welfare system may have on families. Additionally, psychosocial interventions, best practices in psychiatric treatment, and child and family engagement efforts are discussed. Challenges and barriers to attaining mental health services for children and adolescents in the adoption and foster care system, along with efforts to address these challenges, are presented.

Overview of Foster Care System and Adoption in the United States

The child welfare system is composed of a large network of public and private agencies that were established to receive and investigate reports of child maltreatment, in addition to providing coordination of care services, social supports for families, and out-of-home placements when needed. These services are managed by a public child welfare agency in coordination with private agencies, community-based organizations, and other child-serving systems, such as schools and health care providers (Mallon and Hess 2014). The child welfare system has been continuously plagued with concerns about its ability to meet stated objectives in a way that promotes the physical, mental, and emotional well-being of the children it is meant to serve.

More than 110,000 domestic adoptions occur annually; more than a third of them are adoptions by a relative (Jones and Placek 2017). A large majority of the domestic nonrelative adoptions are processed through public agencies, whereas less than a fourth are completed through private entities (Jones and Placek 2017). Infant adoptions make up about a fourth of domestic nonrelative adoptions (Jones and Placek 2017). Intercountry, or international, adoptions totaled just under 3,000 in the United States in 2019 (Bureau of Consular Affairs 2019). This reflects a decline from previous years, with international policies playing a significant role in trends of adoption from particular countries. For example, most children adopted through international adoptions in the United States are born in China, but there has been a progressive decline in the number of adoptions from China over the past decade because of improvements in the Chinese economy and changes in laws affecting the operation of adoption agencies (Bureau of Consular Affairs 2019). With the implementation of a ban on international adoptions, Ethiopia has also decreased its number of U.S. adoptions. Colombia has developed policies to promote domestic adoptions in an effort to decrease intercountry adoptions. In 2019, following China, India, Colombia, Ukraine, and South Korea have the greatest number of adoptions into the United States (Bureau of Consular Affairs 2019).

Families become involved with the child welfare system because of concerns for child maltreatment, most commonly neglect (Lee et al. 2015; Mallon and Hess 2014; U.S. Department of Health and Human Services 2018). Other reasons for entering the foster care system include parental substance use, parental incapacity, physical abuse, housing instability, child behavioral problems, parental incarceration, and sexual abuse. In 2017, there were more than 440,000 children in the child welfare system (52% male, 48% female) (U.S. Department of Health and Human Services 2018). Annually, about 1% of children in the United States are involved with the child welfare system (U.S. Department of Health and Human Services 2018). Lifetime prevalence of involvement with child welfare is estimated to be 5%–6%, with an average time in foster care of about 28 months (Briggs 2012).

Children of color are disproportionately represented in the foster care system. Data from 2017 show that 23% of children in foster care were Black, 21% were Hispanic, 44% were white, and 2% were American Indian or Alaskan Native; in comparison, the general population demographics are 14% Black, 25% Hispanic, 51% white, and 1% Native American (U.S. Department of Health and Human Services 2018). Black children are more likely to be removed from their homes, remain in foster care longer than the average length of placement, and are least likely to be adopted (Harris 2014; Roberts 2012; U.S. Department of Health and Human Services 2018). Although disparities in foster care involvement among Hispanic families are often masked by the population-level data, previous studies have shown that allegations of abuse are more often substantiated; however, the rate of substantiated allegations is mediated by immigration and socioeconomic status (Johnson-Motoyama et al. 2012).

Following investigation of reports of suspected abuse, only a minority of the children who experience maltreatment enter the foster care system (Lee et al. 2015; U.S. Department of Health and Human Services 2018). Foster care is one form of out-of-home placement for children whose home has been determined to be an unsafe environment. Most children in foster care live either in private homes of state-certified nonrelative caregivers or with a relative assisted by the state. Other placement settings include group homes, residential programs, and supervised independent living. In 2017, just under 248,000 children left the child welfare system: half of them returning to their primary caregivers; a fourth leaving the system through adoption; and the rest leaving through guardianship, kinship care, or emancipation (U.S. Department of Health and Human Services 2018).

Children who are not adopted from the foster care system remain until they are 18–24 years old, at which age they are deemed to "age out" of the system. Studies following youth after they aged out found higher rates of unemployment and involvement with the criminal justice system and lower educational attainment when compared with youth of similar age who had not been in the foster care system (Font et al. 2018). Higher prevalence of mental and physical health issues also continues into adulthood for youth aging out of the foster care system (Zlotnick et al. 2012). Efforts to alleviate some of these undesirable outcomes include financial support for 2- and 4-year college education, extended foster care services beyond age 18, and housing support programs (Fernandes-Alcantara 2019; Russ and Fryar 2014).

Historical Perspective

The foundation of the child welfare and foster care system dates back to the seventeenth century, when poverty and neglect were viewed as functionally one and the same. Children were taken from poor families or from the streets to prevent further economic strife and were either indentured or placed in orphanages or with other families (Mallon and Hess 2014; Schene 1998). In the late nineteenth century, the need for formal child welfare services began to grow with the recognition of unsafe and unsanitary conditions in some of the orphanages and workhouses. With a growing population, economic changes, and urban settlements for industrial work, the prevalence of child maltreatment rose (Mallon and Hess 2014; Schene 1998).

In 1875, the New York Society for Prevention of Cruelty to Children was established to investigate and intervene when child abuse was suspected. Under the structure of the American Humane Society, more than 300 societies, run by public and private entities, were formed across the country. As societies began to recognize the role of environmental deprivation, they began to advocate for governmental investment in the protection of children and vulnerable families (Schene 1998). Promotion of a national child welfare system led to the establishment of the Child Welfare League of America in 1921 (Mallon and Hess 2014; Schene 1998). The Social Security Act of 1935 provided funds for vulnerable families by establishing the Aid to Dependent Children program, which continued until major welfare reform in 1996 (Schene 1998).

The Child Abuse Prevention and Treatment Act of 1974 (CAPTA; P.L. 93-247) established a minimum standard on the federal level for the reporting of child maltreatment. States determined the definition of abuse and neglect on the basis of these federal guidelines (Child Abuse Prevention and Treatment Act 1974; Harris 2014; Schene 1998). CAPTA defines child abuse or neglect as "physical or mental injury, sexual abuse, negligent treatment, or maltreatment of a child...by a person who is responsible for the child's welfare..." (Child Abuse Prevention and Treatment Act 1974, p. 5). The legislation has since been amended to include provisions for addressing sex trafficking and exposure to substances in utero (Child Welfare Information Gateway 2019). Child protective services (CPS) agencies use the state's definition of abuse to investigate allegations of abuse and neglect.

Several pieces of legislation have been passed since CAPTA to address the needs of particular populations or concerns related to the structure and function of the child welfare system. Major legislation is summarized in Table 18–1. Each policy has been implemented with a goal of moving toward a more effective and standardized system; however, each has been met with the challenge of serving families with unique needs as well as financial and political constraints.

The Personal Responsibility and Work Opportunity Reconciliation Act of 1996, a welfare reform legislation, although not directly a child welfare legislation, replaced a previous financial assistance program known as Aid to Families with Dependent Children. This new legislation established work requirements and time limits on welfare assistance. Some people argue that as a result of these new rules, mothers were forced to take low-wage jobs that took them away from their children and kept them in poverty (Harris 2014).

The Fostering Connections to Success and Increasing Adoptions Act of 2008, an amendment to the Social Security Act that expanded adoption incentives, extended eligibility for foster care and adoption assistance to age 21, providing additional support for American Indian tribal entities. Requirements for monitoring and coordinating health care services for children within foster care were included in the Child and Family Services Improvement and Innovation Act, signed into law in 2011. Additionally, this law sought to shorten the time during which children younger than 5 years remain within the foster care system. With the increasing emphasis on promotion of permanency, critics have expressed concerns that families more vulnerable to engagement with the child welfare system, mostly poor, Black, and American Indian families, could be unjustly at greater risk of removal of children from their homes and termination of parental rights (Roberts 2014).

The disproportionate representation of families of color in the foster care system can be attributed in great part to the structural effects of poverty and systemic racism in the United States. Child protective cases and adoption of American Indian children were specifically addressed in the Indian Child Welfare Act of 1978 (Williams et al. 2015), which was enacted in response to the disproportionate removal of American Indian children from their families. Unfortunately, data have continued to show that in some states, American Indian children stay in foster care longer than white children do, and they are less likely to return to their families (Harris 2014). In 1994, Congress passed the Multiethnic Placement Act, which was later amended to the Inter-Ethnic Adoption Provisions of 1996 (U.S. Department of Health and Human Services 2008). The objective of this legislation was to prevent discrimination against children and adoptive parents on the basis of race or ethnicity. It also required agencies to recruit adoptive parents of color to reflect the demographics of children eligible for adoption (Harris 2014; Mallon and

TABLE 18-1. Major child welfare legislation in the United States

Child Abuse Prevention and Treatment Act of 1974

- Foundation for identification, reporting, and investigating child maltreatment
- Legislation under which child abuse is prosecuted
- Funding for child abuse prevention and training of child protective services (CPS) workers
- Defines the federal government's role in child welfare policy
- Amended by the Justice for Victims of Trafficking Act of 2015 to improve training for CPS workers and increase identification of children at risk for being victims of sex trafficking
- Amended by the Comprehensive Addiction and Recovery Act of 2016 and Substance Use-Disorder Prevention that Promotes Opioid Recovery and Treatment for Patients and Communities Act (also known as the SUPPORT for Patients and Communities Act) of 2018 to assist children and families affected by substance abuse

Indian Child Welfare Act of 1978

- Special protection for American Indian children within the child welfare system because of disproportionate removal from homes
- Provisions for tribal sanctions in child welfare cases

Multiethnic Placement Act (MEPA) of 1994, later amended as the Inter-Ethnic Adoption Provisions of 1996

- Prohibits delay or denial of placement based on race, color, or nationality
- Promotes recruitment of foster parent and adoptive families that reflect the demographics of children in the foster care system

Adoption and Safe Families Act of 1997

- Promotes permanency through reunification with family, adoption, legal guardianship, or kinship care
- Set standards for concurrent permanency planning
- Established the 15/22 rule to terminate parental rights if a child has been in foster care for 15 of the previous 22 months

John H. Chafee Foster Care Independence Program, Title I of 1999

- Provides funds to states, territories, and Indian tribal entities (states) to support current and former foster youth transitioning into adulthood
- Renewal included the Education and Training Voucher program to assist with educational costs

Source. Adapted from Child Welfare Information Gateway 2011, 2019; Fernandes-Alcantara 2019; Setting the Record Straight 2015; U.S. Department of Health and Human Services 2008, 2012; Williams et al. 2015.

Hess 2014). Critics argued that the legislation did not address contextual factors such as socio-economic disadvantages inextricably tied to race that resulted in a disproportionately higher rate of Black children in foster care and limited availability of Black adoptive parents.

Families of color living in low-income neighborhoods are often familiar with the foster care system, with some neighborhoods having rates of child involvement in the foster care system as high as 1 in 10 (Roberts 2007). The association between poverty and maltreatment has long been established (Drake and Jonson-Reid 2014; Paxson and Waldfogel 2002). Poverty contributes to interpersonal stress, housing instability, and food insecurity, which in turn can result in missed doctor appointments, school absenteeism, and malnourishment, all causes for alerting child welfare agencies. Disproportionate surveillance of parents in low-income neighborhoods increases detection of maltreatment, which could explain in part, but not entirely, the higher rates of out-of-home placement of children of color. The role of implicit bias and lack of culturally sensitive policies within the child welfare and affiliated systems is increasingly recognized as a contributor to decisions on out-of-home placement and lower rates of reunification (Roberts 2014).

Families often have conflicting perspectives of the child welfare system as a source of support while also viewing regulatory expectations and involvement with the family as intrusive and punitive. The child welfare system can serve as a space for parents to connect with a case worker to discuss parental stressors or connect with other needed community resources. However, engagement can be due to other sources of institutional control (Roberts 2012). For example, disproportionate incarceration of Black men and women, with women being the fastest-growing population in prisons, also contributes to the number of Black children engaging with the child welfare system. Additionally, if parents are not able to comply with recommendations set by the child welfare system, removal of the children is ultimately the feared consequence. The data related to immigration and engagement in child welfare for Latinx youth are limited, but isolated trends suggest increasing involvement of immigrant Latinx families with child welfare (Rivera-Rodríguez 2014). Stress of a new environment, family disruption, and the immigration journey are unique experiences CPS workers and other service providers must be aware of as they are engaging with immigrant families (Rivera-Rodríguez 2014).

Transracial Adoption

Race and adoption have long been a controversial topic given the history of race relations, racism, and the role of Eurocentrism in the United States. In the United States, families that adopt are predominantly white and middle class, making up more than 75% of adoptive parents (Jones and Placek 2017). As research has emerged about racial identity development, transracial adoption continues to be an area in which it is important to explore how immersed children feel in their identified culture and their adoptive culture. Children's racial identity can affect their social interaction, perception of social acceptance, self-esteem, and ego development. Dissonance may manifest as problems with emotional regulation, symptoms of depression, or symptoms of anxiety.

Clinicians' Roles When Caring for Youth in the Foster Care System

Child and adolescent mental health clinicians are often involved in the evaluation and treatment of children and adolescents in the foster care system. In addition to understanding the historical context and current state of the child welfare system, psychiatrists often have three tasks when working with youth involved in the foster care system: 1) identify ongoing safety concerns, 2) establish a comprehensive treatment plan with evidence-based psychotherapeutic and psychopharmacological treatment, and 3) advocate for services that are in the best interest of the child (Lee et al. 2015).

Because clinicians are mandated reporters, awareness of the forms of child maltreatment is critical. Neglect is the most common form of maltreatment and is the hardest to identify. Most concerns regarding neglect become apparent as a pattern of failure to meet basic needs (e.g., attending school, obtaining required immunizations, providing appropriate personal care) or as signs of significant malnourishment. These cases are often identified by teachers, health care providers, or other adults who come in contact with children outside the home. Identifying neglect among infants and toddlers can be particularly challenging because they may not regularly engage in structured programs outside the home. Physical abuse includes hitting, punching, physically dropping, shaking, throwing, or kicking a child. Physical abuse is usually reported by the child or is evident from bruising on the child's body. States vary on the distinction between physical abuse and acceptable forms of physical punishment. Sexual abuse includes engagement in sexual acts with or without force, coerced sexual acts with another person, providing sexually explicit material to children, touching of genitalia, and/or exposure of a child for the sexual gratification of others (Sedlak et al. 2010).

The work of Rutter et al. (2004) in Romanian orphanages and the continually expanding data on toxic stress and adverse childhood experiences have provided evidence that children exposed to chronic stress are at higher risk for mental and physical health problems (Felitti et al. 1998; Sonuga-Barke et al. 2017). Chronic stress and deprivation can affect neurocognitive development, leading to learning difficulties, developmental delay, and impairment in social interactions (Pears and Fisher 2005; Pears et al. 2007). Physical health problems include asthma, infections, obesity, and dental caries (Turney and Wildeman 2016). Risk of physical health problems are seen into adulthood, with studies showing higher rates of asthma, hypertension, stroke, heart disease, and smoking in adults with a history of foster care placement (Zlotnick et al. 2012).

Children who have experienced maltreatment often display behavioral symptoms, including aggression, defiance, and anger, whereas others may present as withdrawn, inattentive, passive, or detached. Children within the child welfare system have often been exposed to multiple, chronic traumatic experiences over time. This can lead to symptoms of complex trauma that span traditional diagnostic categories, making diagnosis and treatment difficult (Spinazzola et al. 2005).

Children within the foster care system are most commonly diagnosed with ADHD, oppositional defiant disorder (ODD), and conduct disorder (Maher et al. 2015; McCue et al. 2012; Tan and Marn 2013). Mood and anxiety disorders are also prevalent (McCue et al. 2012; Hambrick et al. 2016; Turney and Wildeman 2016). PTSD and reactive attachment disorder are two trauma-specific disorders commonly diagnosed among youth within the child welfare system that can often be misdiagnosed as ADHD or ODD during initial assessments because of trauma-related behavioral manifestations such as hyperarousal and emotional reactivity. Suicide assessment and screening for substance use are essential components of the mental health evaluation because adolescents placed in foster care are four times more likely to have a history of suicide attempts and five times more likely to have a history of substance abuse (Hambrick et al. 2016).

Assessment for adopted children or those within foster care can sometimes be limited by a fractured history of care, multiple placements, and limited knowledge of family or birth history (Hoagwood et al. 2001). Complex system involvement often requires a multidisciplinary treatment approach; it is important to communicate with all parties involved, including service agencies. Some cases may require a community-based team approach with access to wraparound services and team members, such as an assertive community treatment team instead of a solo physician practice. Psychiatrists also may serve as consultants to agencies and other systems that support children in the foster care system (e.g., schools); doing so may provide additional information to better understand a child's presentation and how to support children with trauma-informed practices.

Use of psychotropic medication must be taken into consideration when developing a comprehensive treatment plan. However, overprescribing, in particular when prescribing antipsychotics, for children within the foster care system has been an issue of concern. It is estimated that 21%–39% of children in foster care receive psychotropic medications, compared with 10% of children in the general population (U.S. Government Accountability Office 2017). In a study examining prescribing practices for children with Medicaid services, children within foster care were prescribed two or more antipsychotics for longer duration for nonindicated diagnoses such as ADHD and conduct disorder (dosReis et al. 2011). Black children in the foster care system were more likely than white children to receive two or more antipsychotics (dosReis et al. 2011).

Use of psychotropic medication must be taken into consideration when developing a comprehensive treatment plan. However, overprescribing, in particular when prescribing antipsychotics, for children within the foster care system has been an issue of concern. It is estimated that 21%–39% of children in foster care receive psychotropic medications, compared with 10% of children in the general population (U.S. Government Accountability Office 2017). In a study examining prescribing practices for children with Medicaid services, children within foster care were prescribed two or more antipsychotics for longer duration for nonindicated diagnoses such as ADHD and conduct disorder (dosReis et al. 2011). Black children in the foster care system were more likely than white children to receive two or more antipsychotics (dosReis et al. 2011). Practices aimed at preventing overprescribing include comprehensive screening and assessment, protocols for consent for treatment, and monitoring ongoing treatment with recommended laboratory tests or periodic medication review (U.S. Government Accountability Office 2017). Several states have implemented oversight for prescribing of children within the foster care system.

Psychotherapeutic Interventions

Psychotherapeutic interventions are the mainstay of treatment for children who experience trauma, and several have been evaluated specifically for children within the foster care system. The treatments are primarily based in addressing trauma-related symptoms through engagement with caregivers and/or service systems. Although there is overlap with symptoms of depression and anxiety, evidence supporting the use of medications for trauma-related symptoms in children is limited (Kaminer et al. 2005). In this section, I briefly review a select number of evidence-based psychotherapeutic treatments for children who have experienced abuse and trauma.

Attachment and Biobehavioral Check-Up

Attachment and Biobehavioral Check-Up (ABC) was developed by Mary Dozier, Ph.D., to help caregivers of children who have been maltreated respond in a nurturing manner when the child becomes distressed. This modality also teaches caregivers how to provide a consistent and caring response when interacting with the child, as well as how to avoid behaviors that may be frightening or threatening to the child. The intervention is composed of 10 sessions within the family's home during which a facilitator or *parent coach* provides real-time feedback, guiding the caregiver's behavior toward the goals of the intervention. Sessions are recorded, and "in the moment" comments are reviewed with the parent so as to identify behaviors. ABC has been evaluated in randomized control trials with foster parents and primary caregivers referred by CPS, usually as part of a foster care diversion program, which has a goal of keeping children with their families instead of placing them in foster care. Postintervention assessments include the Strange Situation, which showed that CPS-involved children who had received the ABC intervention were less likely to show signs of disorganized attachment compared with control subjects (Bernard et al. 2010). ABC also seems to have positive effects on executive functioning skills of children who complete the intervention (Lewis-Morrarty et al. 2012; T. Lind, K. Bernard, A. Wallin, and M. Dozier, "The Effects of an Attachment-Based Intervention on Children's Expression of Negative Affect in a Challenging Task," University of Delaware, Newark, unpublished manuscript, 2012).

Multidimensional Treatment Foster Care for Preschoolers

Multidimensional Treatment Foster Care for Preschoolers (MTFC-P), a treatment modality derived from Multidimensional Treatment Foster Care, was developed to address behavioral problems among children within the juvenile justice and foster care systems (Gilliam and Fisher 2014). The intervention is delivered in a home setting and is composed of parent training in responsive parenting techniques for primary caregivers and foster parents, individual therapy for children, and work with a behavioral specialist. The adapted intervention, MTFC-P, incorporates a developmental framework and includes a therapeutic play group with three primary target areas: behavioral problems, emotional regulation, and developmental delays. As part of MTFC-P, foster parents complete a 20-hour parent training in behavioral management. In addition to parent training, foster parents receive daily phone calls to assess children's behaviors and parental stress. MTFC-P also provides weekly support groups and 24-hour crisis support available through a team consisting of a program supervisor, foster parent consultant, behavior support specialist, family therapist, consulting psychiatrist, and play group staff; each team services 12–15 children. MTFC-P has been shown to improve problem behaviors, increase placement stability, and promote secure attachment (Fisher et al. 2009).

Trauma Systems Therapy

Trauma systems therapy (TST) was developed to meet the needs of children who experience trauma by addressing how patterns of survival, or maladaptive coping strategies, may manifest in the child's social environments (Navalta et al. 2013). The treatment has three phases: safety-focused treatment, regulation-focused treatment, and beyond-trauma treatment. TST includes a clinical component and a system component. Individual therapy focuses on emotional regulation, trauma exposure, and cognitive processing; social environment interventions include advocating services that meet children's needs and promote behaviors that increase feelings of safety while decreasing environmental triggers. An initial assessment process is conducted in order to identify links between the child's behavior, emotional dysregulation, and stimuli in the environment. The TST model has been adapted for child welfare systems and culturally diverse groups, primarily populations of low socioeconomic status. Studies evaluating implementation of TST in foster homes and kinship placement showed improvement in placement stability (Brown et al. 2013).

Trauma-Focused Cognitive-Behavioral Therapy

Trauma-focused cognitive-behavioral therapy (TF-CBT) is a treatment for children who have experienced trauma and their caregivers. It focuses on building skills of affect and behavioral regulation, cognitive coping, trauma processing, and establishing safe and supportive environments (Cohen and Mannarino 2015). TF-CBT effectiveness has been established among children exposed to sexual abuse, domestic violence, and traumatic grief (Cohen et al. 2012). The components of the treatment model are spelled out in the PRACTICE acronym: **P**sychoeducation and parenting skills, **R**elaxation skills, **A**ffective regulation skills, **C**oping strategies, **T**rauma narration and cognitive processing, **I**n vivo mastery of trauma reminders, **C**onjoint child-parent sessions, and **E**nhancing safety and future development (Cohen and Mannarino 2015).

Parent-Child Interaction Therapy

Parent-child interaction therapy (PCIT) is a 14- to 20-week intervention designed for children exhibiting externalizing behaviors (Timmer and Urquiza 2014). This manualized treatment includes a didactic component and real-time coaching. Treatment is conducted in two phases. The first phase is the child-directed interaction, during which the goal of the therapist is to enhance the parent-child relationship. The second phase, parent-directed interaction, focuses on improving child compliance with parental guidance. PCIT has been shown to reduce disruptive behavior and reduce the risk of subsequent abuse in families with a history of trauma (Timmer and Urquiza 2014).

Clinical Vignette

Stacey is a 7-year-old African American girl who presents to the clinic because of concerns about her behavior at school over the past month. She is having difficulty staying focused in class and has been having behavioral outbursts—hitting, kicking, and biting other students. Her maternal grandmother, Mrs. Wilson, reports that Stacey has been having trouble sleeping at night for the past month and has been wetting the bed when she finally does fall asleep. She also cries easily. Mrs. Wilson reports that Stacey is easily upset by minor disappointments but never had behavioral problems in preschool. Mrs. Wilson has been working with Stacey's case manager to find Stacey a therapist, but the child's teacher feels she has ADHD and cannot be managed in the classroom without medication. Mrs. Wilson states that Stacey is very smart and met all developmental milestones on time.

Stacey's mother lost her job about a year ago after she divorced Stacey's father. Mrs. Wilson states that Stacey's mother then got involved with the "wrong crowd" and was ultimately arrested about 6 months ago for possession of cocaine. Stacey was present at the time of her mother's arrest, and although she initially lived with her biological father, she was removed from his home 1 month later after being physically abused by her father's girlfriend. Stacey was then placed in foster care with her grandmother, who brought her in for evaluation today. Mrs. Wilson denies a history of parental substance abuse.

On evaluation, Stacey is small for her age but well groomed. She initially sat very close to her grandmother but separated without difficulty. She speaks quietly. She states that she misses her mom and gets scared at night because her grandmother does not leave a light on in the hallway. She is afraid to wake her grandmother to go to the bathroom and is often tired in the mornings. Stacey admits to getting into trouble at school during recess because she yells when the other kids try to force her to play a game of tag. "I just don't like playing that game," she says. Stacey reports that she often thinks about her mom while at school and at night. When she hears noises, she worries that the police are surrounding the house; she denies nightmares. She reports that she feels safe living with her grandmother and talks to her mother on the phone when she calls.

On the basis of caregiver and teacher report, Stacey was started on an α_2-adrenergic agonist medication for ADHD and ODD. Engagement with a therapist who specializes in TF-CBT was recommended. During the initial appointments, Mrs. Wilson gained a greater understanding of how Stacey's experiences might be affecting her, and she subsequently placed a night light in the hallway. She also spoke with the teacher about what Stacey has been experiencing and how her reactions to physical play on the playground are due to the way her body and mind respond to situations that she might perceive as threatening, even if no threat is intended. Stacey began sharing her narrative with her mother and grandmother, which revealed that she witnessed the police officers holding a gun on her mother during the arrest. Stacey's mother was eventually released, and Stacey was able to continue her therapy with her mother. The legal case is expected to be dismissed, and as a result reunification with her mother is a goal of Stacey's therapy.

Clinical Pearls

- It is important to understand the history of the child welfare system and its procedures because this history may affect rapport building, establishing treatment goals, and continuity of care.

- Racial and ethnic minorities have a fundamentally different relationship with the child welfare system because of disproportionate effects of poverty and racism.

- Early engagement in psychotherapeutic treatments may result in less reliance on medication and can promote improvement of emotional and behavioral symptoms.

Self-Assessment Questions

1. What is the most common form of abuse reported to child protective services?

    A. Physical abuse
    B. Sexual abuse
    C. Neglect
    D. Parental drug use

2. When establishing treatment with a child who has been placed in foster care, which of the following is a key component of the assessment?

    A. Safety assessment
    B. Determining custody and medical decision-making authority
    C. Gathering history from collateral sources
    D. Assessing symptoms
    E. All of the above

3. An effective therapeutic approach to working with children within the child welfare system is based on which of the following?

    A. Psychopharmacological management
    B. Family-centered, trauma-informed care
    C. Primary focus on eliminating problematic behavior
    D. Disregard of the input of biological parents

4. What specific questions will you add to your usual base of interview questions to include content from this chapter?

5. How might you adjust your current rubric for patient conceptualization to include these concepts?

6. As you reflect, how does the information in this chapter inform your future practice?

Answers

1. C
2. E
3. B

References

Bernard K, Butzin-Dozier Z, Rittenhouse J, et al: Young children living with neglecting birth parents show more blunted daytime patterns of cortisol production than children in foster care and comparison children. Arch Pediatr Adolesc Med 164:438–443, 2010

Briggs L: Somebody's Children: The Politics of Transnational and Transracial Adoption. Durham, NC, Duke University Press, 2012

Brown AD, McCauley K, Navalta CP, et al: Trauma systems therapy in residential care: improving emotion regulation and the social environment of traumatized children and youth in congregate care. J Fam Violence 28:693–703, 2013

Bureau of Consular Affairs: FY 2018 annual report on intercountry adoption. Washington, DC, U.S Department of State, March 2019. Available at: https://travel.state.gov/content/dam/NEWadoptionassets/pdfs/Tab%201%20Annual%20Report%20on%20Intercountry%20Adoptions.pdf. Accessed March 14, 2019.

Child Abuse Prevention and Treatment Act, Pub L No 93-247, 1974

Child Welfare Information Gateway: Adoption Assistance for Children Adopted From Foster Care. Washington, DC, Children's Bureau, Administration for Children and Families, U.S. Department of Health and Human Services, 2011

Child Welfare Information Gateway: About CAPTA: A Legislative History. Washington, DC, Children's Bureau, Administration for Children and Families, U.S. Department of Health and Human Services, 2019

Cohen JA, Mannarino AP: Trauma-focused cognitive behavior therapy for traumatized children and families. Child Adolesc Psychiatr Clin N Am 24(3):557–570, 2015

Cohen JA, Mannarino AP, Deblinger E (eds): Trauma-Focused CBT for Children and Adolescents: Treatment Applications. New York, Guilford, 2012

dosReis S, Yoon Y, Rubin DM, et al: Antipsychotic treatment among youth in foster care. Pediatrics 128(6):e1459–e1466, 2011

Drake B, Jonson-Reid M: Poverty and child maltreatment, in Handbook of Child Maltreatment (Child Maltreatment: Contemporary Issues in Research and Policy, Vol 2). Edited by Korbin JE, Krugman RD. Dordrecht, Netherlands, Springer, 2014, pp 131–148

Felitti FV, Anda RF, Nordenberg D, et al: Relationship of childhood abuse and household dysfunction to many of the leading causes of death in adults: the Adverse Childhood Experiences (ACE) study. Am J Prev Med 14(4):245–258, 1998

Fernandes-Alcantara A: John H. Chafee Foster Care Program for Successful Transition to Adulthood. Washington, DC, Congressional Research Service, January 15, 2019. Available at: https://fas.org/sgp/crs/misc/IF11070.pdf. Accessed September 12, 2019.

Fisher PA, Kim HK, Pears KC: Effects of multidimensional treatment foster care for preschoolers (MTFC-P) on reducing permanent placement failures among children with placement instability. Child Youth Serv Rev 31(5):541–546, 2009

Font SA, Berger LM, Cancian M, et al: Permanency and the educational and economic attainment of former foster children in early adulthood. Am Sociol Rev 83(4):716–743, 2018

Gilliam KS, Fisher PA: Multidimensional treatment foster care for preschoolers: a program for maltreated children in the child welfare system, in Evidence-Based Approaches for the Treatment of Maltreated Children: Considering Core Components and Treatment Effectiveness (Child Maltreatment: Contemporary Issues in Research and Policy, Vol 3). Edited by Timmer S, Urquiza A. Dordrecht, Netherlands, Springer, 2014, pp 145–164

Hambrick EP, Oppenheim-Weller S, N'zi AM, et al: Mental health interventions for children in foster care: a systematic review. Child Youth Serv Rev 70:65–77, 2016

Harris M: Racial Disproportionality in Child Welfare. New York, Columbia University Press, 2014

Hoagwood K, Burns BJ, Kiser L, et al: Evidence-based practice in child and adolescent mental health services. Psychiatr Serv 52(9):1179–1189, 2001

Johnson-Motoyama M, Dettlaff AJ, Finno-Velasquez M: Parental nativity and the decision to substantiate: findings from a study of Latino children in the second National Survey of Child and Adolescent Well-being (NSCAW II). Child Youth Serv Rev 34(11):2229–2239, 2012

Jones J, Placek P: Adoption: by the numbers. Alexandria, VA, National Council for Adoption, February 2017. Available at: www.adoptioncouncil.org/publications/2017/02/adoption-by-the-numbers. Accessed May 12, 2020.

Kaminer D, Seedat S, Stein DJ: Post-traumatic stress disorder in children. World Psychiatry 4(2):121–125, 2005

Lee T, Fouras G, Brown R; American Academy of Child and Adolescent Psychiatry (AACAP) Committee on Quality Issues (CQI): Practice parameter for the assessment and management of youth involved with the child welfare system. J Am Acad Child Adolesc Psychiatry 54(6):502–517, 2015

Lewis-Morrarty E, Dozier M, Bernard K, et al: Cognitive flexibility and theory of mind outcomes among foster children: preschool follow-up results of a randomized clinical trial. J Adolesc Health 51 (2 suppl):S17–S22, 2012

Maher EJ, Darnell A, Landsverk J, et al: The well-being of children in the child welfare system: an analysis of the Second National Survey of Child and Adolescent Well-Being (NSCAW-II). Seattle, WA, Casey Family Programs, April 8, 2015. Available at: www.casey.org/nscaw. Accessed May 12, 2020.

Mallon GP, Hess PM: Child Welfare for the Twenty-First Century: A Handbook of Practices, Policies, and Programs, 2nd Edition. New York, Columbia University Press, 2014

McCue HS, Hurlburt MS, Heneghan A, et al: Mental health problems in young children investigated by U.S. child welfare agencies. J Am Acad Child Adolesc Psychiatry 51(6):572–581, 2012

Navalta CP, Brown AD, Nisewaner A, et al: Trauma systems therapy, in Treating Complex Traumatic Stress Disorder in Children and Adolescents: Scientific Foundations and Therapeutic Models. Edited by Ford JD, Courtois CA. New York, Guilford, 2013, pp 329–347

Nickman SL, Rosenfeld AA, Fine P, et al: Children in adoptive families: overview and update. J Am Acad Child Adolesc Psychiatry 44(10):987–995, 2005

Paxson C, Waldfogel J: Work, welfare, and child maltreatment. J Labor Econ 20(3):435–474, 2002

Pears K, Fisher PA: Developmental, cognitive, and neuropsychological functioning in preschool-aged foster children: associations with prior maltreatment and placement history. J Dev Behav Pediatr 26(2):112–122, 2005

Pears KC, Fisher PA, Bronz KD: An intervention to promote social emotional school readiness in foster children: preliminary outcomes from a pilot study. School Psych Rev 36(4):665–673, 2007

Rivera-Rodríguez H: Engaging Latino families, in Child Welfare for the Twenty-First Century: A Handbook of Practices, Policies, and Programs, 2nd Edition. Edited by Mallon GP, Hess PM. New York, Columbia University Press, 2014, pp 86–93

Roberts DE: Child welfare's paradox. William Mary Law Rev 49(3):881–902, 2007

Roberts DE: Prison, foster care, and the systemic punishment of black mothers. UCLA Law Review 59(6)1474–1500, 2012

Roberts DE: Child protection as surveillance of African American families. J Soc Welfare Family Law 36(4):426–437, 2014

Russ E, Fryar G: Creating access to opportunities for youth in transition from foster care: an AYPF policy brief. Washington, DC, American Youth Policy Forum, December 2014. Available at: www.aypf.org/wp-content/uploads/2014/12/FOSTER-CARE-BRIEF-12.10-2nd-Draft.pdf. Accessed May 12, 2020.

Rutter M, O'Connor TG; English and Romanian Adoptees (ERA) Study Team: Are there biological programming effects for psychological development? Findings from a study of Romanian adoptees. Dev Psychol 40(1):81–94, 2004

Schene PA: Past, present, and future roles of child protective services. Future Child 8(1):23–38, 1998

Sedlak AJ, Mettenburg J, Basena M, et al: Fourth National Incidence Study of Child Abuse and Neglect (NIS-4): Report to Congress. Washington, DC, Administration for Children and Families, U.S. Department of Health and Human Services, January 15, 2010

Setting the Record Straight: The Indian Child Welfare Act. Portland, OR, National Indian Child Welfare Association, 2015. Available at: www.nicwa.org/wp-content/uploads/2017/04/Setting-the-Record-Straight-ICWA-Fact-Sheet.pdf. Accessed June 26, 2019.

Sonuga-Barke EJS, Kennedy M, Kumsta R, et al: Child-to-adult neurodevelopmental and mental health trajectories after early life deprivation: the young adult follow-up of the longitudinal English and Romanian Adoptees study. Lancet 389(10078):1539–1548, 2017

Spinazzola J, Ford JD, Zucker M, et al: Survey evaluates complex trauma exposure, outcome, and intervention among children and adolescents. Psychiatric Annals 35(5):433–439, 2005

Tan TX, Marn T: Mental health service utilization in children adopted from US foster care, US private agencies and foreign countries: data from the 2007 National Survey of Adoption Parents (NSAP). Child Youth Serv Rev 35(7):1050–1054, 2013

Timmer S, Urquiza A (eds): Evidence-Based Approaches for the Treatment of Maltreated Children: Considering Core Components and Treatment Effectiveness (Child Maltreatment: Contemporary Issues in Research and Policy, Vol 3). Dordrecht, Netherlands, Springer, 2014

Turney K, Wildeman C: Mental and physical health of children in foster care. Pediatrics 138(5):e20161118, 2016

U.S. Department of Health and Human Services: Ensuring the best interest of children through compliance with The Multiethnic Placement Act of 1994, as amended, and Title VI of the Civil Rights Act of 1964. Washington, DC, Administration for Children and Families, Office for Civil Rights, U.S. Department of Health and Human Services, 2008. Available at: www.hhs.gov/sites/default/files/ocr/civilrights/resources/specialtopics/adoption/mepatraingppt.pdf. Accessed May 12, 2020.

U.S. Department of Health and Human Services: John H. Chafee Foster Care Independence Program. Washington, DC, Children's Bureau, Administration for Children and Families, U.S. Department of Health and Human Services, June 28, 2012. Available at: www.acf.hhs.gov/cb/resource/chafee-foster-care-program. Accessed August 1, 2019.

U.S. Department of Health and Human Services: The AFCARS Report: Preliminary FY 2017 Estimates as of August 10, 2018—No 25. Washington, DC, Children's Bureau, Administration for Children and Families, Administration on Children, Youth and Families, U.S. Department of Health and Human Services, 2018. Available at: www.acf.hhs.gov/sites/default/files/cb/afcarsreport25.pdf. Accessed May 12, 2020.

U.S. Government Accountability Office: Foster care: HHS has taken steps to support states' oversight of psychotropic medications, but additional assistance could further collaboration (Report to Congressional Requesters, GAO-17-129). Washington, DC, U.S. Government Accountability Office, January 2017

Williams JR, Maher EJ, Tompkins J, et al: Indian Child Welfare Act: measuring compliance, a research and practice brief: measuring compliance with the Indian Child Welfare Act. March 2015. Available at: https://caseyfamilypro-wpengine.netdna-ssl.com/media/measuring-compliance-icwa.pdf. Accessed August 18, 2019.

Zlotnick C, Tam TW, Soman LA: Life course outcomes on mental and physical health: the impact of foster care on adulthood. Am J Public Health 102(3):534–540, 2012

CHAPTER 19

Microaggressions

Effects in Early Life and Strategies to Overcome

Ranna Parekh, M.D., M.P.H., DFAPA
Auralyd Padilla, M.D.
Maria Jose Lisotto, M.D.
Sejal Patel, M.P.H.
R. Dakota Carter, M.D., Ed.D.
Cheryl S. Al-Mateen, M.D., FAACAP, DFAPA

THE field of medicine continues to give significant attention to the influence and impact of social determinants of health and mental health, including discrimination and racism (Braveman et al. 2011; Paradies et al. 2015). Furthermore, attention to the contribution of discrimination to health disparities (Williams and Mohammed 2009) has led national medical associations such as the American Academy of Child and Adolescent Psychiatry, American Academy of Pediatrics, and American Psychiatric Association, to come forward with policy statements condemning unequal treatment based on a person's identity (American Academy of Child and Adolescent Psychiatry 2009; American Academy of Pediatrics 2018; American Psychiatric Association 2018; Trent et al. 2019). Although the literature shows robust research on discrimination based on race, emerging evidence highlights other forms of discrimination based on gender, sexual orientation, weight, and physical (Conover and Israel 2019) or cognitive (Bowleg 2012; Garnettt et al. 2014; Seaton et al. 2010) abilities.

Additionally, there is a growing interest in understanding the effect of more subtle forms of discrimination such as microaggressions. The concept of microaggression has gained increasing recognition, becoming part of the daily vernacular, in part as the definition has expanded to include more vulnerable groups. Intersectionality, including the overlap between an individual's racial/ethnic identity and other socioeconomic and gender identities, increases one's risk of experiencing a microaggression. As diversity in the United States continues to grow and become complex, health care providers, educators, school officials, and caregivers working with children, adolescents, and young adults will become more exposed to patients who have experienced microaggressions and may even have personal experiences with microaggression themselves.

In this chapter, we review the literature on microaggression and other forms of discrimination, offering a developmental perspective on the impact that such psychological injuries can have on vulnerable youth populations. In this discussion, the term *youth* is used to describe children, preadolescents, adolescents, and transitional-age youth (TAY); when we use the term *vulnerable*, we are referring to African American; American Indian; Asian American; Latinx; and lesbian, gay, bisexual, transgender, and queer/questioning (LGBTQ) groups. Other aspects of social identities related to gender, religion, and ability or disability also make one vulnerable. We review historical as well as evolving definitions of microaggressions and their subtypes, focusing on differences between microaggression and other types of discrimination. We then review the consequences that microaggressions can have on the physical and mental health as well as the overall well-being of vulnerable populations. An overview of typical development is presented to show youth vulnerability to these consequences. Last, we present specific strategies that can be used by individuals, school teachers, administrators, caregivers, and health care providers to mitigate the negative consequences of microaggressions. A concluding example demonstrates how an adolescent might experience an episode of microaggression.

Microaggressions and Other Forms of Mistreatment

In 1970, the late Harvard psychiatrist and educator Chester Pierce first wrote about *microaggression*, a term he coined to describe the ongoing discrimination experienced by African Americans (Pierce 1970). Dr. Pierce defined microaggressions as "subtle, stunning, often automatic, and non-verbal exchanges" that can "infringe on a person's time, space, energy, and mobility" (Sue 2010, p. xvi). Although the term initially was specific to African American experiences, other researchers later built on Pierce's work to describe similar exchanges experienced by other marginalized groups. Psychologist Derald Wing Sue described microaggressions as "brief, everyday exchanges that send denigrating messages to certain individuals because of their group membership" (Sue 2010, p. xvi) and further subclassified microaggressions as microinsults, microassaults, and microinvalidations. *Microinsults* are subtle verbal or nonverbal discriminatory acts that convey contempt and disrespect for someone for their identity, such as when a peer tells a Latinx student that she doesn't sound Latina (Sue 2010). *Microassaults* are defined as explicit and intentional discriminatory behaviors, such as openly displaying a racist symbol (e.g., a swastika or a Confederate flag) (Sue 2010). Finally, Sue and colleagues categorized *microinvalidations* as "communications that exclude, negate or nullify people's psychological thoughts, feelings, and experiences of people of color or other marginalized groups," such as asking someone "Where are you from?" (Sue 2010, p. 29).

It is important to differentiate microaggressions from overt forms of mistreatment. For example, teasing is a common social interaction for adolescents in which an "intentional provocation is accompanied by playful markers" (Douglass et al. 2016, p. 72). In contrast, bullying is "harassment perpetrated multiple times by another youth more powerful than the victim" (Jones et al. 2018, pp. 50–51). Youth from vulnerable groups are at increased risk of bias-based bullying, a specific type of bullying, in which individuals are targeted or demeaned because of their perceived race, ethnicity, immigration status, religion, sexual or gender identity, disability, or weight (Jones et al. 2018). In addition, microaggressions should be distinguished from the two most overt forms of mistreatment: discrimination and racism. *Discrimination* is defined as "any behavior which denies individuals or groups of people equality of treatment they may wish" (Benner et al. 2018, p. 856). The term *racism* refers to "an organized system that categorizes population groups into 'races' and uses this ranking to preferentially allocate societal goods and resources to groups regarded as superior" (Williams and Mohammed 2009, p. 2).

Mistreatment can be subtle and covert, stemming from stereotypes and implicit bias (Blume et al. 2012). Perceived discrimination is "a behavioral manifestation of a negative attitude, judgment, or unfair treatment toward members of a group" (Szaflarski and Bauldry 2019, p. 174). Scholars describe microaggression as a form of daily discrimination for vulnerable groups and often use the two terms interchangeably. Although perceived discrimination is different from microaggressions, both terms share a focus on the perception of the recipient rather than the perpetrator, which is why some scholars often use these terms interchangeably. Where relevant, literature will be cited when perceived discrimination is applicable to microaggressions.

Consequences of Perceived Discrimination and Experiences of Microaggressions

Over the past decade, there has been an increase in research examining the impact of racial discrimination on the health of children and young adults. Although the pathways in which racial discrimination influences health may differ in children and young adults, commonalities with the adult literature on racial discrimination and its effects on health have been observed (Priest et al. 2013), and there is a clear connection between the additive experiences of discrimination and negative health outcomes. In the first international systematic review of this topic, Priest et al. (2013) found that the most commonly reported health-related outcomes associated with racial discrimination among youth ages 0–18 were mental health outcomes such as anxiety, depression, and negative self-esteem. Weaker relationships existed between discrimination and physical health outcomes (Priest et al. 2013). Nadine Burke Harris, a pediatrician known for her study of adverse childhood experiences (ACEs) in an urban population, developed a primary care screening measure for ACEs (Purewal et al. 2016). This measure includes experiencing racism and discrimination as an ACE along with sexual and physical abuse and exposure to domestic violence, three of the original ACEs first reported by Felitti et al. (1998).

Perceived discrimination and microaggressions can be conceptualized as forms of stress (Conover and Israel 2019; Pascoe and Smart Richman 2009). Studies of stress have shown that unpredictable and uncontrollable stressors, such as perceived discrimination, may be particularly harmful (Pascoe and Smart Richman 2009; Williams and Mohammed 2009). Similar to other types of stress, perceived discrimination may lead to an increased stress response, causing continuously elevated levels of cortisol and other catecholamines that can affect multiple biological systems (Adam et al. 2015). At baseline, the human body is equipped to return to balance following an acute stressor; however, repeated levels of stress can take a biological toll, with long-term health implications. Researchers have defined this toll from chronic physiological stress through a marker known as *allostatic load* (Brody et al. 2014; Pascoe and Smart Richman 2009). Repeated exposure to experiences of discrimination may prepare the body to become more physically reactive when confronted with stressful or potentially stressful social situations (Brody et al. 2014). Routine discrimination, such as daily, repeated experiences of microaggressions experienced by vulnerable groups, can become a chronic stressor that may increase vulnerability to physical illness (Brody et al. 2014).

Interestingly, there may be racial/ethnic differences in terms of the effect that perceived discrimination can have on cortisol levels. For example, in a prospective study of 112 individuals, Adam et al. (2015) examined developmental histories of perceived discrimination and cortisol profiles in adulthood. The study measured whether developmental histories of perceived discrimination were associated with adult diurnal cortisol profiles. The results demonstrated that multiple aspects of the diurnal cortisol rhythm were affected by perceived discrimination among Blacks, making the effect more pervasive for this group. Results also showed that the impact of perceived discrimination on stress biology was most sensitive during adolescence when compared with adulthood (Adam et al. 2015).

Another proposed pathway to the detrimental physical and psychological health effects of perceived discrimination is increased participation in unhealthy behaviors, such as substance use, and decreased participation in healthy ones (Pascoe and Smart Richman 2009). Older adolescents with a history of frequent microaggressions sometimes turn to illicit substance use as an ineffective way of coping with distress, which subsequently further decreases their overall well-being.

Data comparing the physical and mental health effects of perceived discrimination are conflicting. Paradies (2006) found that the impact of discriminatory experiences was more pronounced for mental than physical health. However, Pascoe and Smart Richman (2009) found that this difference was not statistically significant (Lewis et al. 2015). Studies of children and TAY showed a stronger relationship between discrimination and mental health than between discrimination and physical health (Priest et al. 2013). One hypothesis for the weaker association between racial discrimination and physical health outcomes in younger populations could be the delayed onset between exposure to racial discrimination and such outcomes as blood pressure, obesity, and other chronic illnesses (Priest et al. 2013).

Consequences of Microaggressions on Well-Being and Mental Health

Research has shown a positive association between microaggressions and psychopathology among racial/ethnic minority groups (Blume et al. 2012; Hollingsworth et al. 2017; Huynh 2012). Seemingly innocuous forms of discrimination are associated with elevated levels of anxiety, anger, and stress (Huynh 2012; Noh et al. 2007). The subtleness of microaggressions is thought to be a key contributor to their detrimental psychological effects. For the victim, it is unclear if the microaggression was intentional or not, which leads to rumination (Solorzano et al. 2000; Sue et al. 2007), poor self-esteem (Greene et al. 2006), anger, internalization (Huynh 2012), depression (Basáñez et al. 2013; Huynh 2012), anxiety, and substance use (Basáñez et al. 2013; Noh et al. 2007; Respress et al. 2013).

Although an isolated experience of a microaggression may be perceived as mild, the accumulation of microaggressions leads to anger, helplessness, and frustration (Huynh 2012; Solorzano et al. 2000). Dr. Pierce described microaggressions as worse for African Americans because they are most likely to experience them daily, every day, leading to accumulative lifetime burden (Pierce 1970). Studies suggest that other marginalized groups experience daily microaggressions as well (Sue et al. 2007). Noh et al. (2007) found that subtle discrimination, rather than overt discrimination, was associated with more anger and depressive symptoms among a sample of Korean immigrants. For adolescents and TAY, this anger may stem from the ambiguity of the situation (Huynh 2012; Noh et al. 2007). Studies have found consistent associations between interpersonal discrimination and a range of DSM-based psychiatric diagnoses, such as anxiety disorders, eating disorders, and even psychotic disorders (American Psychiatric Association 2013; Lewis et al. 2015).

Certain minorities, such as African Americans, experience microaggressions more frequently than others, which could make them more vulnerable to health and mental health disorders (Huynh 2012). Most of the research on racism and discrimination has focused on African Americans, so it is not clear how diverse racial/ethnic groups and other vulnerable groups may react to specific types of microaggressions. Huyhn (2012) studied Latinx and Asian American adolescents to examine the implications of microaggressions specifically on adolescents' depressive and somatic symptoms. This study showed ethnic differences in the frequency and type of microaggressions. Latinx individuals reported a higher experience of denial of racial reality (being told they are too sensitive about racial matters) and negative treatment (e.g., being ignored by a store clerk) compared with Asian Americans.

Exposure to discrimination in early childhood may result in problem health behaviors later in development (Purewal et al. 2016). In one study, perceived discrimination was shown to influence alcohol and drug consumption in American Indian youth (Pachter and Coll 2009; Whitbeck et al. 2001) and alcohol, drug, and tobacco use among African American youth (Gibbons et al. 2004; Pachter and Coll 2009). Binge drinking among college students is thought to be associated with school-related stress, including the potential stressor of experienced microaggressions (Blume et al. 2012). Because high frequency of microaggressions has been associated with elevated levels of stress among racial and sexual minority students, it is crucial to consider the relationship between microaggressions and alcohol use in college populations, especially among transitional-age minorities. Blume et al. (2012) studied 594 college students, ages 18–20 years, at a historically white institution to examine the relationship between frequency of microaggressions, alcohol use, and anxiety. They determined that students of color who experience higher numbers of microaggressions than do their white counterparts may be at increased risk of anxiety and underage binge alcohol use (Blume et al. 2012). Similarly, microaggressions related to sexual orientation are associated with depression, anxiety, suicidal ideation, self-destructive behaviors, substance use, and PTSD symptoms (Conover and Israel 2019). Other studies have shown that experiencing LGBQ microaggressions is a risk factor for LGBQ college students smoking cigarettes (Ylioja et al. 2018).

According to the 2017 Youth Risk Behavior Surveillance System, 19% of students enrolled nationwide in grades 9–12 reported having been bullied on school property within the preceding 12 months (Centers for Disease Control and Prevention 2018). Youth from vulnerable groups are more likely than nonminority youth to experience bullying (Maynard et al. 2016). The mental health, academic, interpersonal, behavioral, and societal consequences of bullying have been well established in the literature (Maynard et al. 2016). Bias-based bullying is associated with adverse health and mental health consequences for adolescents and adults from minority groups (Maynard et al. 2016; Walton 2018). Although minority youth experience both bias-based bullying and microaggressions, the connection between the two is not yet well defined. Garnett et al. (2014) conducted a study of the intersectionality between multiple attributes of discrimination and bullying in ethnically diverse adolescents and found that specific combinations of discrimination attributes and bullying were associated with increased depressive symptoms, suicidal ideation, and deliberate self-harm. Sanders-Phillips (2009) argued that exposure to specific racial discrimination could represent a form of violence and a constant source of trauma, influencing mental and physical outcomes as well as parent and community support and functioning. Further research on the relationship between bullying and microaggressions is needed.

Few studies have looked at the relationship between microaggression and suicide. O'Keefe et al. (2015) and Hollingsworth et al. (2017) found a positive relationship between microaggression and suicidal ideation in college-age racial and ethnic minority students. Specific types of racial microaggressions, such as invisibility, low-achievement/undesirable culture, and environmental invalidations, were associated with higher levels of perceptions of being a burden on others, which in turn related to higher levels of suicidal ideation in a sample of African Americans (Hollingsworth et al. 2017).

Consequences on Academics and Social Relationships

Microaggressions can impact not only health but also other aspects of a youth's life, such as academics (Benner and Graham 2011; Huynh and Fuligni 2010; Le and Stockdale 2011). Benner et al. (2018) correlated racial/ethnic discrimination with lower academic achievement and engagement, less motivation, externalizing behaviors, and associations with deviant peers (e.g. peer deviance, peer substance use). These behaviors are often influenced by students' perception of the school's climate (e.g., perceived lower school belonging and less supportive teaching environments). Assari and Caldwell (2018) showed an association between perceived discrimination, lower grades, and absenteeism in Latinx students and their perceptions of the school. In the same study, teachers' discrimination and use of biased language were directly associated with low grade point average, student self-reported low grades, and school dropout. Similarly, the 2017 National School Climate Survey showed that of the total number of LGBT students who had been considering dropping out of school, 33.9% were doing so because of the hostile climate created by gendered school policies and practices (Kosciw et al. 2018).

Microaggressions can also have an impact on youth's social behaviors. For example, forms of discrimination have been associated with externalizing behaviors and delinquency among Asian and Latino middle school adolescents (Huynh 2012). The subtleness of microaggressions may keep youth from articulating their emotions, which could make them avoid peers and activities that would heighten the sense of being the "other," impacting youth's interpersonal relationships. Furthermore, anticipation of discrimination leads to mistrust of others, perpetuating the risk of isolation and apprehensiveness. The impact of racism on health and well-being through implicit biases, institutional structures, and interpersonal relationships is clear (Trent et al. 2019).

Youth Development and Effects of Microaggressions

Developmental Milestones

Developmental theorists, including Piaget and Erikson, shed light on critical aspects of physical, cognitive, and emotional transformations in youth. Studies have shown that experiences in early life affect children's development, influencing health outcomes (Karoly et al. 2005). Youth at different developmental stages have specific vulnerabilities and abilities to process the experience of microaggressions. If a microaggression persists, it carries the risk of affecting progression to the next developmental stage. Therefore, it is important to review the key developmental milestones to understand the impact on youth of early and recurring exposures to microaggressions (Table 19–1).

Developmental Stages and Effects of Microaggressions

The latency phase (ages 6–10 years) marks a significant shift in the importance of social relationships. According to Erikson's industry vs. inferiority stage, children experience increased pressure to get along with their peers and become more concerned with how they compare with others. When children perceive themselves as equal to peers, their sense of self-agency and confidence strengthens (Gilmore and Meersand 2014). Children's sense of worth is related to their sense of competence and their ability to master skills. This sense of competence is also influenced by how others evaluate their performance, making children vulnerable to the opinion of others (Gilmore and Meersand 2014). Feelings of inferiority carry the risk of being internalized, affecting the child's self-esteem; this is especially true for minority youth. During Piaget's concrete operational phase, children become more logical and have the ability to take the perspective of others; hence, at this stage, perpetrators of microaggressions may be able to minimize their behavior by putting themselves in the other person's shoes.

The first hormonal and physical changes in the onset of puberty characterize the preadolescent phase (ages 10–12). These changes are accompanied by an increase in body awareness, which explains why experiencing a microaggression related to appearance or weight at this

TABLE 19–1. **Cognitive, physical, and emotional milestones per developmental stage**

Developmental stage	Age range	Milestones
Latency	6–10 years	Cognitive milestones: Piaget's concrete operational stage • Gain the ability to classify objects on the basis of similarities • Begin to think logically Physical milestones • Improved strength and muscle coordination Emotional milestones: Erikson's industry vs. inferiority stage • Increase in social comparison and social network • Heightened importance of sense of competence and having a place in a group
Preadolescence	10–12 years	Cognitive milestones • Growing flexibility and abstract thinking • Heightened ability for self-reflection Physical milestones: hormonal and physical changes associated with puberty • Increase in height and weight • Development of breasts and testicular organs Emotional milestones • Stronger need for autonomy • Stronger need for closeness to peer groups
Early and mid-adolescence	11–17 years	Cognitive milestones: Piaget's formal operational stage • Increased ability to solve problems • Increased capacity for abstraction Physical milestones: hormonally charged puberty • Muscle growth • Sebaceous gland activity Emotional milestones: Erikson's identity vs. role confusion stage • Identity formation is a key component • Growth in peer influence • Increased participation in risky behaviors
Transitional-age youth	18–26 years	Cognitive milestones: Piaget's formal operational stage • Complex strategic planning ability Physical milestones • Maturation of body mass • Continuation of neurobiological development Emotional milestones: Erikson's intimacy vs. isolation stage • Individuation • Continued exploration of identity • Continued development of personality traits

stage may increase the child's self-consciousness. Preadolescents also have an increased need for autonomy and social relationships, which heightens their experiences of *otherness* when they feel different or left out of mainstream peer groups. For example, when a peer tells an African American girl that her hair is "exotic," it can make her more aware of her physical appearance and otherness, potentially contributing to feelings of inadequacy or shame, which are already common among preadolescent youth undergoing bodily changes. This could potentially lead to social isolation, thwarting the healthy need for social interactions and belongingness to same age groups.

During the early and mid-adolescence years (11–17 years), a child's physical development continues to mature rapidly, and hormonal changes may affect emotional stability. Social relationships continue to strengthen, and sexual orientation usually becomes established, although sexual orientation is a continuum and can become more fluid and change throughout adolescence. At this stage, peer influence grows, bringing along an increase in the potential for risky behaviors (King and Rutherford 2017). Adolescents may be especially vulnerable to microaggressions based on their cultural, ethnic, and/or sexual identity. The common belief that their experiences are unique and that others are focused on their appearance and behavior can make it particularly challenging for adolescents to process a microaggression.

During adolescence, youth go through the process of formation of their identity through identification with others. This process can be threatened and thwarted by experiences of microaggressions, potentially leading to identity confusion. For example, when a group of teenagers describe something as being "so gay," they could inadvertently be sending the message that there is something wrong with being gay. For gay adolescents overhearing these peers, the idea that being gay is wrong can further exacerbate their sense of otherness, potentially even increasing thoughts of thwarted belongingness (i.e., social disconnection or alienation, loneliness). Thwarted belongingness, along with perceived burdensomeness (i.e., feeling as though one is a burden to others), are the two interpersonal risk factors shown to be connected with an increase in suicidal ideation according to the interpersonal theory of suicide (Chu et al. 2017; Joiner 2007; Van Orden et al. 2010).

Microinsults such as asking an Asian American adolescent "What are you?" (referring to racial/ethnic heritage) may be associated with worse depressive and somatic symptoms in adolescents because at this developmental stage, they are concerned about the negative evaluation of peers (Huynh 2012). Some authors have proposed that experiences of discrimination may undermine youth's identification with their culture, leading to internalization of negative, harmful stereotypes (Jones and Galliher 2015). Others have suggested that a positive sense of ethnic identification may serve as a protector against stressors faced by minority youth (Jones and Galliher 2015).

The transitional age (ages 18–26) marks an ongoing process of individuation and exploration of identity. At this stage, TAY tend to develop religious and moral values and establish their political value system. According to Erikson's intimacy vs. isolation stage, interest in intimate relationships peaks at this time, which is why recurring episodes of microaggressions can lead to avoidance of intimacy and/or fear of relationships, which, in turn, leads to social isolation.

The impact of microaggressions may vary according to the developmental stage of the recipient and the type and degree of the microaggression. Variants in microaggression themes have been reported across racial groups (Torres-Harding et al. 2012). In a study that measured experiences of racial microaggressions using the Racial Microaggressions Scale (RMAS), Torres-Harding et al. (2012) categorized microaggressions into six types: invisibility (being dismissed or ignored), criminality (being treated as dangerous or aggressive or assumed to have a criminal status), low achieving (being treated as intellectually inferior), sexualization (being exoticized), being a foreigner (being treated as if one does not belong), and environmental invalidations (absence of people from one's race in school or work settings) (Torres-Harding et al. 2012). Table 19–2 shows daily microaggressions experienced by minority groups discussed throughout this book. These examples are depicted from the perspective of the recipient as a reminder that the concept of microaggression is a subjective one.

Strategies

Studies of adverse childhood experiences, bullying, and social determinants of mental health have shown that children are resilient and that high-quality early interventions can mitigate the effects of adversity on their development (Braveman et al. 2011). A study by Li et al. (2017) of the impact of microaggressions in youth postulated that the degree of reactivity to the experience of microaggressions might be associated with higher depressive and somatic symptoms. Thus, strategies that can help an individual cope with the effects of microaggressions could moderate their effects. For example, individuals can use strategies such as naming their experience as a microaggression and objectively evaluating the event with the use of supportive networks. Individuals can then decide if they want to speak up and confront the perpetrator, hence empowering the person subjected to the microaggression. Therefore, health care providers, teachers, and school administrators need to be familiar with how to recognize the presence and effects of microaggressions in order to support youth in using these coping strategies. Caregivers, providers, and teachers can serve as a support network to help youth recognize microaggressions, validate their emotional reactions, and provide context to the experience, thus helping youth boost their self-acceptance (Li et al. 2017) and understand the effects of microaggressions (see Table 19–1). The following case demonstrates how an adolescent might experience a microaggression and use effective strategies to overcome it.

Clinical Vignette

Stephan is a 14-year-old African American boy who lives with his parents and 12-year-old brother in a predominantly white neighborhood. His parents are professors at a nearby university. He is good at sports and has always excelled in academics. A typical adolescent, Stephan is exploring his identity and learning about his interests and abilities. His new teacher asked him what he planned to do after graduating from high school, to which he replied that he wanted to become a doctor. His teacher then said, "That's impressive. Will you be the first in your family to attend college?" Stephan was not sure what the comment was supposed to mean and wondered if the teacher was implying that he was not smart enough or that something about his identity made him unlikely to become a doctor. He was hesitant to discuss this incident with anyone because he was not sure if other people would understand. Instead, he ruminated on it and began feeling anxious. Eventually, Stephan consulted with his school counselor and shared what happened. The counselor told him he had heard other African American students sharing similar experiences of subtle discrimination. Stephan identified with what the counselor described and began to understand his experi-

TABLE 19–2.   Everyday microaggressions experienced by minority groups

Minority group	Example of microaggression	Consequences
African American	David is a 17-year-old adolescent who studies at an Ivy League school. He is concerned about doing well academically because he repeatedly hears that he was "admitted only because of affirmative action."	David begins to wonder if he is not intelligent enough to be a doctor. Adolescents are concerned about their identity and future, as well as fitting in with peer groups. Interactions like this one can threaten minority youth's self-esteem and aspirations.
American Indian	Jim is a 16-year-old adolescent who approaches the football coach to say that he feels the use of an American Indian image as the school mascot is disrespectful to his cultural heritage. The coach replies, "Don't be so sensitive. It's just a mascot."	Jim might feel that his feelings are being negated by the coach and that others do not think his cultural heritage and identity are important. This is an example of microinvalidation. As described by Erikson, such experience can lead to role/identity confusion. Cultural identity is important to American Indian youth, and Jim's minority youth cultural identity is important and can be a source of strength and resilience.
Asian American	Nhi-Ha is a 9-year-old Vietnamese American child who is on an Individualized Educational Program for a specific learning disorder with impairment in mathematics. Her teacher says, "You should be good at this; all Asians are good at math."	A comment like this one likely heightens Nhi-Ha's self-doubt and feelings of being different. During latency stage, children are preoccupied with how they compare with others and achieve competence, which can subsequently lead to feelings of inferiority being internalized.
Latinx/ Hispanic	María is a 10-year-old Hispanic girl. She is playing on the playground with a peer and says, "*Pásame la bola*" (pass me the ball). A boy says to her, "Speak English; you're in America!"	A hallmark of microaggression is the intention of segmenting others. During latency, children want to fit in and are more susceptible to a microaggression intended to make them feel like an outsider.
Arab	Bilal is a 12-year-old Arab boy who is often asked by his schoolteachers, peers, and security guards, "What's in your backpack?"	Bilal does not understand why his peers are not asked the same question. Sometimes he thinks people might be joking, but other times he wonders if they might be afraid of him. He feels singled out, criminalized, and not part of the group. At this preadolescent stage, Bilal is prone to self-consciousness and preoccupation with social relationships as he transitions into the identity formation stage of adolescence.

TABLE 19–2. Everyday microaggressions experienced by minority groups (continued)

Minority group	Example of microaggression	Consequences
LGBTQ+	Tom is a 14-year-old self-identified gay male youth. His peers continually ask him when he is getting a girlfriend.	This experience could send the message that there is something wrong about Tom's sexual identity. As postulated by Erikson, this may lead to role confusion and social isolation, which inherently can place adolescents at higher risk for depression.
Religious groups	Azadeh is a 20-year-old Muslim female pursuing a bachelor's degree in political science. Her professors and peers often say to her how they are "surprised that you are so progressive as a Muslim."	Comments like this one make Azadeh wonder what other professional colleagues think of her. As Erickson notes, transitional-age youth are concerned with finding their place in society and developing their professional, moral, and personal identity. This microaggression could lead Azadeh to believe that her religious identity is in conflict with her professional identity. She may feel different from her peers and may isolate herself, which could consequently affect her social relationships and self-esteem.

ence as being a microaggression. Together, the counselor and Stephan brainstormed the benefits and risks of confronting the teacher. The counselor suggested using nonjudgmental language and focusing on his experience and how the comments made him feel. The counselor also suggested a mentor who could help Stephan process this experience further. The mentor could be a peer, a senior, or a teacher at the school, preferably belonging to the African American community.

Conclusion

Research shows that microaggressions adversely impact physical and mental health, as well as the academic performance of youth, especially among vulnerable populations. Latency-age children, preadolescents, adolescents, and TAY are particularly sensitive to the consequences of microaggressions as they navigate their cognitive, physical, emotional, and social development. Increasing awareness among teachers, caregivers, and health care professionals may help reduce incidences of microaggression and support youth in dealing with the negative impact of microaggressions. Strategies to address microaggression include, but are not limited to, recognition of microaggressions, validation of the emotions associated with microaggressions, confrontation of microaggression behaviors, and use of community support.

Although several studies are under way to understand the impact of microaggressions on the health and mental health of underserved populations, there is a need for further in-depth and longitudinal research on the presence of microaggressions and their impact on developing youth.

First, a deeper understanding of the differential impact of recurring microaggressions on youth of different racial, ethnic, religious, and sexual minority groups is required. This may help practitioners understand how different variables such as racial and ethnic identities, adherence to cultural values, and gender identity may impact the experience of microaggressions. Second, a comprehensive analysis of the available strategies and the development of new strategies specific for youth in diverse settings such as classrooms, college campuses, and health care provider offices will help reduce the exposure to and negative impact of microaggressions in minority youth. Last, there is a need for additional research focusing on developing interventions that can raise awareness among children, teachers, and health care providers who regularly interact with minority youth. Examining protective factors specific to different communities can also help foster resilience among youth.

Clinical Pearls

- Vulnerable youth populations may be at increased risk of experiencing microaggressions.

- The cumulative experience of microaggressions can have mental, physical, academic, and social implications for children, adolescents, transitional-age youth, and families.

- Health care providers such as pediatricians, therapists, and psychiatrists, as well as school staff and caregivers, can be the first line in helping youth recognize experiences of microaggressions, foster resilience, and identify developmentally appropriate strategies to better cope with such complicated experiences.

Self-Assessment Questions

1. Who originally coined the term *microaggression*?

    A. Chester M. Pierce, M.D.
    B. Mary Rowe, Ph.D.
    C. Sigmund Freud, M.D.
    D. Derald Wing Sue, Ph.D.

2. Microaggression can be defined as which of the following?

    A. A delusion that someone or something is dangerous, likely to cause pain, or a threat.
    B. Minor intentional acts that cause pain, with the hope of positive change.
    C. An aggression toward someone that is acceptable because it is micro (or small) in magnitude.

    D. A verbal or nonverbal denigrating message that can result in a negative emotional response in certain individuals because of their group membership.

3. Studies have shown that mental health consequences of microaggression include which of the following?

    A. Psychosis
    B. Depression, low self-esteem, social isolation, and symptoms of trauma
    C. Autism
    D. Mania

4. The object of microaggression can include which groups of people?

    A. Females
    B. LGBTQ+ populations
    C. People of color
    D. Anyone

Answers

1. A
2. D
3. B
4. D

Recommended Readings

Griffith E: Race and Excellence: My Dialogue With Chester Pierce. Iowa City, University of Iowa Press, 1998

Ong AD, Burrow AL: Microaggressions and daily experience. Perspect Psychol Sci 12(1):173–175, 2017

Pierce CM: Stress analogs of racism and sexism: terrorism, torture, and disaster, in Mental Health, Racism, and Sexism. Edited by Willie C, Rieker P, Kramer B, et al. Pittsburgh, PA, University of Pittsburgh Press, 1995, pp 277–293

Shahrokh NC, Hales RE: American Psychiatric Glossary, 8th Edition, Washington, DC, 2003

Williams MT, Kanter JW, Ching TW, et al: Anxiety, stress, and trauma symptoms in African Americans: negative affectivity does not explain the relationship between microaggressions and psychopathology. J Racial Ethn Health Disparities 5(5):919–927, 2017

Wong-Padoongpatt G, Zane N, Okazaki S, et al: Decreases in implicit self-esteem explain the racial impact of microaggressions among Asian Americans. J Couns Psychol 64(5):574–583, 2017

References

Adam EK, Heissel JA, Zeiders KH, et al: Developmental histories of perceived racial discrimination and diurnal cortisol profiles in adulthood: a 20-year prospective study. Psychoneuroendocrinology 62:279–291, 2015

American Academy of Child and Adolescent Psychiatry: Sexual orientation, gender identity, and civil rights. Washington, DC, American Academy of Child and Adolescent Psychiatry, 2009. Available at: www.aacap.org/aacap/Policy_Statements/2009/Sexual_Orientation_Gender_Identity_and_Civil_Rights.aspx. Accessed May 14, 2020.

American Academy of Pediatrics: AAP diversity and inclusion statement. Itasca, IL, American Academy of Pediatrics, April 2018. Available at: https://pediatrics.aappublications.org/content/141/4/e20180193. Accessed May 14, 2020.

American Psychiatric Association: Diagnostic and Statistical Manual of Mental Disorders, 5th Edition. Arlington, VA, American Psychiatric Association, 2013

American Psychiatric Association: Position statement on resolution against racism and racial discrimination and their adverse impacts on mental health. Washington, DC, American Psychiatric Association, May 2018.

Assari S, Caldwell CH: Teacher discrimination reduces school performance of African American youth: role of gender. Brain Sci 8(10):E183, 2018

Basáñez T, Unger JB, Soto D, et al: Perceived discrimination as a risk factor for depressive symptoms and substance use among Hispanic adolescents in Los Angeles. Ethn Health 18(3):244–261, 2013

Benner AD, Graham S: Latino adolescents' experiences of discrimination across the first 2 years of high school: correlates and influences on educational outcomes. Child Dev 82(2):508–519, 2011

Benner AD, Wang Y, Shen Y, et al: Racial/ethnic discrimination and well-being during adolescence: a meta-analytic review. Am Psychol 73(7):855–883, 2018

Blume AW, Lovato LV, Thyken BN, et al: The relationship of microaggressions with alcohol use and anxiety among ethnic minority college students in a historically white institution. Cultur Divers Ethnic Minor Psychol 18(1):45–54, 2012

Bowleg L: The problem with the phrase women and minorities: intersectionality—an important theoretical framework for public health. Am J Public Health 102(7):1267–1273, 2012

Braveman P, Egerter S, Williams DR: The social determinants of health: coming of age. Annu Rev Public Health 32:381–398, 2011

Brody GH, Lei MK, Chae DH, et al: Perceived discrimination among African American adolescents and allostatic load: a longitudinal analysis with buffering effects. Child Dev 85(3):989–1002, 2014

Centers for Disease Control and Prevention: Youth Risk Behavior Surveillance System (YRBSS). Atlanta, GA, Adolescent and School Health, Centers for Disease Control and Prevention, August 22, 2018. Available at: www.cdc.gov/HealthyYouth/yrbs/index.htm. Accessed May 14, 2020.

Chu C, Buchman-Schmitt JM, Stanley IH, et al: The interpersonal theory of suicide: a systematic review and meta-analysis of a decade of cross-national research. Psychol Bull 143(12):1313–1345, 2017

Conover KJ, Israel T: Microaggressions and social support among sexual minorities with physical disabilities. Rehabil Psychol 64(2):167–178, 2019

Douglass S, Mirpuri S, English D, et al: "They were just making jokes": ethnic/racial teasing and discrimination among adolescents. Cultur Divers Ethnic Minor Psychol 22(1):69–82, 2016

Felitti VJ, Anda RF, Nordenberg D, et al: Relationship of childhood abuse and household dysfunction to many of the leading causes of death in adults: the Adverse Childhood Experiences (ACE) study. Am J Prev Med 14(4):245–258, 1998

Garnett BR, Masyn KE, Austin SB, et al: The intersectionality of discrimination attributes and bullying among youth: an applied latent class analysis. J Youth Adolesc 43(8):1225–1239, 2014

Gibbons FX, Gerrard M, Cleveland MJ, et al: Perceived discrimination and substance use in African American parents and their children: a panel study. J Pers Soc Psychol 86(4):517–529, 2004

Gilmore KJ, Meersand P: Normal Child and Adolescent Development: A Psychodynamic Primer. Arlington, VA, American Psychiatric Publishing, 2014

Greene ML, Way N, Pahl K: Trajectories of perceived adult and peer discrimination among black, Latino, and Asian American adolescents: patterns and psychological correlates. Dev Psychol 42(2):218–236, 2006

Hollingsworth DW, Cole AB, O'Keefe VM, et al: Experiencing racial microaggressions influences suicide ideation through perceived burdensomeness in African Americans. J Couns Psychol 64(1):104–111, 2017

Huynh VW: Ethnic microaggressions and the depressive and somatic symptoms of Latino and Asian American adolescents. J Youth Adolesc 41(7):831–846, 2012

Huynh VW, Fuligni AJ: Discrimination hurts: the academic, psychological, and physical well-being of adolescents. J Res Adolesc 20(4):916–941, 2010

Joiner T: Why People Die by Suicide. Cambridge, MA, Harvard University Press, 2007

Jones ML, Galliher RV: Daily racial microaggressions and ethnic identification among Native American young adults. Cultur Divers Ethnic Minor Psychol 21(1):1–9, 2015

Jones LM, Mitchell KJ, Turner HA, et al: Characteristics of bias-based harassment incidents reported by a national sample of U.S. adolescents. J Adolesc 65:50–60, 2018

Karoly LA, Kilburn RM, Cannon JS: Early childhood interventions: proven results, future promise. Santa Monica, CA, RAND Corporation, 2005. Available at: www.rand.org/pubs/monographs/MG341.html. Accessed May 13, 2020.

King RA, Rutherford HJV: Adolescence, in Lewis's Child and Adolescent Psychiatry: A Comprehensive Textbook, 5th Edition. Philadelphia, PA, Lippincott Williams & Wilkins, 2017

Kosciw JG, Greytak EA, Zongrone AD, et al: The 2017 National School Climate Survey: The Experiences of Lesbian, Gay, Bisexual, Transgender, and Queer Youth in Our Nation's Schools. New York, GLSEN, 2018

Le TN, Stockdale G: The influence of school demographic factors and perceived student discrimination on delinquency trajectory in adolescence. J Adolesc Health 49(4):407–413, 2011

Lewis TT, Cogburn CD, Williams DR: Self-reported experiences of discrimination and health: scientific advances, ongoing controversies, and emerging issues. Annu Rev Clin Psychol 11:407–440, 2015

Li MJ, Thing JP, Galvan FH, et al: Contextualising family microaggressions and strategies of resilience among young gay and bisexual men of Latino heritage. Cult Health Sex 19(1):107–120, 2017

Maynard BR, Vaughn MG, Salas-Wright CP, et al: Bullying victimization among school-aged immigrant youth in the United States. J Adolesc Health 58(3):337–344, 2016

Noh S, Kaspar V, Wickrama KA: Overt and subtle racial discrimination and mental health: preliminary findings for Korean immigrants. Am J Public Health 97(7):1269–1274, 2007

O'Keefe VM, Wingate LR, Cole AB, et al: Seemingly harmless racial communications are not so harmless: racial microaggressions lead to suicidal ideation by way of depression symptoms. Suicide Life Threat Behav 45(5):567–576, 2015

Pachter LM, Coll CG: Racism and child health: a review of the literature and future directions. J Dev Behav Pediatr 30(3):255–263, 2009

Paradies Y: A systematic review of empirical research on self-reported racism and health. Int J Epidemiol 35(4):888–901, 2006

Paradies Y, Ben J, Denson N, et al: Racism as a determinant of health: a systematic review and meta-analysis. PloS One 10(9):e0138511, 2015

Pascoe EA, Smart Richman L: Perceived discrimination and health: a meta-analytic review. Psychol Bull 135(4):531–554, 2009

Pierce C: Offensive mechanisms, in The Black Seventies. Edited by Barbour F. Boston, MA, Porter Sargent, 1970, pp 265–282

Priest N, Paradies Y, Trenerry B, et al: A systematic review of studies examining the relationship between reported racism and health and wellbeing for children and young people. Soc Sci Med 95:115–127, 2013

Purewal SK, Bucci M, Wang LG, et al: Screening for adverse childhood experiences (ACEs) in an integrated pediatric care model. Zero to Three 37(1):10–17, 2016

Respress BN, Small E, Francis SA, et al: The role of perceived peer prejudice and teacher discrimination on adolescent substance use: a social determinants approach. J Ethn Subst Abuse 12(4):279–299, 2013

Sanders-Phillips K: Racial discrimination: a continuum of violence exposure for children of color. Clin Child Fam Psychol Rev 12(2):174–195, 2009

Seaton EK, Caldwell CH, Sellers RM, et al: An intersectional approach for understanding perceived discrimination and psychological well-being among African American and Caribbean black youth. Dev Psychol 46(5):1372–1379, 2010

Solorzano D, Ceja M, Yosso T: Critical race theory, racial microaggressions, and campus racial climate: the experiences of African American college students. Journal of Negro Education 69(1/2):60–73, 2000

Sue DW: Microaggressions in Everyday Life: Race, Gender and Sexual Orientation. Hoboken, NJ, Wiley, 2010

Sue DW, Bucceri J, Lin AI, et al: Racial microaggressions and the Asian American experience. Cultur Divers Ethnic Minor Psychol 13(1):72–81, 2007

Szaflarski M, Bauldry S: The effects of perceived discrimination on immigrant and refugee physical and mental health. Adv Med Sociol 19:173–204, 2019

Torres-Harding SR, Andrade AL, Romero Diaz CE: The racial microaggressions scale (RMAS): a new scale to measure experiences of racial microaggressions in people of color. Cultur Div Ethnic Minor Psychol 18(2):153–164, 2012

Trent M, Dooley DG, Dougé J: The impact of racism on child and adolescent health. Pediatrics 144(2):e20191765, 2019

Van Orden KA, Witte TK, Cukrowicz KC, et al: The interpersonal theory of suicide. Psychol Rev 117(2):575–600, 2010

Walton LM: The effects of "bias based bullying" (BBB) on health, education, and cognitive-social-emotional outcomes in children with minority backgrounds: proposed comprehensive public health intervention solutions. J Immigr Minor Health 20(2):492–496, 2018

Whitbeck LB, Hoyt DR, McMorris BJ, et al: Perceived discrimination and early substance abuse among American Indian children. J Health Soc Behav 42(4):405–424, 2001

Williams DR, Mohammed SA: Discrimination and racial disparities in health: evidence and needed research. J Behav Med 32(1):20–47, 2009

Ylioja T, Cochran G, Woodford M, et al: Frequent experience of LGBQ microaggression on campus associated with smoking among sexual minority college students, Nicotine Tob Res 20(3):340–346, 2018

CHAPTER 20

Cultural Aspects of College Mental Health

Ludmila De Faria, M.D.

COLLEGE students are the human capital of a nation, and ensuring their well-being is investing in the economic and social growth of the country. In a 2016 "Position Statement on College and University Mental Health" (American Psychiatric Association 2016), the American Psychiatric Association (APA) recognized the importance of addressing the challenges that might arise when treating this population. The APA position statement emphasizes the importance of access to timely and culturally sensitive mental health care, as well as health and wellness education, for college students, their parents, and university staff. This has become a difficult task because of high demand and changing demographics within college campuses. There has been a steady increase in numbers and severity of college students with mental illness over the past decade (Locke et al. 2016; Martel et al. 2018), and institutions of higher education around the country have struggled to facilitate access to care. Moreover, college campuses today are diverse, technologically advanced, and globally connected, foreshadowing the future of America's demographics and highlighting the importance of cultural competence in mental health.

For the purposes of this chapter, *college student* refers to individuals ages 18–25 years who entered college immediately after finishing high school and who predominantly live on campus. They are transitioning from adolescence to adulthood, going through the developmental period known as emerging adulthood or transitional age. For clarity and consistency, they will be referred to as *emerging adults* throughout this chapter. I acknowledge the existence of nontraditional college students (i.e., older, married, commuter, part-time working, graduate or professional degree students), but although some of the issues covered in this chapter also apply to them, they are not the primary focus of this chapter. The primary focus is the emerging adult college student who belongs to a racial/ethnic or sexual/gender minority group.

Other important definitions pertinent to this chapter include the following:

- *Minority groups* are defined by their lack of power or representation relative to other groups within a society
- *Race* is defined as how an individual self-identifies with one or more social groups (e.g., white, Black or African American, Asian, American Indian and Alaskan Native, Native Hawaiian and other Pacific Islander)
- *Ethnicity* is a term that describes shared culture and national origin (e.g., Hispanic, non-Hispanic, Chinese)
- *Sexual and gender minority* is used to refer to sexual orientation and/or gender identity that differ from that of the mainstream population

Early adulthood remains a crucial period when major developmental tasks such as individuation from family, accepting responsibility for one's self, making independent decisions, and establishing an adult relationship with parents take place. It is also a time when most major psychiatric disorders can initially manifest (Alonso et al. 2018; Kessler et al. 2005). Distinguishing between stress associated with developmental milestones and clinical syndromes that may impair functioning is an essential skill when working in college mental health. In the case of minority students, being sensitive and attentive to their cultural background and environment can help clinicians distinguish between pathology and accepted cultural behaviors (Alarcón 2013).

The spring of 2020 brought about two events that underscore the daily experiences of young adults of color. First, the novel coronavirus SARS-CoV-2 (COVID-19) pandemic unleashed a wave of abusive behavior toward Asian Americans, with college students reporting several instances of verbal and physical abuse on campus (Levien and Li 2020) and exposed the health and economic disparities that affect minority communities (Laurencin and McClinton 2020). Second, the police-involved deaths of several African American individuals highlighted the state of terror that young Black men and women live with daily. The protests that ensued triggered several university and colleges to start, continue, or expand a dialogue about racism (Collins 2020). The psychological burden resulting from these daily experiences of racism may result in or exacerbate poor functioning and clinical symptoms of distress in this population (Benner et al. 2018; Litam 2020).

Of note, the Cultural Formulation Interview delineated in the *Diagnostic and Statistical Manual of Mental Disorders,* 5th Edition (American Psychiatric Association 2013) is an excellent tool to help providers organize culturally relevant clinical information and enhance clinical understanding as well as decision-making. I recommend using it as an integral part of any clinical interview.

In this chapter, I present three important and emerging concepts that shape cultural psychiatry in today's college mental health systems: emerging adulthood, globalization, and social media. The use of technology and social media has changed not only *how* but *when* emerging adults achieve developmental milestones, and it also has changed *how* and *when* they reach out for help and get treatment. Cultural backgrounds and globalization affect how emerging adults understand and respond to each other and to environmental stressors, therefore impacting their mental health. After illustrating a frequently encountered clinical presentation in today's college setting with a brief case vignette, I conclude the chapter by offering guidance on best practices in providing culturally informed and sensitive mental health services to vulnerable college populations.

Emerging Adults and Minority Stress

College, to paraphrase the author Charles Dickens, can be the best of times and the worst of times. It can pose significant challenges during a developmental stage marked by important milestones. Emerging adults must individuate from their family, explore their sexuality, discover and coalesce their identity, establish and maintain new relationships, assert themselves in the world, succeed academically, and take the first steps toward career success (Hunt and Eisenberg 2010; Leebens and Williamson 2017)—all with relatively little support and in an environment that can be quite demanding, both academically and socially. It is not surprising that several researchers have noticed an increase in stress and mental illness starting before college and peaking in early adulthood (Alonso et al. 2018; Bruffaerts et al. 2018; Leebens and Williamson 2017). Over the past 25 years, more young adults have reported feeling anxious and stressed, and overall rates of suicide in the college-age population have increased by 43%, from 10.1 per 100,000 in 2010 to 14.46 per 100,000 in 2017 (American Foundation for Suicide Prevention 2020).

College also introduces a wide array of cultural and social experiences. Students are still struggling to find their "group" in a period characterized by strong peer influence and opinion, making them susceptible to social exclusion and possible prejudice. They may also experience a decrease in healthy behaviors (e.g., less exercise, poor eating habits, lapses in or no preventive care) and an increase in risky behaviors (e.g., substance use, sexual experimentation). For those coming from more homogeneous cultural backgrounds who have had minimal exposure to other cultures, being exposed to so many new experiences can be anxiety provoking (Ahmed et al. 2017).

These stressors pose additional risks because they happen during the developmental stage when most major psychiatric illnesses emerge. Stress has been known to accelerate or precipitate severe mental illness (Shah and Malla 2015; Shalev et al. 2013). Vulnerable populations, such as those with genetic predisposition (family history), history of childhood exposure to adverse environmental factors (obstetric and perinatal complications), and/or early consumption of drugs such as cannabis during a crucial period for brain development, are at elevated risk for early onset of different mental illness (Leebens and Williamson 2017; Shalev et al. 2013). Additional exposure to stress related to minority status and school may tip the scale even further (Cooke et al. 2014).

Emerging adults belonging to racial/ethnic or gender/sexual minority populations who are entering college must cope with added stressors of meeting family and/or cultural expectations of success and dealing with acculturative stress and discrimination (Carrera and Wei 2014; Gaydosh et al. 2018; Pittman et al. 2017). Those who belong to multiple minority groups (racial/ethnic *and* sexual/gender) experience even more discrimination and negative mental health outcomes (Kulick et al. 2017), fully understood only through an intersectional framework. According to recent data, racial/ethnic minorities comprise about 40% of the general population ages 18–24 years (Rivas-Drake and Stein 2017; U.S. Census Bureau 2019), and sexual minorities comprise 4.5% of the general population, with about one-third between ages 18–24 years (Williams Institute 2019).

As this cohort develops their identity (racial/ethnic, gender, sexual orientation) and solidifies their place in the world, they also become more aware of how social marginalization affects and potentially limits their lives, from career choices to upward mobility. Minority youth are more likely to encounter personal and structural barriers to success even before seeking postsecondary education, including perceived, felt, or internalized bias; immigration status; access to mentoring; and bullying (Hurd et al. 2016; Siemons et al. 2017; Wilson et al. 2016). Recent data indicate that a significant portion of racial/ethnic and of sexual/gender minority youth have reported experiencing some form of discrimination throughout their lifetime (Benner et al. 2018). The psychological burden may result in poor functioning and clinical symptoms of distress (Benner et al. 2018). In fact, most emerging adults belonging to any minority group report feeling down or sad and having difficulty with sleep (Cooke et al. 2014). Some of these experiences of discrimination are so traumatic that they can lead to PTSD, severe depression, or anxiety (Cooke et al. 2014; Cheng and Mallinckrodt 2015; Hwang and Goto 2009; Lowe et al. 2019; Marx and Sloan 2003; Wilson et al. 2016).

Recently, the COVID-19 pandemic and protests for racial justice have significantly disrupted college life and increased mental health needs for all college students (Lee 2020; Zhai 2020). The protests against police brutality toward African Americans and the recent waves of discrimination against Asian Americans following the spread of the pandemic have pushed the conversation about race and ethnicity in America into the mainstream. College students have not only participated in the conversation on campuses; they have also driven the discussion. The cathartic experience of sharing stories of microaggressions associated with their college experience (#BlackInTheIvory) comes at a price, including heightened anxiety and mood symptoms. When students reach out for help to counseling centers and student health clinics, they need providers who understand and are ready to address their symptoms in a culturally sensitive manner.

In addition to discrimination, for college students who are children of immigrants (or may be immigrants themselves), competing expectations and values between their culture of origin and the host culture increase the likelihood of acculturative stress. The struggle between acculturation and assimilation is associated with increased vulnerability and decreased self-efficacy. As a result, emerging adults are likely to engage in high-risk behaviors that increase the possibility of developing psychiatric and substance use disorders and lead to poor health outcomes (Ahmed et al. 2017; Claudat et al. 2016; Corona et al. 2017; Kim and Cronley 2020; Kwan et al. 2018; Pittman et al. 2017). First-generation college students or those who do not speak English as their primary language may be unable to access financial aid because of their immigration status or limited knowledge of the system. The need to work part or full time to support themselves and their families while attending college may contribute to academic struggle (Stephens et al. 2012). Eventually, they feel isolated and inadequate and are at risk of dropping out of school without completing their degrees. For the ones who stay and finish, the associated stress results in long-lasting health issues (Gaydosh et al. 2018).

Another important aspect of providing care to emerging adults of minority backgrounds is being cognizant of the fact that many lacked appropriate access to health and psychiatric care throughout childhood and adolescence and subsequently enter college with undiagnosed mental illnesses such as ADHD and anxiety (Chen et al. 2019; Cheng and Mallinckrodt 2015; Cooke et al. 2014; Hwang and Goto 2009; Marx and Sloan 2003). This lack of early access is a result of both structural and personal barriers that will be discussed further later in the chapter. These barriers often persist during the college years and need to be addressed systemically. Improving access to and quality of health care services in college is beneficial for all but can be especially important for minority student retention and success (Ciotoli et al. 2018).

Once in college, minority students seek mental health care at similar rates as their nonminority counterparts but usually present with higher levels of distress (Locke et al. 2016). According to the 2018 spring survey by the American College Health Association (2018), 43%–50% of students seeking help are first-generation students struggling to navigate higher education without the aid of intergenerational information. Out of the 88,178 students at 140 schools that participated in the survey, about 45% defined themselves as a racial or ethnic minority, 17.3% as sexual minority, and 6% as international students. Mental health remained a frequent complaint, with 33% reporting stress, 26.5% anxiety, and 18.7% depression as factors affecting their academic performance within the past 12 months (American College Health Association 2018).

In summary, minority stress has serious effects on emerging adults' mental health and academic progress. To better understand and address such effects, college mental health providers need to familiarize themselves with and appreciate the cultural background of their patients. Integrating the DSM-5 Cultural Formulation Interview as a regular component of assessment helps differentiate illness from culturally normal behaviors so that providers can suggest treatment options that align better with a student's culture of origin.

Globalization and Diversity

Globalization has increased diversity in U.S. colleges and universities. Institutions of higher education offer a unique opportunity for different cultures to interact and merge. Whether students are born and raised in the United States or come from elsewhere in the pursuit of higher education, the U.S. college population is increasingly mobile and culturally diverse.

Over the past 15 years, students from racial/ethnic populations that are disproportionately represented in higher education, also known as underrepresented students, are enrolling in higher numbers because of the economic and social costs associated with not achieving a bachelor's degree (de Bray et al. 2019; Garriott et al. 2015). Unfortunately, higher enrollment rates have not affected the graduation gap. Except for Asians, only half of underrepresented students go on to complete their degree (compared with two-thirds of white students) (de Bray et al. 2019). This trend was published in a document by the U.S. Department of Education (2016) that highlighted key data on race and ethnicity in college. According to this document, attrition and graduation gaps between minority and nonminority students remain a problem, leading institutions to establish different programs to reduce this gap. Some of the programs, such as student support services, have existed since 1968 as part of the federal administration's "War on Poverty" efforts and currently serve students attending more than 1,000 colleges and universities. These programs were established to assist disadvantaged students, and many of those currently served are from minority and underserved populations. These students benefit from access to a variety of services, including academic tutoring, personalized counseling, and housing and financial aid (Thayer 2000).

Simultaneously, the college population has become international and highly mobile, with international students becoming a key force in shaping globalization and diversity on college campuses. According to the U.S. Department of State survey of international exchange activity in the United States published in the Open Doors Fast Facts 2019 (Institute of International Education 2019), foreign students attending American universities represent 5.5% of all students enrolled, about 1.1 million international students. Most of them come from Asia (63%), especially China and India (Institute of International Education 2019).

International students' diverse backgrounds shape their view of the world and how they interact with American students and faculty. At the same time, they face challenges with acculturation and developmental milestones similar to those of American college students, and their attempts to "fit in" may cause them significant stress (Geary 2016; Kim and Cronley 2020). Recently, international students experienced significant environmental stressors as a result of the COVID-19 pandemic. Many found themselves stranded and unable to return home and were exposed to abuse because of their race and ethnicity. They had to deal with the threat of losing their visas after U.S. Immigration and Customs Enforcement announced that it would strip the visas of foreign students whose entire courses were moved online (Kausar 2020; Lee 2020; Litam 2020; Zhai 2020).

As a result, international students can develop clinical symptoms that require assessment and treatment by campus providers, highlighting the need for cultural sensitivity in clinicians providing care. The diversity of college campuses in the United States exposes all students to different cultural and identity politics and stretches the definition of what constitutes the *cultural norm* (Werneke and Bhugra 2018). Over the past decade, several universities have developed programs to educate staff and faculty on cultural competency and social justice and to offer training on how to apply these concepts not only to research and teaching (see "Resources for Providers" at the end of the chapter) but also to clinical practice.

Unfortunately, despite widespread adoption by institutions as part of a commitment to excellence, college programs and promoted values of equity and diversity often do not change the campus climate in a tangible way. Thus, students of color continue to face racial profiling, including a disproportionate number of police citations, arrests, and incidents of campus police brutality perpetrated against them (Greenlee 2016). Students who are beneficiaries of the Deferred Action Child Arrivals (DACA) policy are unable to access some of the support service programs described above (Siemons et al. 2017), and students who are lesbian, gay, bisexual, transgender, or queer/questioning still face high rates of discrimination and violence on campus (Evans et al. 2017). These differences have led many student activist groups to denounce the misalignment of stated institutional values and messaging and institutional actions and initiatives (Hoffman and Mitchell 2016).

As mentioned previously, the toll that minority stress takes on students is tangible and often leads to an increase in chronic stress and anxiety, poor physical health outcomes, and an increase in mental illness (Claudat et al. 2016; Cooke et al. 2014; Corona et al. 2017; Gaydosh et al. 2018; Kim and Cronley 2020; Kwan et al. 2018; Pittman et al. 2017). Because minority students may lack access to both medical and mental health care, untreated illness plays a significant role in higher attrition rates for that segment of the college population (Alonso et al. 2018; Leebens and Williamson 2017; O'Keeffe 2013; Pittman et al. 2017).

For many minority students, the achievements of higher education elicit significant loyalty conflicts. Should they leave home and their community in pursuit of further career success? Or should they risk stagnation by staying in their communities to "pay back" the sacrifices made by their families? Should they adopt the mainstream culture in order to fit in socially and academically, even when this may result in accusations of "selling out"? Should they push back against microaggressions or stay quiet to avoid accusations of preferential treatment and reverse discrimination? The answers are often complex and require difficult choices. For racial/ethnic minority students, the struggle to develop an identity that incorporates their culture of origin and the mainstream culture causes significant acculturation stress. They understand their unique social, political, and economic position in society, which shapes their unique attitudes, perspectives, and behaviors in response to racial discrimination. However, the relationship between racial/ethnic identity and acculturation stress is not linear. A recent study by Woo et al. (2019) found that racial/ethnic identity seems to modulate response to stress differently for different groups. Specifically, strong racial/ethnic identity amplifies the psychological burden associated with racial discrimination for whites, American Natives, and Latinx/Hispanics, whereas a moderate level of racial/ethnic identity functions as a buffer for African Americans and Asians. This is explained by the researchers as different identity development statuses exhibited by different racial/ethnic groups. Internalized bias, or what Versey et al. (2019) call *wearing the mask* and *trying to fit in*, increases feelings of shame and guilt related to being associated with a specific group and negatively affects their response to stress.

Overall, students who belong to racial/ethnic minorities face sustained exposure to stressors that require continued coping strategies. The very characteristics that promote well-being and achievement, such as self-control, grit, and perseverance, also result in sustained activation of the stress system, which can worsen health outcomes (Gaydosh et al. 2018). Furthermore, exposure to acculturative stress and discrimination trigger or exacerbate clinical symptoms of depression, anxiety, PTSD, metabolic syndrome, and eating disorders in college students (Claudat et al. 2016; Hwang and Goto 2009; Kwan et al. 2018; Lowe et al. 2019; Marx and Sloan 2003; Woo et al. 2019).

The 2% of all enrolled American students who choose to study abroad (Institute of International Education 2019) are also exposed to acculturative stress. They experience an array of stressful conditions, including language difficulties, discrimination, identity threat, opportunity deprivation, poor self-confidence, values conflict, lack of cultural competence, and homesickness. These stressors increase vulnerability and decrease self-efficacy, leading to high-risk behaviors and poor health outcomes and higher incidence of depression, anxiety, and substance use (Kim and Cronley 2020). Once back at home, they require mental health care that can contextualize their acculturative stress. Institutions and students alike often focus on the positive aspects of exposure to new cultures and identities, including increased diversity, but exposure to stress and discrimination are also more prevalent in diverse environments.

One way to mitigate minority student attrition and to decrease the effects of minority stress is to promote diversity of college faculty and providers in counseling centers (Rodríguez et al. 2014). Recruiting and retaining a diverse workforce results in long-lasting changes to the pipeline within institutions (Rubio et al. 2018). It creates a campus culture of diversity and inclusion that promotes student success and decreases barriers to seeking help. Diversity among faculty and providers can facilitate support and mentorship (Hurd et al. 2016; Rodríguez et al. 2014) and decrease students' feelings of alienation, especially in view of recent stressors of rising xenophobia in the country (Lowe et al. 2019). Mental health providers' cultural experiences and background are equally important for identifying and understanding patients' needs. How mental health symptoms are described, experienced, and reported by patients, and the way they are understood and formulated by the provider, are directly affected by each provider's cultural background.

Clinicians working with this international and multicultural college population, which is at high risk for developing mental illness, should also be culturally competent, regardless of their own cultural background, because "understanding culture is a prerequisite for understanding people" (Werneke and Bhugra 2018, pp. S1–S2). College mental health providers must be able to understand patients' individual cultural experiences and their significance for social functioning (American Psychiatric Association 2016) as well as identify when a behavior becomes pathological. Diagnosis and treatment in a college setting means assessing and evaluating specific minority stressors. Some examples of specific minority stressors can be found in Table 20–1.

Social Media and Cultural Psychiatry in College

Social media has recently been conceptualized as a unique social context and environment that shapes individuals' thoughts, behaviors, and relationships (Nesi et al. 2018). It can improve global citizenship and social identity (Lee et al. 2017) and increase connectivity. The use of social network sites is now widespread among college students, with more than 95% of them reporting daily usage across all cultural backgrounds. This presence is facilitated by smartphones, laptops, and personal tablets, all required tools for learning.

Social media use has been particularly influential among the current generation matriculating for college, sometimes referred to as iGen (Twenge 2018). This population was born from 1995 to 2012 and grew up with smartphones and tablets. They had a social media presence even before they started high school and do not remember a time before the Internet. As these students reach college, there has been an increase in the use of technology on campus, which has led to a paradigm shift in how college-age students relate to and communicate with each other. It has also changed how and when these students access help. In order to communicate with them and assess their mental health, providers must understand how modern technology shapes the distinct culture and language of college students.

Several studies describing the effect of technology and social media use on social and mental well-being are discussed in detail in Chapter 14, "Digital Media, Culture, and Child and Adolescent Mental Health," and Chapter 15, "Culture of Technology." In this section, I focus on recent research on how use of social media and technology devices affects the college population. In brief, research has connected the use of social media to higher rates of mood and anxiety disorders, disturbances in sleep and time management, and increases in risky behaviors such as substance use (Levenson et al. 2016; Richards et al. 2015; Steers et al. 2019; Twenge 2018). Data collected by the American College Health Association (2018) show that college students themselves are aware of the issue, with about 10% of college students reporting that Internet or computer use significantly affected their academic performance within the past year and 21% reporting sleep problems within the same period. As these students seek help, providers need to become familiar with social media and technology and how to assess and treat clinical issues resulting from their use by this technologically informed population.

TABLE 20–1. Examples of specific minority stressors

Minority population in college	Example of specific stressor
Latinx students	Balancing familial obligations with college expectations
Asian American students	The struggle between interdependency and independence
African American students	Feelings of being unsafe around campus police
Muslim students	Negotiating Islamic beliefs with the secular curricula and maintaining their religious and cultural identities in a predominantly American cultural environment
Transgender students	Fear of being "outed" by being misgendered or called by the name used prior to transitioning (deadname)

However, this cultural shift has not happened without difficulty. Nesi et al. (2018) highlighted how the use of social media and technology facilitates alienation by creating a homogeneous, less rich social network and increases harmful behaviors such as reassurance seeking (as opposed to self-soothing), negative feedback seeking, and co-rumination. The use of social media has caused the current college generation to develop relationships that are more superficial and may not provide the protective factors that come with a well-developed social network. Most importantly, by offering increased comfort in interactions and creating so-called echo chambers and bubbles in which individuals interact only with people who mirror their beliefs, social media has fundamentally changed conflict and problem-solving. Most students, regardless of their cultural background, tend to gravitate toward online groups that reflect and reaffirm their own perceptions and cultural identities. Students who spend longer periods of time online, including minority students, have only limited, if any, exposure to different points of view and opportunities for establishing connections with people who think and look different from themselves. Ultimately, this may cause further stress when students are exposed to campus diversity because such exposure accentuates inequalities and creates obstacles for establishing and nurturing a strong and diverse social support network. Other potentially negative effects include cyberbullying and feelings of exclusion, especially among minority groups (Lee 2017; Ramsey et al. 2016), resulting in reduced self-image and self-esteem.

On the other hand, using social media and technology has beneficial aspects for college students. Minority student populations often explore racial/ethnic, sexual, and gender self-identification through their online presence (Lee 2012; Nesi et al. 2018). Studies have found a positive correlation between the number of social networks of which students are members and global citizenship identification (Lee et al. 2017). The latter is defined by improved interconnectedness with others in the world and participation in social movements via *hashtag activism* such as #MeToo, #BlackLivesMatter, #NoBanNoWall, #BlackInTheIvory, and #TimesUp. Technology may benefit minority students by helping them establish cultural identity, reducing isolation, and decreasing acculturative stress (Lee 2012; Lee et al. 2017). Social media use can also provide frequent, immediate social support, which can be important for minority students who feel isolated. Technology and social media facilitate help seeking through the availability of telecounseling and information about services (Heron et al. 2019) and by minimizing stigma surrounding mental health. Several organizations (e.g., The Steve Fund, Crisis Text Line) have fully integrated the use of technology into their outreach programs to improve college students' mental health. The Steve Fund caters specifically to students of color. Providers need to be familiar with these resources in order to share information about them with students.

Use of technology and social media is now part of college culture, and monitoring this use and its impact is a necessary part of clinical assessment and treatment of college students. During clinical assessments, providers can use existing tools such as the Problematic and Risky Internet Use Screening Scale (PRIUSS) that include questions about time, frequency, and impact of technology and social media use. Harmful effects can be addressed in the treatment plan.

Clinical Vignette

Gavin is a 19-year-old African American male who came in for initial evaluation at the request of his academic adviser, who was concerned with changes in his behavior since the previous semester. He was starting his sophomore year at the state university and had done relatively well during his freshman year. However, his academic performance was now inconsistent, with failing grades and multiple absences. Gavin is the first in his family to attend college. He lives at home with his mother, who raised him as a single parent, and a younger half-brother who is in middle school. Gavin had no previous psychiatric history and visited the doctor's office only for immunizations. Significant issues included "anger outbursts" and heavy cannabis use since his senior year in high school. Aggressive behaviors had escalated recently, culminating with an incident in which he threatened his younger brother with a kitchen knife and his mother called the police. Gavin tried to look for help by visiting the campus counseling center but gave up after a few visits because he felt his white counselor "doesn't get me." He was particularly upset at her insistence that he see a psychiatrist for possible medication because he did not want his family and friends to think he was "crazy." Unfortunately, his condition deteriorated until he could no longer function, and he had to come in for crisis intervention.

During evaluation, Gavin was guarded, selectively mute, and uncooperative. He admitted to occasional thoughts that others were talking about him and said he had been able to "catch" random people on campus making derogatory comments about his appearance and academic performance. He admitted to hearing voices a couple of times. Self-assessment tools completed during the visits indicated moderately severe depressive symptoms and severe anxiety symptoms. He was diagnosed with bipolar disorder and cannabis use disorder.

Gavin was started on medications to treat both depression and psychosis. He was also instructed to abstain from cannabis. Initially, treatment resulted in improved symptoms within a couple of months. Unfortunately, Gavin was unable to establish a good rapport with his psychiatrist, who focused solely on substance use as a perpetuating factor for symptoms. He relapsed and was lost for follow up. Not long after that, Gavin dropped out of school.

Gavin's case is all too common in colleges. The stress of entering postsecondary education coupled with substance use can trigger possible genetic predisposition for severe mental illness. Differential diagnosis might be confusing because of multiple precipitating and perpetuating factors. Existing stigma surrounding the diagnosis of a severe and persistent mental illness results in ambivalence about treatment from both patients and families. This translates to poor compliance and frequent relapses and exacerbations. Treatment plans for college students like Gavin should include support and education through groups and counseling, medications (ideally using long-acting injectable formulations for improved compliance), and substance use treatment. After acute stabilization, students can be referred to the campus disability services office for academic accommodations and case management for ongoing support and education. When symptoms are well managed, students can function well and successfully complete school.

Access to Care and the Role of Providers

Many schools have implemented programs to support and retain minority and underrepresented students in college, including cultural training for faculty and staff, workshops for leadership training for minority students, and cultural sensitivity training for health care providers. However, there is still much to be done to improve access to care. First and foremost, it is important to remember that health inequalities start before students arrive at college; racial/ethnic minority youth receive very different mental health services than those given to their white counterparts (Stewart et al. 2012). This is equally true for sexual and gender minorities (Institute of Medicine of the National Academies 2011; Romanelli and Hudson 2017).

The reasons for access inequalities include structural barriers (lack of insurance, limited number of providers, inadequate access to specialist care, lack of transportation to attend visits), cultural barriers (beliefs and attitudes, health literacy, preference for use of family and community resources in cases of distress), and provider barriers (referral bias, lack of knowledge about different cultural manifestations of disorders or explanations for symptoms). Limited or delayed access to care prior to entering college often results in minority students coming into college counseling centers and clinics with more severe symptoms than those of their nonminority counterparts (Locke et al. 2016). They are less likely to self-refer and may agree to meet with mental health providers only when their academic performance is affected. Therefore, training staff institution-wide to identify and refer students at risk for assessment and treatment is critical (Ciotoli et al. 2018).

Of equal importance is ensuring that when the student is seen, mental health providers exercise cultural humility and consider integrating cultural formulation into their assessment. The 2016 APA position statement on college mental health (American Psychiatric Association 2016), mentioned earlier in the chapter, specifically addresses the need to provide culturally appropriate care and ongoing education regarding health and wellness to staff, students, and parents, identifying the importance of "recognizing mental health problems and understanding appropriate interventions, including how to respond to disturbing behavior or apparent distress, whom to contact and how to access services both for routine care and for urgent and emergency interventions." Similarly, health accreditation organizations such as the Accreditation Association for Ambulatory Health Care and the Joint Commission are mandating cultural training for all providers in the institution seeking accreditation.

Unfortunately, cultural training is sometimes inadequate and does not provide practical guidelines on how to create an inclusive environment. This training may create a false sense of proficiency among providers, who are often unaware of their own lack of knowledge and implicit biases when caring for minority populations, and it may foster complacency regarding further need for cultural competency training. Community mental health providers, who often treat college students in their clinics or solo practices, have even less access to cultural mental health training. One possible way to increase access to and quality of such trainings is having state agencies promote trainings by making them a mandatory requirement for relicensing.

Providers can improve patient counseling and treatment by using concepts that align with the patient's cultural, family, and social environment. In addition to providing cultural sensitivity training, institutions can also improve culturally appropriate care by promoting a campus culture of inclusiveness that will increase retention of minority population students. This can be achieved by hiring and retaining a diverse staff and transforming the environment with culturally appropriate cues that make it more welcoming for minority populations. Examples of this include multilingual signs and brochures, gender-neutral bathrooms, and designated areas for religious practices.

There is no accredited specialization in college mental health, and a significant portion of mental health providers seeing college-age students lack familiarity with emerging adults' developmental milestones. Offering opportunities for providers to be trained on the developmental needs of this population can improve the quality of care. Different agencies and organizations provide training modules and other resources that address diversity and inclusion in mental health care and in college specifically. Some of these resources can be found at websites listed under "Resources for Providers" at the end of the chapter.

How to Provide Culturally Competent College Mental Health Services

Culturally competent college mental health involves what psychiatrists Renato Alarcon and Jerome Frank call "the common ingredients of all psychotherapies" (Alarcón 2013): hope, trust, faith, respect, and support. An institution that promotes and supports different cultural identities can develop policies that minimize environmental stressors and facilitate help-seeking behavior. Likewise, practitioners who recognize that cultural dissonance in any aspect of college experience can impact patient outcomes (Jongen et al. 2017) will work toward developing congruent behaviors and attitudes. Culturally informed college mental health providers must be prepared to advocate for cultural competency and to disseminate information on best practices while also maintaining their own cultural curiosity. Table 20–2 summarizes best practices that will ensure culturally competent mental health care in college.

Conclusion

The college cultural landscape is shifting rapidly, fueled by changing demographics and increasing use of technology. At the same time, there is a worsening in the mental well-being of college students. In order to meet these challenges, colleges and universities need to change how they deliver care. Part of the change must include addressing specific needs of the growing minority (soon to be a majority) population on campuses because untreated mental health severely hampers these students' ability to succeed and graduate. Meeting their needs includes decreasing environmental stress (e.g., by increasing faculty diversity, by decreasing student debt); developing a more inclusive campus culture; and providing effective cultural sensitivity training for faculty,

TABLE 20–2. Best practices in providing culturally competent mental health care in college

Who	What	How
Individual provider	Perform assessment that contextualizes culture and setting • Include familial/gender role • Consider issues of self-determination and autonomy when assessing symptoms and developing a treatment plan	• Familiarize yourself with the DSM-5 Cultural Formulation Interview and American Academy of Child and Adolescent Psychiatry Practice Parameter for Cultural Competence in Child and Adolescent Psychiatric Practice
Individual provider	Address immigration-related traumas, acculturation stress, and identity conflicts (internal or generational) • Be aware of culturally based transference and countertransference • Be open about differences in values and beliefs	• Have cultural humility and curiosity: ask questions and avoid assumptions • Examine perceptions and biases of therapist and student • Identify and promote cultural values and traditions that can increase resiliency
Individual provider	Use evidence-based approaches with cultural modifications	• Promote healthy coping skills • Encourage and facilitate help seeking that is culturally appropriate • Be familiar with culturally specific modalities as expected by the student and know where to refer if not familiar with those modalities
Institution	Go beyond culture matching • Create an environment of hope, trust, faith, respect, and institutional support	• Provide resources and information to families, especially those with limited English skills • Address discrimination by advocating for campus policies that promote diversity and inclusion • Create on-campus support groups that help students explore their ethnic, sexual, and/or gender identity • Coordinate care with other campus services (e.g., case management, disability services) that can provide further resources

Source. Adapted from Karnik and Dogra 2010; Pumariega 2019.

providers, and staff. Effectively addressing diversity on campus can reduce the risk of poor outcomes for minority and underrepresented students by decreasing attrition and improving graduation rates.

This chapter offers a primer in college mental health for clinicians who treat college students on campus and in the community, with practical advice on how to improve cultural sensitivity.

Including cultural assessment helps ensure that treatment plans are aligned with students' cultural and sexual/gender experiences and improves clinical outcomes. Better mental health can, in turn, improve graduation rates.

It is important for providers to advocate within their institutions for changes that promote diversity, ranging from hiring multicultural staff to having patient education literature available in different languages. It is also important for providers to practice cultural humility and seek to improve their cultural sensitivity in a continuous manner. Most important, new care delivery systems need to be monitored to ensure that they do not create further access barriers to minority students.

Finally, more research is needed on the mental health problems of minority students. Minorities, including racial/ethnic and sexual/gender minorities, are often treated as a monolithic block, but there are enormous intrapopulation variability and intersectionality. It is important to design research studies that address cultural nuances and guide further clinical recommendations.

Clinical Pearls

- Students' time in college coincides with the age when most major mental illnesses emerge, potentially disrupting their ability to succeed.

- Students from racial/ethnic minorities are enrolling in college at higher rates. Exposure to minority stress puts them at high risk for poor mental and physical health and compromises their ability to succeed.

- Globalization and technology contribute to increased exposure to diversity on campus.

- Colleges and universities can positively impact graduation rates for all minority students by improving access to culturally sensitive mental health services on campus and promoting education for families, staff, and community psychiatrists.

- Incorporating cultural formulation when treating minority students can improve clinical outcomes and improve adherence to treatment.

Self-Assessment Questions

1. Researchers have noticed an increase in stress and mental illness starting in adolescence and peaking in college/early adulthood. Which of the following statements regarding minority stress may be a reason why?

    A. Learning how to care for themselves in an environment that is academically and socially demanding can be very taxing for emerging adults.

     B. Colleges introduce a wide array of cultural and social experiences that make young adults susceptible to strong peer influence and opinion, social exclusion, and possible prejudice.

     C. Adolescents and emerging adults belonging to racial/ethnic, gender, or sexual minority populations must cope with added stressors of meeting family and/or cultural expectations of success and dealing with acculturative stress and discrimination.

     D. All of the above.

2. True or false: Emerging adults who belong to racial/ethnic minorities face sustained exposure to stressors that require continued coping strategies. Ironically, the characteristics that promote well-being and achievement, such as self-control, grit, and perseverance, also result in sustained activation of the stress system, which can worsen health outcomes.

     A. True.

     B. False.

3. All of the following statements about cultural aspects of college mental health are true except which of the following?

     A. Exposure to acculturative stress and discrimination can trigger or worsen clinical symptoms of depression, anxiety, PTSD, metabolic syndrome, and eating disorders in this population.

     B. Technology and social media have no beneficial aspects for college students struggling with minority stress.

     C. One way to mitigate minority student attrition and to decrease the effects of minority stress among them is to promote diversity within school faculty and providers in the counseling centers and communities.

     D. Clinicians working with children and adolescents should be culturally competent, regardless of their own cultural background.

4. What specific questions will you add to your usual base of interview questions to include content from this chapter?

5. How might you adjust your current rubric for patient conceptualization to include these concepts?

6. As you reflect, how does the information in this chapter inform your future practice?

Answers

1. D
2. A
3. B

Resources for Providers
Cultural Sensitivity Training Examples

Academic Senate: Faculty diversity training programs and best practices, preliminary draft. Los Angeles, University of Southern California, 2016. Available at: https://academicsenate.usc.edu/files/2015/08/Climate-Committee-Faculty-Diversity-Best-Practices-11-10-16.pdf.

Office of Minority Health: A physician's practical guide to culturally competent care. Rockville, MD, Office of Minority Health, U.S. Department of Health and Human Services, 2019. Available at: www.thinkculturalhealth.hhs.gov/education/physicians.

Websites Containing Helpful Training

American Psychiatric Association: Mental health disparities: diverse populations. Washington, DC, American Psychiatric Association, 2018. Available at: www.psychiatry.org/psychiatrists/cultural-competency/education/mental-health-facts.

Center of Excellence for Cultural Competence: Demonstration of Cultural Formulation Interview [video]. New York, Center of Excellence for Cultural Competence, 2014. Available at: www.youtube.com/watch?v=IqFrszJ6iP8andfeature=youtube.

Center of Excellence for Cultural Competence: Using the DSM-5 Cultural Formulation Interview: online training module. New York, Center of Excellence for Cultural Competence, 2014. Available at: http://nyculturalcompetence.org/cfionlinemodule.

Mathai C, Lewis-Fernández R, Jiménez-Solomon O: Using the Cultural Formulation Interview to support recovery. Rockville, MD, Substance Abuse and Mental Health Services Administration, 2016. Available at: www.samhsa.gov/sites/default/files/programs_campaigns/recovery_to_practice/using-cultural-formulation-interview-support_recovery.pdf.

References

Ahmed SR, Amer MM, Killawi A: The ecosystems perspective in social work: implications for culturally competent practice with American Muslims. J Relig Spiritual Social Work 36(1–2):48–72, 2017

Alarcón RD: Cultural psychiatry: a general perspective. Adv Psychosom Med 33:1–14, 2013

Alonso J, Mortier P, Auerbach RP, et al: Severe role impairment associated with mental disorders: results of the WHO World Mental Health Surveys International College Student project. Depress Anxiety 35(9):802–814, 2018

American College Health Association: National College Health Assessment II: reference group executive summary spring 2018. Silver Spring, MD, American College Health Association, 2018. Available at: www.acha.org/documents/ncha/NCHA-II_Spring_2018_Reference_Group_Executive_Summary.pdf. Accessed May 14, 2020.

American Foundation for Suicide Prevention: Suicide statistics: March 1, 2020. New York, American Foundation for Suicide Prevention, 2020. Available at: https://afsp.org/about-suicide/suicide-statistics. Accessed May 14, 2020.

American Psychiatric Association: Diagnostic and Statistical Manual of Mental Disorders, 5th Edition. Arlington, VA, American Psychiatric Association, 2013

American Psychiatric Association: Position statement on college and university mental health. Arlington, VA, American Psychiatric Association, 2016. Available at: www.psychiatry.org/psychiatrists/practice/helping-patients-access-care/position-statements. Accessed October 15, 2019.

Benner AD, Wang Y, Shen Y, et al: Racial/ethnic discrimination and well-being during adolescence: a meta-analytic review. Am Psychol 73(7):855–883, 2018

Bruffaerts R, Mortier P, Kiekens G, et al: Mental health problems in college freshmen: prevalence and academic functioning. J Affect Disord 225:97–103, 2018

Carrera SG, Wei M: Bicultural competence, acculturative family distancing, and future depression in Latino/a college students: a moderated mediation model. J Couns Psychol 61(3):427–436, 2014

Chen JA, Stevens C, Wong SHM, et al: Psychiatric symptoms and diagnoses among U.S. college students: a comparison by race and ethnicity. Psychiatr Serv 70(6):442–449, 2019

Cheng HL, Mallinckrodt B: Racial/ethnic discrimination, posttraumatic stress symptoms, and alcohol problems in a longitudinal study of Hispanic/Latino college students. J Couns Psychol 62(1):38–49, 2015

Ciotoli C, Smith AJ, Keeling RP: Call to action: better care, better health, and greater value in college health. J Am Coll Health 66(7):625–639, 2018

Claudat K, White EK, Warren CS: Acculturative stress, self-esteem, and eating pathology in Latina and Asian American female college students. J Clin Psychol 72(1):88–100, 2016

Collins S: Why these protests are different. Vox, June 4, 2020. Available at: www.vox.com/identities/2020/6/4/21276674/protests-george-floyd-arbery-nationwide-trump. Accessed August 3, 2020.

Cooke CL, Bowie BH, Carrère S: Perceived discrimination and children's mental health symptoms. ANS Adv Nurs Sci 37(4):299–314, 2014

Corona R, Rodriguez VM, McDonald SE, et al: Associations between cultural stressors, cultural values, and Latina/o college students' mental health. J Youth Adolesc 46:63–77, 2017

de Bray C, Musu L, McFarland J, et al: Status and trends in the education of racial and ethnic groups 2018 (NCES 2019-038). Washington, DC, U.S. Department of Education, National Center for Education Statistics, 2019. Available at: https://nces.ed.gov/pubs2019/2019038.pdf. Accessed May 14, 2020.

Evans R, Nagoshi JL, Nagoshi C, et al: Voices from the stories untold: lesbian, gay, bisexual, trans, and queer college students' experiences with campus climate. Journal of Gay and Lesbian Social Services 29(4):426–444, 2017

Garriott PO, Hudyma A, Keene C, et al: Social cognitive predictors of first- and non-first-generation college students' academic and life satisfaction. J Couns Psychol 62(2):253–263, 2015

Gaydosh L, Schorpp KM, Chen E, et al: College completion predicts lower depression but higher metabolic syndrome among disadvantaged minorities in young adulthood. Proc Natl Acad Sci USA 115(1):109–114, 2018

Geary D: How do we get people to interact? International students and the American experience. Journal of International Students 6(2):527–541, 2016

Greenlee C: Safety zone: issues surrounding policing on campus raise questions about security and profiling. Diverse Issues in Higher Education 33(suppl):16–21, 2016

Heron KE, Romano KA, Braitman AL: Mobile technology use and mHealth text message preferences: an examination of gender, racial, and ethnic differences among emerging adult college students. Mhealth 5:2, 2019

Hoffman GD, Mitchell TD: Making diversity "everyone's business": a discourse analysis of institutional responses to student activism for equity and inclusion. Journal of Diversity in Higher Education 9(3):277–289, 2016

Hunt J, Eisenberg D: Mental health problems and help-seeking behavior among college students. J Adolescent Health 46 (1):3–10, 2010

Hurd NM, Tan JS, Loeb EL: Natural mentoring relationships and the adjustment to college among underrepresented students. Am J Community Psychol 57(3–4):330–341, 2016

Hwang WC, Goto S: The impact of perceived racial discrimination on the mental health of Asian American and Latino college students. Asian Am J Psychol 1(suppl):15–28, 2009

Institute of International Education: Fast facts 2019. New York, Open Doors, Institute of International Education, 2019. Available at: https://opendoorsdata.org/fast_facts/fast-facts-2019. Accessed August 7, 2020.

Institute of Medicine of the National Academies: The health of lesbian, gay, bisexual, and transgender people: building a foundation for better understanding. Washington, DC, Institute of Medicine of the National Academies, 2011. Available at: www.nap.edu/catalog/13128/the-health-of-lesbian-gay-bisexual-and-transgender-people-building. Accessed August 5, 2020.

Jongen CS, McCalman J, Bainbridge RG: The implementation and evaluation of health promotion services and programs to improve cultural competency: a systematic scoping review. Front Public Health 5:24, 2017

Kausar H: New US visa rule leaves Indian, Chinese students in panic. Al Jazeera, July 10, 2020. Available at: www.aljazeera.com/news/2020/07/visa-rule-leaves-indian-chinese-students-panic-200709091726735.html. Accessed August 3, 2020.

Karnik NS, Dogra N: The cultural sensibility model: a process-oriented approach for children and adolescents. Child Adolesc Psychiatr Clin N Am 19(4):719–737, 2010

Kessler R, Berglund P, Demler O, et al: Lifetime prevalence and age-of-onset distributions of DSM-IV disorders in the National Comorbidity Survey Replication. Arch Gen Psychiatry 62(6):593–602, 2005

Kim YK, Cronley C: Acculturative stress and binge drinking among international students in the United States: resilience and vulnerability approaches. J Am Coll Health 68(2):207–218, 2020

Kulick A, Wernick LJ, Woodford MR, et al: Heterosexism, depression, and campus engagement among LGBTQ college students: intersectional differences and opportunities for healing. J Homosex 64(8):1125–1141, 2017

Kwan MY, Gordon KH, Minnich AM: An examination of the relationships between acculturative stress, perceived discrimination, and eating disorder symptoms among ethnic minority college students. Eat Behav 28:25–31, 2018

Laurencin CT, McClinton A: The COVID-19 pandemic: a call to action to identify and address racial and ethnic disparities. J Racial Ethn Health Disparities 7(3):398–402 2020

Lee EB: Young, black, and connected: Facebook usage among African American college students. J Black Stud 43(3):336–354, 2012

Lee EB: Cyberbullying: prevalence and predictors among African American young adults. J Black Stud 48(1):57–73, 2017

Lee J: Mental health effects of school closures during COVID-19. Lancet Child Adolesc Health 4(6):421, 2020

Lee RB, Baring R, Maria MS, et al: Attitude towards technology, social media usage and grade-point average as predictors of global citizenship identification in Filipino university students. Int J Psychol 52(3):213–219, 2017

Leebens PK, Williamson ED: Developmental psychopathology: risk and resilience in the transition to young adulthood. Child Adolesc Psychiatr Clin N Am 26(2):143–156, 2017

Levenson JC, Shensa A, Sidani JE, et al: The association between social media use and sleep disturbance among young adults. Prev Med 85:36–41, 2016

Levien SJ, Li AW: Harvard Ph.D. students map incidents of anti-Asian aggression. Harvard Crimson, April 16, 2020. Available at: www.thecrimson.com/article/2020/4/16/asian-aggression-map-coronavirus. Accessed August 3, 2020.

Litam SDA: "Take your kung-flu back to Wuhan": counseling Asians, Asian Americans, and Pacific Islanders with race-based trauma related to COVID-19. The Professional Counselor, 2020. Available at: https://tpcjournal.nbcc.org/take-your-kung-flu-back-to-wuhan-counseling-asians-asian-americans-and-pacific-islanders-with-race-based-trauma-related-to-covid-19/. Accessed September 10, 2020.

Locke B, Wallace D, Brunner J: Emerging issues and models in college mental health services. New Directions for Student Services 2016(156):19–30, 2016

Lowe SR, Tineo P, Young MN: Perceived discrimination and major depression and generalized anxiety symptoms: in Muslim American college students. J Relig Health 58(4):1136–1145, 2019

Martel A, Derenne J, Leebens PK (eds): Promoting Safe and Effective Transitions to College for Youth With Mental Health Conditions. Cham, Switzerland, Springer International, 2018

Marx BP, Sloan DM: The effects of trauma history, gender, and race on alcohol use and posttraumatic stress symptoms in a college student sample. Addict Behav 28(9):1631–1647, 2003

Nesi J, Choukas-Bradley S, Prinstein MJ: Transformation of adolescent peer relations in the social media context: part 1—A theoretical framework and application to dyadic peer relationships. Clin Child Fam Psychol Rev 21(3):267–294, 2018

O'Keeffe P: A sense of belonging: improving student retention. College Student Journal 47(4):605–613, 2013

Pittman DM, Cho Kim S, Hunter CD, et al: The role of minority stress in second-generation black emerging adult college students' high-risk drinking behaviors. Cultur Divers Ethnic Minor Psychol 23(3):445–455, 2017

Pumariega A: Ethical and legal issues in the management of high-risk patients in college. Lecture presented at the annual meeting of the American Psychiatric Association, San Francisco, CA, May 2019.

Ramsey JL, DiLalla LF, McCrary MK: Cyber victimization and depressive symptoms in sexual minority college students. Journal of School Violence 15(4):483–502, 2016

Richards D, Caldwell PHY, Go H: Social media and the health of young people. J Paediatr Child Health 51(12):1152–1157, 2015

Rivas-Drake D, Stein GL: Multicultural developmental experiences: implications for resilience in transitional age youth. Child Adolesc Psychiatr Clin N Am 26(2):271–281, 2017

Rodríguez JE, Campbell KM, Mouratidis RW: Where are the rest of us? Improving representation of minority faculty in academic medicine. South Med J 107(12):739–744, 2014

Romanelli M, Hudson KD: Individual and systemic barriers to health care: perspectives of lesbian, gay, bisexual, and transgender adults. Am J Orthopsychiatry 87(6):714–728, 2017

Rubio DM, Mayowski CA, Norman MK: A multi-pronged approach to diversifying the workforce. Int J Environ Res Public Health 15(10):E2219, 2018

Shah JL, Malla AK: Much ado about much: stress, dynamic biomarkers and HPA axis dysregulation along the trajectory to psychosis. Schizophr Res 162(1):253–260, 2015

Shalev I, Entringer S, Wadhwa PD, et al: Stress and telomere biology: a lifespan perspective. Psychoneuroendocrinology 38(9):1835–1842, 2013

Siemons R, Raymond-Flesch M, Auerswald CL, et al: Coming of age on the margins: mental health and well-being among Latino immigrant young adults eligible for deferred action for childhood arrivals (DACA). J Immigr Minor Health 19(3):543–551, 2017

Steers MN, Neighbors C, Wickham RE, et al: My friends, I'm #SOTALLYTOBER: a longitudinal examination of college students' drinking, friends' approval of drinking, and Facebook alcohol-related posts. Digit Health 5:2055207619845449, 2019

Stephens NM, Fryberg SA, Markus HR, et al: Unseen disadvantage: how American universities' focus on independence undermines the academic performance of first-generation college students. J Pers Soc Psychol 102(6):1178–1197, 2012

Stewart SM, Simmons A, Habibpour E: Treatment of culturally diverse children and adolescents with depression. J Child Adolesc Psychopharmacol 22(1):72–79, 2012

Thayer PB: Retention of Students from First Generation and Low Income Backgrounds. Washington, DC, Council for Opportunity in Education, 2000

Twenge J: iGen: Why Today's Super-Connected Kids Are Growing Up Less Rebellious, More Tolerant, Less Happy—and Completely Unprepared for Adulthood—and What That Means for the Rest of Us. New York, Atria, 2018

U.S. Census Bureau: QuickFacts: United States, 2019. Available at: www.census.gov/quickfacts/fact/table/US/PST045218. Accessed May 14, 2020.

U.S. Department of Education: Advancing diversity and inclusion in higher education: key data highlights focusing on race and ethnicity and promising practices. Rockville, MD, Office of Planning, Evaluation, and Policy Development and Office of the Under Secretary, 2016. Available at: www2.ed.gov/rschstat/research/pubs/advancing-diversity-inclusion.pdf. Accessed May 14, 2020.

Versey HS, Cogburn CC, Wilkins CL, et al: Appropriated racial oppression: implications for mental health in whites and blacks. Soc Sci Med 230:295–302, 2019

Werneke U, Bhugra D: Culture makes a person. Nord J Psychiatry 72 (suppl 1):S1–S2, 2018

Williams Institute: LGBT data and demographics. Los Angeles, CA, UCLA School of Law, January 2019. Available at: https://williamsinstitute.law.ucla.edu/visualization/lgbt-stats/?topic=LGBT#demographic. Accessed May 14, 2020.

Wilson EC, Chen YH, Arayasirikul S, et al: The impact of discrimination on the mental health of trans*female youth and the protective effect of parental support. AIDS Behav 20(10):2203–2211, 2016

Woo B, Fan W, Tran TV, et al: The role of racial/ethnic identity in the association between racial discrimination and psychiatric disorders: a buffer or exacerbator? SSM Popul Health 7:100378, 2019

Zhai Y, Du X: Addressing collegiate mental health amid COVID-19 pandemic. Psychiatry Res 288:113003, 2020

PART V
Applied Concepts

CHAPTER 21

DSM-5 Outline for Cultural Formulation and Cultural Formulation Interview

Complex Case Examples

Kathryn L. Jones, M.D., Ph.D.
Pratik Jain, M.D.
Collin Weintraub, B.S.
Cheryl S. Al-Mateen, M.D., FAACP, DFAPA

PSYCHIATRY, by way of the *Diagnostic and Statistical Manual of Mental Disorders*, now in its fifth edition (DSM-5; American Psychiatric Association 2013), has long struggled to account for the contribution of cultural differences to diagnosis and conceptualization. The development of the Outline for Cultural Formulation (OCF) in DSM-IV (American Psychiatric Association 1994) and its evolution over later iterations of DSM (currently DSM-5) represent attempts to operationalize and standardize the characterization of these effects. Four key elements were identified for consideration: 1) the cultural identity of the individual, 2) cultural explanations of the individual's illness and help-seeking experience (in DSM-5, this element is termed *cultural conceptualizations of distress*), 3) cultural factors related to the psychosocial environment and functioning (in DSM-5, these factors are termed *psychosocial stressors* and *cultural features of vulnerability and resilience*), and 4) cultural elements of the relationship between the individual and the clinician (Table 21–1).

TABLE 21–1. Elements of the DSM-5 Outline for Cultural Formulation

Cultural identity of the individual

Cultural conceptualizations of distress

Psychosocial stressors and cultural features of vulnerability and resilience

Cultural features of the relationship between the individual and the clinician

Overall cultural assessment

Information from the OCF is used to better understand the expression of mental illness and can potentially influence diagnosis. For example, a study that reviewed medical records of culturally diverse patients found that almost half of those with an initial diagnosis of a psychotic disorder were rediagnosed with nonpsychotic disorders after consideration of cultural factors (Adeponle et al. 2012). The impact of the OCF on clinical outcomes is still being studied. It has been underutilized because of time constraints in real practice, and efforts are being made to promote its widespread use (Fortuna et al. 2009; Leseth 2015; Lewis-Fernández 2009; Lewis-Fernández and Aggarwal 2013). After the publication of the OCF, Rousseau et al. (2008) noted that it required adaptation for use with children and youth. They emphasized the importance of cultural expectations in attaining developmental milestones, parenting, discipline, and independence in sleeping or eating.

The Cultural Formulation Interview (CFI) is a semistructured interview introduced in DSM-5 as an attempt to increase the utility and acceptance of the OCF. As the first standardized method of obtaining the needed information for the OCF, the utility of the CFI has been studied in adults, but field testing has excluded children and youth and is recommended (Ang 2017; Rousseau and Guzder 2016).

However, several case reports regarding use of the OCF in children and youth have been published (Table 21–2). The topics of these reports include the developmental nature of cultural identity, the effect of acculturative stress on ethnic identity development, idioms of distress, and suicidality (Chartonas and Bose 2015; Fang et al. 2013; Novins et al. 1997; Schofield et al. 2013; Shaffer and Steiner 2006; Takeuchi 2000). There have also been articles that provide sociocultural knowledge to improve culturally informed care of Muslim and Turkish children and families (Al-Mateen and Afzal 2004; Yilmaz et al. 2013).

Aggarwal (2010) noted differences in assessing culture in child and adolescent mental health, many of which are included in the DSM-5 supplemental modules (American Psychiatric Association 2013). He recommended asking children how they self-identify in comparison to their parents or caregivers, as well as asking about any differences in preferred language when determining salient features in the child's own cultural identity. Acceptance or rejection of parents' cultural identity may relate to developmental, cultural, or psychological factors. Consideration of the family context (i.e., how parents and children explain the child's and/or relative's illnesses and treatment) is key in understanding the cultural conceptualization or explanation of the illness.

Similarly, both the child and caregivers should be asked about others involved in the family's decision-making process. Aggarwal (2010) noted that the child's psychological environment and level of functioning relate to characteristics of the primary household and the family's sources of support. This includes an understanding of the child's ability to achieve cultural milestones or to fulfill expected rites of passage and gender role expectations. Birth order, gender, and age all contribute to these expectations.

TABLE 21–2. Case reports regarding cultural psychiatry and youth

Study	Case description	Cultural formulation
Novins et al. 1997	Three American Indian children and the developmental nature of cultural identity	The OCF was useful in providing a cultural formulation, but the study found limitations because not all requested material was available. Researchers noted that the caretakers' cultural identity should be part of the formulation. Additions to the OCF were recommended.
Takeuchi 2000	13-year-old girl with schizoaffective disorder that met criteria for a cultural syndrome	Author noted the usefulness of the OCF and the glossary of culture-bound syndromes in DSM-IV.
Shaffer and Steiner 2006	Acculturative stress and ethnic identity development in a 16-year-old second-generation Mexican American girl	The study used the DSM-IV OCF.
Fang et al. 2013	Idioms of distress and immigration in a 10-year-old first-generation Chinese American boy	Cultural formulation included the following: • Cultural reference group • Language • Cultural factors in development • Involvement with culture of origin • Involvement with host culture • Idioms of distress and local illness categories • Meaning and severity of symptoms in relation to cultural norms • Perceived causes and explanatory models • Help-seeking experiences and plans • Social stressors and supports • Levels of functioning and disability • Cultural elements in the therapist-patient relationship • Overall cultural assessment
Schofield et al. 2013	Cultural factors in a nearly lethal suicide attempt of an exchange student in the United States	The study included cultural formulation using the DSM-IV-TR OCF (American Psychiatric Association 2000). The OCF was useful in understanding the clinical material.

TABLE 21–2. Case reports regarding cultural psychiatry and youth (continued)

Study	Case description	Cultural formulation
Chartonas and Bose 2015	Spirit possession as an idiom of distress in an 8-year-old girl from Eritrea with epilepsy who immigrated to the United Kingdom	Cultural formulation included the following: • Cultural identity • Spirit possession as an idiom of distress • Social stressors and acculturative stress • Perceived causes, explanatory models, and cultural formulation • Treatment, help-seeking plans, and social supports

Note. OCF= Outline for Cultural Formulation.

Cultural factors influence how the patient and family conceptualize events as contributing to vulnerability or resilience. Family, community, and religious leaders (cultural brokers) participate in family decision-making related to mental health treatment, in addition to providing support during stressful times. Cultural features between the patient, family, and clinician may be explicit (e.g., language) or implicit (e.g., stigma) (Aggarwal 2010). Synthesis of these factors is similar to what an ethnographer does (Mezzich et al. 2009); the resulting overall assessment can be critical in fully understanding a patient's clinical presentation and developing a conceptualization and treatment plan.

In 2013, DSM-5 included the CFI to increase the utility and acceptance of the OCF (Tables 21–3 and 21–4). However, although many practitioners recognize the impact of culturally competent treatment in adult psychiatry (Aggarwal et al. 2015; Mills et al. 2017; Paralikar et al. 2019), the literature regarding the use of the CFI for children and adolescents is sparse (La Roche and Bloom 2018). Additionally, the CFI probes abstract concepts that children may not be able to understand sufficiently enough to generate valuable discussion of cultural influences (La Roche and Bloom 2018). Therefore, special considerations are needed when working with children and teenagers. Culturally specific content may not be as obvious to the young. They may not be able to tell us what cultural differences might be present. They may lack the developmental maturity to provide clear history or insight into the contributions of their cultural background and experience to their illness. This may be particularly true for first- and second-generation children of immigrants, who may have been encouraged to assimilate into the majority culture and have done so or who may have intentionally sought to reject their natal culture and have embraced the majority culture as being more socially relevant and acceptable (or as a way of opposing their parents).

The CFI is composed of three tools: the core CFI, the CFI—Informant Version, and 12 supplemental modules to broaden available information (Aggarwal et al. 2016). The core CFI consists of 16 questions, with instructions, to be used with patients who have any diagnosis in any setting. It has been recommended that it be used in all standard clinical assessments, and it was designed to be consistent with the progression of a routine mental health evaluation (Aggarwal et al. 2016). The CFI addresses four domains: cultural definition of the problem; cultural per-

TABLE 21–3. **When to use the DSM-5 Cultural Formulation Interview**

Difficulty in diagnostic assessment owing to significant differences in the cultural, religious, or socioeconomic backgrounds of the clinician and the individual

Uncertainty about the fit between culturally distinctive symptoms and diagnostic criteria

Difficulty in judging illness severity or impairment

Disagreement between the individual and clinician on the course of care

Limited engagement in and adherence to treatment by the individual

Source. Reprinted from American Psychiatric Association: *Diagnostic and Statistical Manual of Mental Disorders,* 5th Edition, Arlington, VA, American Psychiatric Association, 2013, p. 751. Copyright © 2013 American Psychiatric Association. Used with permission.

TABLE 21–4. **Principles for using the DSM-5 Cultural Formulation Interview with children and youth**

Brevity is essential; attention span and concentration increase with age and developmental stage. Resist the urge to get all the information in one sitting. Consider use of additional modalities (e.g., observation, drawing, play).

Adapt the questions to the child's or adolescent's cognitive and linguistic development. Language differences and dislocation experiences influence all aspects of development that are being assessed.

Include collateral information from significant adults.

Source. Adapted from Rousseau and Guzder 2016, p. 158.

ceptions of cause, context, and support; cultural factors affecting self-coping and past help seeking; and cultural factors affecting current help seeking.

The CFI—Informant Version is designed for "the spouse, other family member, or friend" who may also be present, as well as the parent or caregiver of a young child (Aggarwal et al. 2016, p. 33); the clinician determines which questions are most relevant for use with each patient. The informant version may be used in conjunction with the Caregivers supplementary module (see www.psychiatry.org/psychiatrists/practice/dsm/educational-resources/assessment-measures, "Early Development and Home Background").

There are three types of supplementary modules: expansion of core domains, special populations, and informant perspectives (the latter of which is appropriate for caregivers). The special populations modules include School-Age Children and Adolescents, Older Adults, and Immigrants and Refugees. A focus of the CFI and the supplementary modules is to "help the clinician avoid errors of decontextualization that result from neglecting the patient's life situation, sense of belonging to one or more social groups, and understanding of the 'problem' and how to obtain help for it" (Hinton and Hinton 2016, p. 54).

Case Examples

This section includes four blended clinical cases representing diverse child and adolescent patient populations, outlining use of the OCF to generate a cultural formulation. The cases presented here represent amalgamations of several actual patients; all identifying patient health information and other historical elements have been altered in order to protect confidentiality. For each of the following cases, we have provided a synopsis of the clinical case, followed by a brief, focused analysis of case elements through the lens of the OCF, concluding with an overall cultural assessment and formulation.

African American Cultural Formulation

Case Vignette 1: Quentin

Quentin is a 12-year-old boy with a history of depression, anxiety, and autism spectrum disorder. He self-identifies as Black, was born in the United States to African American parents, and was raised in a midsize city. Quentin has an apparent high intellect (full-scale IQ 137) and shows no evidence of developmental delays aside from deficits in social pragmatics. He has a highly reactive and risk-averse temperament and has struggled with disruptive mood dysregulation disorder and parent-child relational problems for years.

Quentin was admitted to the acute inpatient psychiatric unit with suicidal ideation and concern for psychosis after he was observed behaving oddly at school and attempted suicide by hanging himself at home. When the inpatient treatment team met with Quentin, he seemed quiet, withdrawn, and mostly focused on drawing comics of his own invention. The only time he made sustained eye contact with the psychiatrist on the team was to ask if they knew what a *senpai* was. He explained that one reason he had been depressed and suicidal recently was that he liked a girl in his class and he wanted her to be his *senpai*—a term he had embraced ever since hearing it in his favorite animé shows, such as *Ouran High School Host Club* and *Naruto*. This term is defined formally as a senior individual or mentor to a junior, or *kōhai*, but in social media it is most often used to describe a romantic interest. When Quentin built up the courage to ask the girl if she would be this for him, she laughed and rejected him. He was confused and hurt but seemed reassured when the psychiatrist said he was familiar with the term and shared similar interests in multimedia.

When the psychiatrist met with him during rounds, Quentin often talked about animé and seemed to identify closely with different characters. His medications were adjusted during admission, and he was discharged home after 8 days. However, over the next several months, Quentin was readmitted several times to various hospitals. Each admission was longer in duration; his behaviors appeared to be escalating in terms of their bizarreness and aggression toward peers and himself. He started to report hearing satanic voices and having satanic visions, and he was noted to antagonize peers by using crude sexual comments about their family members. After multiple hospitalizations, Quentin met the initial psychiatrist again one weekend, and the clinician was struck by how some of the supposedly psychotic content Quentin described and behaviors he displayed reflected and reenacted storylines and characters of some specific animé, including *Yu Yu Hakusho, Inuyasha*, and *Black Butler*. Using this information, the team was able to facilitate Quentin's discharge to a residential treatment facility for ongoing care.

Quentin's parents met at an historically black university (HBCU), where his father played on the baseball team. They both work in criminal justice. Quentin did not talk about animé with his family because they did not share his interests. His parents knew of, but did not connect to, any Black animé enthusiasts, having grown up in the 1980s when there was a broader fascination with what was then termed *Japanimation*. Even then, it was not thought to be a typical hobby for young Black children or teenagers, and this continues to be the case now despite greater access to certain animé series via online streaming services. For Black boys in particular, the culturally bound belief (among some Black Americans and also some white Americans) that intellectual pursuits are seen as effeminate and discordant with the ideal of the strong Black man who both prefers and excels in physical activities can be limiting, and in Quentin's case, his family struggled to accept that this identity did not fit him.

Quentin engaged most with African American members of the treatment team. He generally did not engage with others on his unit, but he frequently discussed animé with same-age peers. His parents recognized that Quentin exhibited unusual behaviors, and they were focused primarily on his willfulness and occasional explosiveness. Additionally, they did not want him to be "labeled" because of his academic potential. They were reluctant to consider medications but ultimately accepted the recommendation of Quentin's physician, who was African American.

Quentin's diagnoses are complicated by his parents' cultural understanding of his illness as subject only to his will and thereby a sign of internal weakness if he is unable to overcome his symptoms without medications and therapy. Quentin's parents hold certain beliefs common in African American culture (i.e., among individuals descended from West African slaves) (Abdullah and Brown 2011; Buque 2017; Jimenez et al. 2012; Stewart et al. 2012; Sullivan et al. 2020; U.S. Department of Health and Human Services 2001; Ward et al. 2013), and these beliefs affect their understanding of and ability to function with Quentin's illness (Table 21–5). Given these cultural factors, their understanding of the role culture plays in Quentin's life, and the relationship between his culture and his illnesses, it is unsurprising that Quentin's parents initially rejected the diagnoses of autism spectrum disorder, disruptive mood dysregulation disorder, and parent-child relational problems. Quentin's fascination with animé culture was the most salient aspect of his identity during his hospitalizations, and these differences represent the intersectionality that was seen with this family.

Evangelical Christianity and LGBTQ+ Cultural Formulation

Case Vignette 2: Maggie

Maggie is a 15-year-old white girl from a rural area who has a history of depression and multiple medical and surgical interventions for ulcerative colitis, including complete removal of her colon, necessitating a colostomy bag. She has an apparent above average intellect, developmental delays in terms of gross and fine motor milestones, and a high-reactive yet somewhat novelty-seeking temperament. Maggie has struggled with a recurrent, moderate major depressive disorder and psychological factors affecting other medical conditions (her ulcerative colitis) for many years. She was admitted to the inpatient acute psychiatric unit for depressed mood and suicidal ideation after her parents found sexually explicit texts between her and a female friend from school.

Collateral history obtained from Maggie's mother, Mrs. Stone, confirmed that Maggie's relationship with this female peer had triggered an argument with her parents. Mrs. Stone stated that she and Maggie's father did not believe in homosexuality but that they loved family members who were gay despite their sexual orientation. When Maggie's parents overheard her talking to a suicide hotline worker about this relationship, they terminated the phone call. Mrs. Stone shared with the team that she did not think Maggie was truly attracted to girls, or, at least, she was hoping that this was untrue and that it was "just a phase."

TABLE 21–5. Cultural formulation for Quentin

Cultural formulation	Description
Cultural identity	• Black boy born in the United States to African American parents and raised in a midsize city
Cultural conceptualizations of distress	• Descriptions of mental illness have at times been conceptualized as designed by and intended for whites alone and thus may be a tool of oppression and domination of African Americans. Quentin's parents have told him about instances in which the medical profession has engaged in targeted abuse of African Americans (e.g., the Tuskegee syphilis experiments) to better help white Americans. • There is a historical expectation for African Americans to demonstrate resiliency in response to stress because of their struggles in the United States from slavery and civil rights to the current era of heightened white supremacy. Quentin is expected to be a "strong young Black man." This conflicts with the foundational ideals of mental health, that seeking support is not weakness. In particular, he is struggling to find his place in the world as a young Black man with severe, persistent mental illness who does not fit the picture of a strong Black man.
Psychosocial stressors and cultural features of vulnerability and resilience	• Quentin feels isolated from his culture as a young African American man because of severe, persistent mental illness. • He finds strength in Japanese culture but does not belong to it.
Cultural features of the relationship between the individual and the clinician	• Stigma and identity conflicts are barriers to seeking help. • The medical profession is not trustworthy when it comes to the African American community. • Seeking help may be easier with a clinician of similar African American cultural identity and appreciation of Japanese culture.
Overall cultural assessment	Given these cultural factors and his understanding of the role culture plays in his life and his relationship with illness, it is unsurprising that Quentin presents with clinical symptoms consistent with a disruptive mood dysregulation disorder and parent-child relational problems in the setting of autism spectrum disorder.

During her hospitalization, Maggie started taking antidepressant medication and was actively involved in individual and group therapeutic interventions. However, she was reluctant to engage in family therapy because of her belief that her parents would never change and accept her sexuality. Mrs. Stone expressed frustration with the lack of available local mental health services because the family happened to be from an underserved area.

The treatment team recommended individual outpatient therapy for Maggie, as well as family therapy, and Mrs. Stone noted that it would be hard for both parents to accept the possibility that Maggie was bisexual or gay. They wanted to "retrain her brain" in counseling. Mrs. Stone also expressed an interest in home schooling Maggie using a faith-based curriculum approved by their church, with the goal of removing Maggie from public school, where she was exposed to behaviors and lifestyles counter to their faith. Both the psychiatrist and the family therapist explained their concerns about pursuing any kind of conversion therapy, and Mrs. Stone expressed understanding of their perspective. She was willing to engage in family therapy with Maggie, which went better than expected, and Maggie was discharged home thereafter with plans to follow up with her inpatient psychiatrist at the outpatient clinic.

When she returned to see her psychiatrist for their first outpatient appointment, Maggie shared that she had decided "not to force the sexuality issue" with her parents and had ended her relationship with her female friend after they had a falling out at school.

Maggie's diagnoses are complicated by her cultural understanding of her illness as suffering, both physical and existential, intended to help her to become stronger in her faith (Bock et al. 2018; Salwen et al. 2017; Wesselman et al. 2015). Specific aspects of her faith culture (Bock et al. 2018; Salwen et al. 2017; Wesselman et al. 2015) have impacted her general function across multiple domains in both positive and negative ways that have come into conflict with each other (Table 21–6).

Multiracial Cultural Formulation

Case Vignette 3: Scout

Scout is an 8-year-old multiracial boy with a history of extensive trauma, including witnessing his mother shoot her ex-boyfriend, sexual abuse by two close male relatives, and intermittent homelessness. He was raised in multiple settings, from an isolated rural community to a medium-size city, by both biological and foster families. He has apparent average intellect; some history of developmental delays (speech, gross, and fine motor); and a highly reactive, sensitive temperament. He has struggled with reactive attachment disorder and PTSD for many years.

Scout was hospitalized because of mood dysregulation, behavioral dyscontrol, and aggression toward his foster mother, his biological sister who was in foster care with him, and peers and teachers at school. He appears much younger than his stated age and is thin and delicately built, with mild facial dysmorphism and very curly, fluffy hair. Scout was very guarded and answered most questions without much detail or affect but endorsed no acute safety concerns.

The team spoke with Scout's social services guardian to identify a safe discharge plan for him once he was ready. His foster mother, Ms. Grant, would not commit to taking him home without a guarantee that he would not act aggressively against her or Scout's sister if he returned home. She was not willing or able to visit with him while he was in the hospital. She also did not schedule an intake appointment with intensive in-home services, as had been recommended by other outpatient providers over the past several weeks.

In an effort to develop a therapeutic alliance and to gain a better understanding of the nature of the relationship and dynamics between Scout and his foster mother, the team met with Ms. Grant separately. Ms. Grant is a single, middle-age, light-skinned African American woman without children who appears to identify herself primarily by way of her connections with community groups, particularly the local NFL team. She was able to provide the treatment team with a more detailed past history for Scout. His parents were an interracial couple, with a white mother and an African American father, both born in the United States. At one point, Scout had lived in the home of his maternal grandparents, where both he and his younger sister were severely physically and sexually abused and exposed to adult sexual behavior, whereas his older sister, who had a white father, was protected.

When Scout and his sisters returned to their mother's care, they were homeless, sleeping in cars and in a 24-hour fast food restaurant near his foster mother's current home. They were exposed to adult sexual activity. After his mother shot one sexual partner in the face, Scout and his sisters were placed in foster care. Both of Scout's sisters were placed with a white foster mother, and Scout was placed in a different home. Later, all three children were placed with an African

TABLE 21-6. Cultural formulation for Maggie

Cultural formulation	Description
Cultural identity	• White girl born in the United States to parents of European ancestry and raised in the evangelical Christian faith in an underserved rural community • Adolescent girl with a chronic inflammatory bowel disease managed by surgical intervention, with ongoing clinical manifestations and requiring ongoing care
Cultural conceptualizations of distress	• Among evangelical Christians, illness and suffering are generally seen as tests of faith; if tests of faith are gifts from a loving God, then illness and suffering are gifts from God. • Doubt and lack of faith, as evidenced by medical and mental illness, are both personal failings.
Psychosocial stressors and cultural features of vulnerability and resilience	• Among evangelical Christians, generally speaking, nonheterosexual love and desire are sinful. Therefore, Maggie's tentative exploration of her sexual desire is sinful and must be suppressed. Although Maggie finds connection, community, and comfort within the church, her identity as a young queer or questioning woman is not acceptable in her church or in her home with her evangelical Christian parents. • A negative perception of her body and its limitations conflicts with her faith's identification of these limitations as gifts from God for which she should be grateful or at least accepting. As part of her faith, Maggie is expected to have a close and loving connection to God and to find succor in the belief that God loves her. However, the complex medical conditions that her faith tells her are challenges from a loving God test her belief in that same loving God. • Rural Americans are expected to be hardy, to demonstrate resilience in the face of deprivation, and to find comfort in their local community. • Maggie experiences minimal cultural diversity and limited mental health resources in her underserved rural community.
Cultural features of the relationship between the individual and the clinician	• Stigma and identity conflicts are cultural barriers to seeking help. Specific barriers include bias against Maggie's sexual identity and internal conflict between what her faith tells her to believe about her body and her personal experience living in her body. • Seeking help may be easier from a clinician with some understanding of her evangelical Christian faith and her medical history who appreciates the challenges of living in a small, rural community and is either allied with or part of LGBTQ+ culture.
Overall cultural assessment	Given these cultural factors and Maggie's understanding of the role culture plays in her life and her relationship with illness, it is unsurprising that Maggie presents with clinical symptoms consistent with recurrent, moderate major depressive disorder and psychological factors affecting other medical conditions in the setting of postcolectomy ulcerative colitis.

American foster mother, but his older sister eventually returned to live with her first foster mother, and Scout and his younger sister came to live with Ms. Grant.

Ms. Grant noticed that both Scout and his sister had sexually reactive behavior. Additionally, she noted that Scout sometimes hoarded food; stole things from others and hid them; and was occasionally incontinent of stool, even at school. She was committed to keeping his younger sister in the home with her but felt overwhelmed by managing Scout's behaviors and was open to considering a different setting for him, although she wished to continue to be present in his life.

Given Scout's age, both chronologically and developmentally, he has a limited understanding of the impact of culture on his illness, not to mention limited insight into illness itself (Table 21–7). Therefore, the perspective of his current foster mother is particularly useful, even though it is entangled with her own cultural identity as a well-educated, never-married light-skinned African American woman with no biological children and little experience with children with Scout's history. Through his foster mother's lens, Scout's presentation is complicated by her cultural understanding of Scout's illness as conscious, purposeful, and subject to his will, as well as organic and somewhat immutable.

Scout's foster mother finds that certain elements of her own culture affect her understanding of Scout and his ability to function with his illnesses in the following ways:

- African Americans are expected to show strength in the face of adversity and to not show distress, particularly outside their community (Abdullah and Brown 2011; Buque 2017; Jimenez et al. 2012; Stewart et al. 2012; Sullivan et al. 2020; U.S. Department of Health and Human Services 2001; Ward et al. 2013).
- Colorism, or bias for or against other members of the African American community based on lightness or darkness of complexion, is associated with assumptions of beauty, intellect, and success, particularly in the majority white society. Historically, darker-complected African Americans were also believed to have higher pain tolerance than those with lighter skin, an unconscious bias that persists today. Such beliefs are grounded in slave culture, in which slaves with darker skin more often worked in the fields, and slaves with lighter skin more often worked in the house. Despite current understanding that it was the white slave owners' systematic rape of darker-complected slaves that produced the variety in coloration among African Americans, these constructs continue to divide the African American community (Cobb et al. 2016; Laidley et al. 2019; Landor et al. 2013).
- Little boys with African American ancestry are vulnerable to mental health treatment, particularly when they have a history of violence, but more often simply by being little Black boys in a majority white society. They are more likely to be prescribed antipsychotic medications to manage anger and dysregulated behavior and more likely to have their aggressive behaviors attributed to willfulness (U.S. Department of Health and Human Services 2001; Ward et al. 2013).
- Children of interracial relationships have historically struggled with identity and whether to belong to one race/culture or the other, and often they have been isolated from both (Landor et al. 2013; Roberts and Gelman 2017; Schlabach 2013). Within the Black community, where colorism and passing for white has long been a source of conflict, a biracial child may feel pressured to choose sides, and caregivers may choose for them.

TABLE 21-7. Cultural formulation for Scout

Cultural formulation	Description
Cultural identity	• Scout: multiracial boy born to an African American father and a white mother in the United States and raised in multiple settings, from an isolated rural community to a medium-sized city, by biological and foster families • Foster mother: African American woman with fair complexion, born to African American parents in the United States and raised in midsize and large cities
Cultural conceptualizations of distress	• Mental health care is neither designed by nor intended for African Americans. • African Americans are expected to be resilient in response to pain and stress (including abuse and neglect and separation from biological parents).
Psychosocial stressors and cultural features of vulnerability and resilience	• In the African American community, light skin is associated with greater beauty, intellect, and success, whereas darker complexions are associated with higher pain tolerance; this belief persists as unconscious bias among medical professionals. • Violent behavior among African Americans is perceived as indicative of a violent nature, particularly among boys, who are more likely to experience legal consequences, to be diagnosed with severe and persistent mental illness, and to be prescribed heavier medication doses. • The underresourced foster care system provides minimal supports for foster parents caring for children with severe attachment and trauma issues.
Cultural features of the relationship between the individual and the clinician	• Scout's foster mother identifies stigma and identity conflicts as cultural barriers to seeking help. • Seeking help may be easier with a clinician of similar cultural background who has an understanding of the role of color and the challenges of defining identity within the African American community, in addition to a firm understanding of attachment and trauma. • The medical profession is not trustworthy when it comes to the African American community.
Overall cultural assessment	Given these cultural factors and Scout's foster mother's understanding of the role culture plays in her and Scout's life and their relationship with his illness, it is unsurprising that Scout presents with clinical symptoms consistent with his diagnoses of reactive attachment disorder and PTSD in the setting of complex trauma.

Ms. Grant identifies stigma related to her African American identity as a light-skinned Black woman and as a single woman attempting to raise a Black boy and identity conflicts (between her and Scout, her and health care providers, and Scout and providers) as cultural barriers to seeking help. Ms. Grant believes that she and Scout would be best supported in coping with his illness by a clinician of similar cultural background who understands the role of color and the challenges of defining identity in the African American community when one is light skinned or multiracial, and with some understanding of the challenges Scout has faced given his social history.

Muslim and Immigrant Cultural Formulation

Case Vignette 4: Adil

Adil is a 14-year-old Muslim refugee who arrived in the United States 2 months prior to his admission to an inpatient adolescent psychiatric unit after attempting to stab himself. This suicide attempt occurred after he learned that his betrothed had been kidnapped to either be forced to marry or be killed unless a ransom was paid. Adil neither speaks nor understands English; he is fluent only in his native tongue, for which there is only one interpreter within a 3-hour radius of the hospital, with limited availability. The interpreter was able to come in person for only a few hours of Adil's 5-day stay. Adil does speak broken Bengali; although a Bengali interpreter was available via video, this was not adequate. Understandably, Adil seemed skeptical about receiving treatment in a foreign country and involving people who had limited knowledge of his culture.

Despite communication difficulties, Adil is clearly noted to be distraught and guilt ridden about his inability to help his fiancée and his family. Through the interpreter, he endorses suicidal ideations, stating, "If the problem cannot be solved, I will find a way." Adil's somatic symptoms include poor appetite and vomiting. Intermittent auditory hallucinations of his fiancée are attributed to his history of trauma and most likely are a self-soothing coping mechanism. He meets DSM-5 criteria for major depressive disorder and PTSD.

Adil's foster parents of 2 months were able to provide some history of Adil's past trauma. After seeking employment at age 10, he was captured and held hostage by a human trafficking ring for 4 years, during which he was physically and emotionally abused while they extorted his parents for his release. He was rescued and brought to an immigration detention camp, where he was allowed only brief moments of telephone contact with his family. Human rights organizations later deemed that because of his prolonged separation, he would be best served by refugee status and placement with a foster family in the United States.

Adil shared additional stressors, such as being unable to connect well with his foster family, peers in school, and others in general because of significant language and cultural barriers. Difficulty in communicating his thoughts or feelings led to misinterpretation and frustration. Once during his admission, he attempted to calm a younger male peer by touching the peer's chest, shoulder, upper arm, and back. This was misconstrued by staff members as sexualized contact, leading to a brief separation from peers. Effective communication could have prevented this. When asked about the incident, Adil remarked, "You learn after making a mistake."

After Adil learned that his fiancée had been rescued, his suicidal thoughts subsided, and his mood improved. He was able to be safely discharged.

Adil identifies with his countrymen as a devout Muslim male and a caretaker of his biological family whom he had to leave behind (Table 21–8). Adil's strength is grounded in his faith, which offers a tremendous source of reassurance. During his hospital stay, he requested and received a copy of the Qur'an, and although his request to attend *Jumu'ah* (Friday prayers) could not be fulfilled, staff was able to arrange for an Imam to visit him. Adil was noted to have a very fatalistic view about his mortality, vacillating between wanting to live but also claiming that "all is in God's hands" and that nothing could prevent God's will with regard to dying. On learning about his fiancée's kidnapping and the lack of options given his Islamic faith and his situation, Adil felt that suicide was the only honorable option. He conceptualized his obligations and responsibilities as needing to uphold his family's honor. The hospital staff's persistence in obtaining face-to-face interpretation for a limited period after much difficulty not only had a marked positive impact on Adil's mood but also helped to alleviate his distrust of authority figures, and he was more willing to discuss his emotional state.

Adil was confronted with multiple stressors on arrival in the United States. He was placed with a foster family who had no experience with immigrant children and who had limited understanding of his culture. It was difficult for him to accept having a safe place to sleep and food readily available to eat after years of forced deprivation and having a family after he had to leave his own family behind. He began receiving formal high school education in English after having never attended school and having no familiarity with the complex social mores of U.S. adolescent life. Adil was more mature than his same-age peers in some respects because he had endured such horrific trauma, making it even more difficult for him to relate to them.

Adil's initial unwillingness to engage in treatment and single-mindedness with regard to completing suicide were in part due to internal distress but also were due to his distrust of the treatment team on the locked unit. His language barrier limited his involvement in various therapeutic modalities and prevented establishment of rapport with staff and peers. His relationship with the treatment team improved after they acknowledged his request for a copy of the Qur'an, arranged for a live interpreter, and provided an Imam. The team also showed respect by explaining why certain requests went unfulfilled.

Adil was also faced with the stress of his enforced immigration. Being separated from his community significantly affected his mood and behavior. Connecting with an interpreter from his home culture helped to alleviate his feelings of loneliness. The interpreter also agreed to remain in contact with Adil to act as a liaison between Adil and the local expatriate community. Adil's foster family was encouraged to attend services at a local mosque with him to help reaffirm his cultural identity and to help them form a stronger family bond.

Adil demonstrated marked resilience. Once he was able to let his guard down, he was noted to be inquisitive, focused on learning about his situation, and eager to engage in problem-solving. Adil showed promise in improving his mastery of English. Ultimately, Adil worked with the treatment team to formulate a plan for a safe discharge. His short-term goals were to remain connected with his culture and to continue English classes to help with acculturation. In the long term, Adil hoped to reunite with his family and fiancée once they were allowed to join him in the United States.

TABLE 21–8. **Cultural formulation for Adil**

Cultural formulation	Description
Cultural identity	• Strong identity as an East Asian male, a devout Muslim, and caretaker of his extended family • Religion offers a tremendous source of reassurance for him; he is aware that suicide is strongly condemned in Islam
Cultural conceptualizations of distress	• Adil's culture has an abundance of terms to assist with the description of feelings and emotions that do not have a precise translation in the Western lexicon. • Feelings of distress are communicated through facial expression, verbalizations of hopelessness/helplessness, and statements of wanting to die, as well as somatic symptoms of poor appetite and vomiting. • Adil endorses auditory hallucinations of his fiancée, which are conceptualized as a self-soothing means of coping.
Psychosocial stressors and cultural features of vulnerability and resilience	• Adil was brought to the United States and placed with a family who had no prior experience in fostering immigrant children. He was provided formal high school education in a foreign language after having never attended school. • Adil did not speak the language and did not have access to religious supports to help him process these changes. • He struggled with social aspects of U.S. adolescent life, which made it hard for him to connect. • Despite numerous stressors, Adil was very mature and demonstrated marked resilience. He focused his energy on gathering as much information as possible about his situation. He utilized available resources, including interpreters and clergy, to formulate a plan for a safe discharge that included both his foster family and his biological family.
Cultural features of the relationship between the individual and the clinician	• Obtaining an in-person interpreter who spoke Adil's language had a marked positive impact on his mood and helped improve his relationship with hospital staff. • Adil's initial distrust of the treatment team was understandable because of his previous negative experiences with other organizations. Provision of the requested religious text and transparency as to why certain requests could not be honored also served to build trust and mutual respect with staff. • Adil's cultural diet was not available at the hospital. He expressed fears about his food being adulterated with medications and threatened to "never eat again." This resolved somewhat as trust was developed.

TABLE 21–8. Cultural formulation for Adil

Cultural formulation	Description
Overall cultural assessment	Adil is a resilient child who has overcome numerous obstacles. Many changes in Adil's mood and behavior stemmed from feeling detached from his community and being unable to communicate effectively. The use of the interpreter, who also served as a cultural consultant for the treatment team, addressed some immediate feelings of loneliness and ultimately allowed Adil to build a long-term relationship with his native expatriate community for further acculturation and connection. Encouraging the foster family to help him attend the local mosque helped them to form a stronger family bond with him. On a long-term basis, continued development of communication in all settings will assist in effective integration of home and host cultures.

Conclusion

In this chapter, we have discussed the use of the OCF in the child and adolescent population and presented several cases to demonstrate its application in the clinical setting. We reviewed the elements of the OCF and how they can be used. However, the question may remain as to why cultural formulation matters at all.

It has long been presumed by many practitioners that differences between individuals are irrelevant to patient care and that treatment should be blind to color, creed, sexuality, gender, and socioeconomic circumstances or the intersection of these characteristics. If this is the goal, then paying attention to cultural differences would be undesirable. We, and others, find that the opposite is true: if we are to treat our patients in a holistic manner and to provide truly personalized care, then we must consider their cultural context. Every patient we encounter is unique; therefore, ignoring those elements that contribute to their individuality is to deny them truly personalized, patient-centered care. This is not to endorse discriminatory or segregated practices or to privilege cultural factors over others. Rather, this provides us with a lens through which to better understand the thoughts and feelings that drive patients' behaviors. In a more practical sense, it can also prevent clinical errors such as misdiagnosis, overmedication, and polypharmacy.

In the current era of Black Lives Matter and LGBTQ+ Pride, some people have countered these attempts to give voice to traditionally underserved and disenfranchised populations, proclaiming movements such as "Straight Pride" and "All Lives Matter," as if these are mutually exclusive. On the contrary, to affirm that cultural differences matter does not mean that they matter more; rather, it means that within the majority culture, minority cultural identities matter too and matter equally. By thinking critically about the impact that culture has on our patients, we shine a light on what makes them unique and help them to more completely understand themselves (and help others to understand them). Erasure benefits none of us, and to intentionally blind ourselves to culture and its formative role in our lives does a disservice to our patients and to ourselves.

We believe that the case examples in this chapter illustrate the depth and breadth of the cultural impact on child and adolescent mental health and how use of the OCF can improve patient care. More research is needed to determine best practices for use in this population, particularly in very young children and in children and adolescents with intellectual disability or developmental delays. We hope that this work represents a significant step on the path of greater appreciation for the impact of cultural identities and more consistent utilization of the DSM-5 OCF and CFI to improve patient care.

Clinical Pearls

- Culture is everywhere.
- Consider culture when assessment and treatment are not going as you expect.
- Use the DSM-5 Outline for Cultural Formulation to organize your thinking for conceptualization, diagnosis, and treatment.
- Use your experience with the DSM-5 Cultural Formulation Interview (CFI) to generate your own questions to help you develop the cultural formulation for your patient.
- Consider that CFI questions may be most appropriate for follow-up questions for some children and families and as initial questions for others.

Self-Assessment Questions

1. How might you adjust your current conceptualization of patients to include cultural formulation concepts?

2. How can you incorporate ethnographic interviewing into your clinical work?

3. What does this information tell you about your previous practice?

References

Abdullah T, Brown TL: Mental illness stigma and ethnocultural beliefs, values, and norms: an integrative review. Clin Psychol Rev 31(6):934–948, 2011

Adeponle AB, Thombs BD, Groleau D, et al: Using the cultural formulation to resolve uncertainty in diagnoses of psychosis among ethnoculturally diverse patients. Psychiatr Serv 63(2):147–153, 2012

Aggarwal NK: Cultural formulations in child and adolescent psychiatry. J Am Acad Child Adolesc Psychiatry 49(4):306–309, 2010

Aggarwal NK, Desilva R, Nicasio AV, et al: Does the Cultural Formulation Interview for the fifth revision of the Diagnostic and Statistical Manual of Mental Disorders (DSM-5) affect medical communication? A qualitative exploratory study from the New York site. Ethn Health 20(1):1–28, 2015

Aggarwal NK, Jiménez-Solomon O, Lam PC, et al: The core and informant Cultural Formulation Interviews in DSM-5, in DSM-5 Handbook on the Cultural Formulation Interview, Edited by Lewis-Fernández R, Aggarwal NK, Hinton L, Hinton DE, Kirmayer LJ. Arlington, VA, American Psychiatric Publishing, 2016, pp 27–44

Al-Mateen CS, Afzal A: The Muslim child, adolescent, and family. Child Adolesc Psychiatr Clin N Am 13(1):183–200, 2004

American Psychiatric Association: Diagnostic and Statistical Manual of Mental Disorders, 4th Edition. Washington, DC, American Psychiatric Association, 1994

American Psychiatric Association: Diagnostic and Statistical Manual of Mental Disorders, 4th Edition, Text Revision. Washington, DC, American Psychiatric Association, 2000

American Psychiatric Association: Diagnostic and Statistical Manual of Mental Disorders, 5th Edition. Arlington, VA, American Psychiatric Association, 2013

Ang W: Bridging culture and psychopathology in mental health care. Eur Child Adolesc Psychiatry 26(2):263–266, 2017

Bock NA, Hall MEL, Wang DC, et al: The role of attachment to God and spiritual self-awareness in predicting evangelical Christians' appraisals of suffering. Ment Health Relig Cult 21(4):353–369, 2018

Buque M: Is psychotherapy for people of color? Psychology Today, July 10, 2017. Available at: www.psychologytoday.com/us/blog/unpacking-race/201707/is-psychotherapy-people-color. Accessed November 29, 2019.

Chartonas D, Bose R: Fighting with spirits: migration trauma, acculturative stress, and new sibling transition—a clinical case study of an 8-year-old girl with absence epilepsy. Cult Med Psychiatry 39(4):698–724, 2015

Cobb RJ, Thomas CS, Laster Pirtle WN, et al: Self-identified race, socially assigned skin tone, and adult physiological dysregulation: assessing multiple dimensions of "race" in health disparities research. SSM Popul Health 2:595–602, 2016

Fang L, Lee E, Huang FY: A child who sees ghosts every night: manifestations of psychosocial and familial stress following immigration. Cult Med Psychiatry 37(3):549–564, 2013

Fortuna LR, Porche MV, Alegria M: A qualitative study of clinicians' use of the cultural formulation model in assessing posttraumatic stress disorder. Transcult Psychiatry 46(3):429–450, 2009

Hinton DE, Hinton L: Supplementary modules: overview, in DSM-5 Handbook on the Cultural Formulation Interview. Edited by Lewis-Fernández R, Aggarwal NK, Hinton L, Hinton DE, Kirmayer LJ. Arlington, VA, American Psychiatric Publishing, 2016, pp 45–55

Jimenez DE, Bartels SJ, Cardenas V, et al: Cultural beliefs and mental health treatment preferences of ethnically diverse older adult consumers in primary care. Am J Geriatr Psychiatry 20(6):533–542, 2012

Laidley T, Domingue B, Sinsub P, et al: New evidence of skin color bias and health outcomes using sibling difference models: a research note. Demography 56(2):753–762, 2019

Landor AM, Simons LG, Simons RL, et al: Exploring the impact of skin tone on family dynamics and race-related outcomes. J Fam Psychol 27(5):817–826, 2013

La Roche MJ, Bloom JB: Examining the effectiveness of the Cultural Formulation Interview with young children: a clinical illustration. Transcult Psychiatry 1363461518780605, 2018

Leseth AB: What is culturally informed psychiatry? Cultural understanding and withdrawal in the clinical encounter. BJPsych Bull 39(4):187–190, 2015

Lewis-Fernández R: The Cultural Formulation. Transcult Psychiatry 46(3):379–382, 2009

Lewis-Fernández R, Aggarwal NK: Culture and psychiatric diagnosis. Adv Psychosom Med 33:15–30, 2013

Mezzich JE, Caracci G, Fabrega H, et al: Cultural formulation guidelines. Transcult Psychiatry 46(3):383–405, 2009

Mills S, Xiao AQ, Wolitzky-Taylor K: Training on the DSM-5 Cultural Formulation Interview improves cultural competence in general psychiatry residents: a pilot study. Transcult Psychiatry 54(2):179–191, 2017

Novins DK, Bechtold DW, Sack WH, et al: The DSM-IV Outline for Cultural Formulation: a critical demonstration with American Indian children. J Am Acad Child Adolesc Psychiatry 36(9):1244–1251, 1997

Paralikar VP, Deshmukh A, Weiss MG: Qualitative analysis of Cultural Formulation Interview: findings and implications for revising the Outline for Cultural Formulation. Transcult Psychiatry 1363461518822407, 2019

Roberts SO, Gelman S: Multiracial children's and adults' categorizations of multiracial individuals. J Cogn Devel 18(1):1–15, 2017

Rousseau C, Guzder J: Supplementary module 9: School-Age Children and Adolescents, in DSM-5 Handbook on the Cultural Formulation Interview. Edited by Lewis-Fernández R, Aggarwal NK, Hinton L, Hinton DE, Kirmayer LJ. Arlington, VA, American Psychiatric Publishing, 2016, pp 156–164

Rousseau C, Measham T, Bathiche-Suidan M: DSM IV, culture and child psychiatry. J Can Acad Child Adolesc Psychiatry 17(2):69–75, 2008

Salwen ED, Underwood LA, Dy-Liacco GS, et al: Self-disclosure and spiritual well-being in pastors seeking professional psychological help. Pastoral Psychol 66(4):505–521, 2017

Schlabach S: The importance of family, race, and gender for multiracial adolescent well-being. Fam Relat 62(1):154–174, 2013

Schofield DW, Al-Mateen CS, Hardy LT: Management of a mental health crisis in an international high school exchange student: a case study. Adolescent Psychiatry 3(1):52–60, 2013

Shaffer TG, Steiner H: An application of DSM-IV's Outline for Cultural Formulation: understanding conduct disorder in Latino adolescents. Aggression and Violent Behavior 11(6):655–663, 2006

Stewart SM, Simmons A, Habibpour E: Treatment of culturally diverse children and adolescents with depression. J Child Adolesc Psychopharmacol 22(1):72–79, 2012

Sullivan M, Cogavin M, Bajor B, et al: Mental health counseling across cultures: African American Culture. 2020. Available at: https://mentalhealthacrosscultures.weebly.com/african-american-culture.html. Accessed May 18, 2020.

Takeuchi J: Treatment of a biracial child with schizophreniform disorder: cultural formulation. Cultur Divers Ethnic Minor Psychol 6(1):93–101, 2000

U.S. Department of Health and Human Services:Mental Health: Culture, Race, and Ethnicity—A Supplement to Mental Health: A Report of the Surgeon General. Rockville, MD, Center for Mental Health Services, Substance Abuse and Mental Health Services Administration, U.S. Department of Health and Human Services, 2001

Ward EC, Wiltshirt JC, Detry MA, et al: African American men and women's attitude toward mental illness, perceptions of stigma, and preferred coping behaviors. Nurs Res 62(3):185–194, 2013

Wesselman ED, Day M, Graziano WG, et al: Religious beliefs about mental illness influence social support preferences. J Prev Interv Community 43(3):165–174, 2015

Yilmaz HB, Dalkilic A, Al-Mateen C, et al: Culturally informed care of the Turkish-American child, adolescent, and family. Adolesc Psychiatry 3(1):39–45, 2013

CHAPTER 22
Advocacy
Debra E. Koss, M.D., DFAACAP, DFAPA

Clinical Vignette: Maribel and Dr. Walsh

Eight-year-old Maribel was sent to see Ms. Tan, the school guidance counselor, after falling asleep in class for a fifth day in a row. Ms. Tan looked up Maribel's record and learned that she had transferred into district 3 months ago and had missed 10 days of school since enrollment. She also noted that Maribel's primary language was Spanish and that she was assigned to an English as a second language teacher. When Ms. Tan met Maribel, she noticed that the student didn't make eye contact and appeared very sad and withdrawn. Ms. Tan contacted Mrs. Sandoval, Maribel's aunt and guardian, who reported that Maribel had been waking from nightmares most nights, seemed sad most days, and was not playing with her cousins. Ms. Tan received permission to refer Maribel to Dr. Walsh, the child and adolescent psychiatrist working with the school-based mental health program.

Dr. Walsh, fluent in Spanish, first engaged Maribel in drawing pictures of her family and over several appointments invited her to share stories about her family. He learned that Maribel was living with her aunt, uncle, and three cousins. Maribel shared that it had been a long time since she had seen her parents or sisters. The family tried to escape the violence in their hometown in Mexico, but her father and teenage brother were killed in the process. Her mother and two sisters made it safely to the United States, where they spent time in a shelter before Maribel and her sisters were sent to live with different relatives. Maribel had not heard from her mother or sisters since leaving the shelter. Maribel described memories of her hometown, nightmares about gangs and guns, and fears that she would never see her family again.

Dr. Walsh was all too familiar with this story. He had seen a dramatic increase in the number of refugee and immigrant children enrolled in district and was frequently called to evaluate these students. Like Maribel, these children presented with histories of exposure to violence in their countries of origin and then acute distress as their families tried to access asylum in the United States. Dr. Walsh was concerned about the rates of PTSD, depression, and anxiety among these students and found it difficult to access mental health resources for them.

The preceding chapters of this volume have presented the latest scientific research highlighting the unique mental health needs of children, adolescents, and families from diverse cultural backgrounds. This research serves to inform the delivery of culturally competent care. I now invite the reader to move beyond the impact of cultural competency on direct clinical care and next consider the impact on mental health advocacy and the development of health care policy.

In this chapter, I highlight the elements of effective advocacy and provide a road map for how psychiatrists can use their expertise to engage and inform legislators about issues that are critical to the mental health of children, adolescents, and families. I also highlight resources that are available to psychiatrists to support the development of effective advocacy skills. The chapter is directed toward physicians because that is my personal experience. However, the principles are applicable to all mental health professionals through their professional organizations. Case examples pertaining to diverse populations of children, adolescents, and families are included to demonstrate the importance of advocacy efforts for culturally diverse populations.

What Is Advocacy?

According to *Merriam-Webster*, advocacy is the act or process of supporting a cause or proposal. Advocacy generally involves using one's experience and expertise to inform and persuade public opinion as well as legislators' opinions. The role of physician as advocate has been supported by professional organizations. For instance, the American Medical Association states in its "Declaration of Professional Responsibility" that physicians must "advocate for social, economic, educational, and political changes that ameliorate suffering and contribute to human well-being" (American Medical Association 2020). Evidence of the impact of physician engagement in advocacy is seen in multiple domains. Much of the progress that has been made in reducing mental health stigma and improving access to quality evidence-based mental health care has occurred as a result of advocacy involving mental health professionals working jointly with members of the community.

Psychiatrists routinely advocate on behalf of patients within the clinical arena. For instance, psychiatrists may appeal the decision of a health plan denying initiation or maintenance of medication. Psychiatrists may also argue in favor of school-based accommodations for a student with mental illness. This type of advocacy is likely familiar to most psychiatrists, who are able to use the knowledge acquired during medical education and residency training to offer a rationale in support of treatment recommendations. These efforts are impactful and often lead to improving access to evidence-based treatments.

Psychiatrists also have an opportunity to serve as advocates within the legislative arena, upholding important issues that will serve to protect patients and advance the profession. For instance, psychiatrists may advocate in support of mental health parity, funds for research on trauma-informed care for children and adolescents, or reimbursement for depression screening in primary care settings for children and adolescents. These are just several examples of issues that have been addressed with legislative action at the federal and state levels. This type of advocacy may not be as familiar to psychiatrists. However, the same knowledge acquired in medical education and residency training can be used to offer a scientific frame for drafting legislation. In addition, clinical anecdotes can be used to illustrate the impact of legislation on patient outcomes. This type of advocacy may occur at the local, state, or federal level and ultimately can lead to substantive improvements in policy and design of health care delivery systems.

Why Should I Advocate?

"All politics is local." This statement, attributed to former Speaker of the House Tip O'Neill, highlights that legislators are motivated to hear from their constituents who have elected them to leadership. Conversations with constituents keep legislators in touch with priorities that exist within district. These conversations can also influence legislative agendas. In addition, legislators seek individuals who bring subject matter expertise to the table. Legislators are called on to review bills covering a broad range of issues. As a result, they seek professionals who can provide a comprehensive overview of these diverse issues. Constituents who serve as subject matter experts can be particularly valuable as a local resource and can provide recommendations for developing policy initiatives.

"If you're not at the table, you're on the menu." This phrase reminds advocates that it is critical to develop a constituent relationship with one's elected officials and then consistently communicate one's views. Legislators will meet with constituents arguing both sides of an issue and hear compelling reasons to vote both for and against a bill. Advocates must be "at the table" in order to effectively engage and persuade legislators.

Physicians are especially called on to serve as advocates on behalf of children and adolescents because this vulnerable patient population does not otherwise have a voice in the political or legislative process. Children and adolescents cannot vote. Self-advocacy is even less likely in marginalized minority children and adolescents, who experience significant rates of stigma and oppression.

The mental health needs of children and adolescents are of paramount importance, and mental health issues often begin early in life. In fact, half of all mental health problems begin by age 14 (National Institute of Mental Health 2020). Many of the identifiable risk factors for mental illness, including disadvantages in socioeconomic status and exposure to childhood adversity, disproportionately affect minority children. Furthermore, children from racial and ethnic minority groups experience greater disparities in access to and intensity of quality mental health care (Alegria et al. 2010). When left untreated, mental health disorders can lead to devastating consequences, including academic failure; high rates of substance use disorders; involvement in juvenile justice; and suicide, which is now the second leading cause of death in youth ages 10–24 years (National Institute of Mental Health 2019). Moving forward, as research uncovers the many barriers to care, advocacy efforts will need to include steps to promote innovative and culturally relevant solutions to overcome them.

Finally, physicians will recognize that advocacy is incredibly rewarding. Being a part of a process that creates policies that support the mental health of children and youth is impactful on a large scale and enables physicians to step outside their usual clinical roles and find solutions to public health crises. Policies developed through the legislative process with the input of physicians will lead to positive changes in health care delivery systems; improvement in physician workflow; and improved access to quality, evidence-based mental health treatment. Ultimately, the most important reason for getting involved in advocacy is that it works.

How Do I Get Started?

Psychiatrists may engage in advocacy as private citizens and individual constituents of their elected officials. However, engaging in advocacy as a member of a professional organization, such as the American Psychiatric Association (APA) or American Academy of Child and Adolescent Psychiatry (AACAP), can magnify one's voice and increase the impact of one's efforts. Participating through the APA provides access to a wealth of advocacy resources that can improve communication and help organize strategy. These resources include position statements, policy briefings, and talking points.

The APA Division of Government Relations provides advocacy strategy and direction for both federal and state advocacy initiatives. In Washington, D.C., APA leaders and government relations staff advise Congress, the White House, and other federal agencies on issues important to the practice of psychiatry and to patients and families. At the state level, government relations staff provide assistance to APA district branches and state associations on both legislative and regulatory matters.

All psychiatrists seeking opportunities to engage in mental health advocacy will benefit from advocacy training. The APA provides a variety of resources and opportunities for members to receive training. The APA Council on Advocacy and Government Relations, consisting of APA members from across the country with advocacy expertise, works collaboratively with the APA Division of Government Relations to develop advocacy training materials, including webinars, printed materials, and workshops at the APA Annual Meeting. Training materials cover essential advocacy communication skills as well as in-depth reviews of policies and related talking points.

The APA also provides members with opportunities to participate in advocacy efforts to relay APA's advocacy priorities to legislators. For example, APA members may be asked to respond to a call to action, which is an advocacy initiative organized by the Division of Government Relations in advance of a vote on a specific piece of legislation. APA members are able to access Engage, a program available on the APA website, to efficiently contact their elected officials and ask Congressional representatives to take specific action on a bill (American Psychiatric Association 2020). This action takes very little time but can have a significant impact, especially when APA members speak in one united voice. APA members are also encouraged to join the Congressional Advocacy Network (American Psychiatric Association 2020), APA's political grassroots network. APA members who join the network serve as key contacts for their members of Congress. In this role, psychiatrists maintain communication with their elected officials, serve as a resource on mental health issues, and represent the views of organized psychiatry. The APA provides psychiatrists with information on pending legislation and relevant policy resources so they can effectively advocate on the issues.

Opportunities to participate in advocacy also exist at the state level. APA members interested in advocacy can work with their district branch or state association. Psychiatrists can organize at the state level to advance an agenda of mental health priorities that are specific to local constituents through such actions as building a grassroots network of physician advocates or hosting a legislative day at their state capitol. The APA Division of Government Relations assists district branches and state associations with developing an effective advocacy campaign, including tracking health care legislation, serving as a clearing house for best lobbying practices, and offering strategic assistance and grassroots training.

TABLE 22–1.   Steps for an effective advocacy campaign

1. Define the issue
2. Develop an advocacy toolkit
3. Identify allies and opponents
4. Identify legislative champions
5. Identify the best time to communicate your message
6. Remain steadfast in your efforts
7. Be prepared to compromise

The AACAP Department of Government Affairs provides similar resources for members interested in federal and state advocacy. At the federal level, AACAP members are able to access the Legislative Action Center, a program available on the AACAP website, which allows members to contact their members of Congress and ask them to take action on specific bills (American Academy of Child and Adolescent Psychiatry 2020b). In addition, AACAP members are invited to participate in the annual Legislative Conference. This is an opportunity for members to partner with family advocates and meet with legislators on Capitol Hill to raise awareness about children's mental health and offer support for legislation that will improve access to quality evidence-based care.

At the state level, AACAP invites members to join the Advocacy Liaison Network (American Academy of Child and Adolescent Psychiatry 2020a). This group of member advocates participates in monthly phone calls with AACAP Government Affairs staff in which they receive advocacy training and policy briefings on issues specific to children's mental health. Members of the network also learn about strategies to effectively organize grassroots advocacy campaigns at the state level with members of their AACAP regional organizations.

What Are the Elements of an Effective Advocacy Campaign?

Although there is no one path that guarantees the success of all advocacy initiatives, taking certain steps can contribute to effective advocacy campaigns (Table 22–1).

An effective advocacy plan begins with a clear and succinct description of the issue. This should include a brief synopsis of background information that defines the problem as well as a brief synopsis of the data that support the solution. Be careful to avoid using medical jargon or acronyms. Next, develop an advocacy toolkit that is built on policy resources and scholarly articles. Summarize this information in easy-to-read fact sheets that can be used as a resource when advocating with legislators. These fact sheets can also be used as leave-behind materials for legislators to help them remember you and your issue. When developing fact sheets, remember that a picture is worth a thousand words. A map reflecting the distribution of mental health professionals in your state will call attention to critical workforce shortages more clearly than will a list of statistics.

As you develop your advocacy toolkit, identify other stakeholders who will serve as allies in your advocacy campaign. Develop a temporary alliance of organizations that will work together toward a common goal. Having such an alliance will reflect consensus, allow for sharing of resources, and support increased access to legislators. Simply stated, there is strength in numbers. In addition to allies, it is helpful to identify opponents and their concerns about your issues. When working with opponents, advocates should be prepared either to refute their concerns or to consider compromise.

Efforts to advocate for specific legislative solutions will require *champions*, elected officials interested in sponsoring or cosponsoring pieces of legislation. This is not a time for partisan politics. In fact, mental health advocacy is built on the premise that mental health is a bipartisan issue. When seeking legislative champions, it can be particularly powerful to identify sponsors from both sides of the aisle to demonstrate bipartisan support.

A critical component of advocacy strategy involves timing: identifying the best time and how often to deliver your message to legislators in order to have maximum impact. Lobbyists can be instrumental in selecting the best time to act because they are aware of the legislative calendar and political current events. Communicating with legislators early in a session may be the most effective time to influence the writing of a bill. Initiating an advocacy campaign as a Hail Mary pass in the final hours of the game is rarely effective. Communicating often will ensure that your message is heard. Communicating too often may cause legislators to ignore your calls or requests for meeting. Outreach to legislators should provide new and meaningful updates.

Finally, advocates must be steadfast in their efforts. Advocacy requires patience and persistence. Advocacy is often compared to a marathon rather than a sprint. Congress begins a new session every 2 years, and state legislative sessions turn over every year or two. This results in the introduction of new elected officials and new political agendas on a routine basis. It takes time to build new constituent relationships, educate lawmakers on the issues, get support for legislation, and ultimately see a bill become law. Change takes time; commitment to the process is necessary. Furthermore, compromise is often required in order to advance an issue (Ptakowski 2010). Developing an advocacy plan built on agility and short-term goals can lead to consensus and conclusive policy change.

Building a Constituent Relationship

In order to be effective in advocacy, you need to first build a relationship with your elected official. This can occur with federal legislators but may require additional effort. Members of Congress have busy schedules and often are unable to take face-to-face meetings when they are in Washington, D.C. Quite often, meetings on Capitol Hill will actually be assigned to the legislator's staff. You should not be offended if this happens; staff assigned to health care policy are quite knowledgeable on the issues and often are influential in identifying priorities for the legislator. Meeting with one's member of Congress may be easier to accomplish when the legislator is visiting his or her home district. Consider attending a town hall meeting, participating in a local fundraising event, or going to a state fair.

Building a constituent relationship directly with one's state legislator is generally easier to accomplish. State legislators are more approachable, more often in district, and more likely to have time for face-to-face meetings. This can begin simply with a phone call or e-mail, offering to meet to discuss mental health services in district. When planning a face-to-face meeting, contact the legislator's office, speak with the scheduler, and ask for a convenient time. Be patient but persistent; anticipate that it may take several attempts to schedule an appointment. Prepare for the meeting by researching both the issue and your legislator. Learn about the lawmaker's position on key health care issues and identify any committee appointments, especially appointments to committees that have oversight of mental health legislation. Be prepared to thank the legislator for any support of pro-mental health legislation.

Consider beginning a conversation as follows:

> Hello Senator Rivera. My name is Dr. Blake. I am a physician specializing in child and adolescent psychiatry. I live in district, and I'm the Medical Director of Psychiatric Emergency Services at Community Hospital. I attended a recent town hall meeting where you spoke about your interest in addressing the increase in suicide among children and teens. Thank you for your interest in addressing this public health crisis. I'm reaching out today to let you know that we've seen a recent increase in LGBTQ+ teens presenting to our local emergency department with thoughts of suicide. I'd like to share some examples of quality evidence-based treatments for this group of teens and see if we can work together to bring these services to our community.

Face-to-face meetings can take place in the legislator's office. Alternatively, you may invite a legislator to a meeting at your health care facility to see firsthand the importance of having access to developmentally and culturally appropriate services in district. Over time, you can follow up with your elected official and offer updates on local mental health issues, providing factual information such as a recently published scholarly article on adolescent depression and suicide.

Ultimately, you can reach out to your legislator asking for his or her support of a particular bill. This can occur without the previously described efforts to build a constituent relationship. However, the "ask" to support or oppose a bill is generally much more impactful when delivered within the context of a constituent relationship. Consider the following example:

> Hello Senator Rivera. This is Dr. Blake, the psychiatrist from Community Hospital. Thank you for taking the time to meet with me last month to discuss the health care needs of LGBTQ+ teens in our community. I'm reaching out today because I learned that Bill 123 was introduced; this bill would ban conversion therapy for youth questioning their sexuality. I'm reaching out to ask you to vote in support of this bill. I'd like to provide you with several resources highlighting the harmful effects of conversion therapy, including a 2018 Position Statement from the American Psychiatric Association. May we set up a time to meet?

Referring to the APA position statement (American Psychiatric Association 2018a) structures the conversation by providing clear talking points and adds credibility to your recommendation because it reflects the collective wisdom and experience of a national professional organization. However, the ask to support the bill can be made more compelling by sharing a clinical anecdote. Presenting the legislator with a deidentified story that reflects the consequences of treatments that discriminate against LGBTQ+ adolescents will more directly engage the legislator and leave a memorable imprint of the importance of the issue. After the meeting, be sure to send a thank you message summarizing your talking points and providing your contact information.

TABLE 22–2. Preparing your elevator speech

1. Identify yourself as a constituent and a physician with a specialty in psychiatry
2. Clearly identify the issue, including the bill number
3. Provide two or three reasons for your position
4. Include data to highlight scientific evidence, but use data judiciously
5. Tell a story—make it personal, local, and memorable
6. Conclude with the "ask"—ask the legislator to support or oppose the bill

Preparing Your Elevator Speech

Legislators are frequently running between committee hearings and constituent meetings. They may be available for brief in-person meetings, but if a bill is quickly coming up for review, your message may need to be delivered by e-mail through the legislator's website or by telephone to the legislator's staff. Therefore, as an advocate, you need to be prepared to describe and give your position on an issue in 5 minutes or less. This is often referred to as an elevator speech. Following the simple steps in Table 22–2 will help you provide a cohesive structure to your presentation.

Avoid becoming confrontational or personal. A conversation that is confrontational in nature is never productive. Instead, use your elevator speech to impart new information, and you may be able to educate the legislator about the issue even if he or she does not ultimately agree with your position. You may be able to advance the issue without receiving support for all of the elements of the initial bill. Finally, you will want to preserve a good working relationship with your elected official because you likely will meet again to discuss other legislation.

Media Advocacy

Media advocacy can be a powerful way to persuade public opinion, engage allies in advocacy efforts, and inform legislators of priority issues (Ptakowski 2010). Psychiatrists may write letters to the editor or work with journalists to write an editorial. An opinion piece about a mental health bill that is published just before an upcoming committee hearing can provide factual information on the issues, correct myths or misconceptions, and outline recommendations for legislative action. Local television and radio stations will frequently assign reporters to cover health topics or legislative action from the state capitol. Building a working relationship with these reporters and offering to serve as a subject matter expert can also be an effective way to inform and persuade. Increasingly, social media serves as an effective and efficient way to engage a diverse audience, including other stakeholders and legislators. Professional organizations are turning to platforms such as Twitter and Facebook to advance advocacy messaging. Psychiatrists engaged in advocacy may find it useful to establish professional social media accounts to be able to communicate with wider audiences engaged in mental health advocacy.

Advocacy in the Wake of COVID-19

The disproportionate impact of the novel coronavirus SARS-CoV-2 (COVID-19) on minority populations has raised awareness regarding the impact of long-standing patterns of structural racism on health outcomes and equitable access to health care. In addition to general concerns regarding COVID-19, families are experiencing challenges related to the unique needs of children and adolescents. These concerns include access to broadband communication technologies for remote learning, access to special education and school-based mental health services, opportunities for social-emotional learning, and food insecurities. As psychiatrists working with vulnerable children and adolescents, we must inform policy makers and elected officials about the impact of COVID-19 on children and offer recommendations for policies that will minimize health disparities. Although in-person meetings with decision makers have been suspended in response to social distancing and risk mitigation procedures, opportunities for advocacy are plentiful. Legislators are hosting virtual town hall meetings, organizing public health briefings, and scheduling virtual meetings with constituents. Legislative meetings, including committee hearings, are also being held virtually. Members of the scientific and health care communities are especially being called on to give presentations and offer expert testimony. I encourage psychiatrists to seek out these opportunities for virtual meetings in order to persist in advocacy efforts.

Call for Coalitions

As the cultural landscape in the United States continues to diversify and data emerge regarding the health disparities experienced by marginalized and minoritized communities, the need for mental health advocacy and policy reform comes into focus. There is a tremendous amount of work to be done to ensure a strong knowledge base in the area of culturally competent health care systems and public health policies focused on reducing and ultimately eliminating health disparities. Multiple voices are needed in order to effectively communicate with legislators and policy makers. In order to be effective, stakeholders must collaborate and agree to share scientific data, organize advocacy initiatives, and leverage political capital. Physicians, mental health professionals, educators, and other members of child-serving systems all play an important role in advocacy coalitions. Our children are our future, and no greater investment can be made than to ensure their right to health.

Clinical Vignette *(Continued)*

Dr. Walsh, a member of the APA, decided to call his district branch and ask for assistance. He reported on the increase in refugee and immigrant children in his community and the challenges associated with accessing care for these children. His district branch put him in touch with several organizations that had developed resources for psychiatrists and other clinicians working with this vulnerable patient population.

His district branch also let Dr. Walsh know that they were attempting to set up a meeting with a state legislator who had publicly announced her concern about the separation of immigrant children and families. The district branch was working with the APA and other professional organizations to advocate for reform in immigration policies. One of the stated goals included improving access to "trauma-informed, culturally, linguistically, developmentally and structurally competent qualified health professionals" as described in the 2018 APA position statement "Separation of Immigrant Children and Families" (American Psychiatric Association 2018b). Dr. Walsh indicated that he had no experience speaking with legislators or advocating for policy reform. He was referred to a colleague who was chairing the district branch's Council on Legislation who reassured him that no prior experience was required. Dr. Walsh learned that his clinical experience working in the school district would serve as an essential component of the council's advocacy plan. He also learned that he could receive training and mentorship in basic advocacy skills prior to the meeting. Dr. Walsh immediately thought of all the children under his care and knew that he would join this meeting. He had stories to share. His voice mattered.

Self-Assessment Questions

1. Which of the following is true regarding the role of physician as advocate?

    A. It exists only within the clinical arena.
    B. It is generally reserved only for physicians seeking political office.
    C. It has been supported by professional organizations such as the American Medical Association.
    D. It is time-consuming and generally ineffective.

2. Which of the following is *not* considered an element of an effective advocacy campaign?

    A. Identifying allies and opponents.
    B. Identifying legislative champions.
    C. Remaining steadfast in your efforts.
    D. Never compromising.

3. Which of the following statements is true regarding media advocacy?

    A. Physicians should avoid using social media as part of an advocacy campaign.
    B. Media advocacy is an effective way to persuade public opinion and engage allies in advocacy efforts.
    C. Media advocacy is not an effective way to inform legislators.
    D. Physicians should avoid speaking with journalists.

Answers

1. C
2. D
3. B

References

Alegria MA, Vallas M, Pumariega A: Racial and ethnic disparities in pediatric mental health. Child Adolesc Psychiatr Clin N Am 19(4):759–774, 2010

American Academy of Child and Adolescent Psychiatry: How to be an advocate. Washington, DC, American Academy of Child and Adolescent Psychiatry, 2020a. Available at: www.aacap.org/AACAP/Advocacy/How_to_Be_an_Advocate/Home.aspx. Accessed May 19, 2020.

American Academy of Child and Adolescent Psychiatry: Legislative Action Center. Washington, DC, American Academy of Child and Adolescent Psychiatry, 2020b. Available at: www.aacap.org/AACAP/Advocacy/Action_Center/Home.aspx. Accessed May 19, 2020.

American Medical Association: AMA Declaration of Professional Responsibility: medicine's social contract with humanity, Chicago, IL, American Medical Association, 2020. Available at: www.ama-assn.org/delivering-care/public-health/ama-declaration-professional-responsibility#:~:text=Adopted_by_the_AMA_House.trust_in_the_healing_profession. Accessed: August 13, 2020.

American Psychiatric Association: Position statement on conversion therapy and LGBTQ patients. Washington, DC, American Psychiatric Association, 2018a. Available at: www.psychiatry.org/File%20Library/About-APA/Organization-Documents-Policies/Policies/Position-Conversion-Therapy.pdf. Accessed October 5, 2019.

American Psychiatric Association: Separation of immigrant children and families. Washington, DC, American Psychiatric Association, 2018b. Available at: www.psychiatry.org/File%20Library/About-APA/Organization-Documents-Policies/Policies/Position-Separation-of-Immigrant-Children-and-Families.pdf. Accessed October 5, 2019.

American Psychiatric Association: APA Advocacy (including Congressional Advocacy Network). Washington, DC, American Psychiatric Association, 2020. Available at: www.psychiatry.org/psychiatrists/advocacy. Accessed May 19, 2020.

National Institute of Mental Health: Suicide. Bethesda, MD, National Institute of Mental Health, April 2019. Available at: www.nimh.nih.gov/health/statistics/suicide/index.shtml. Accessed September 12, 2019.

National Institute of Mental Health: NIMH-funded National Comorbidity Survey Replication (NCS-R) study: mental illness exacts heavy toll, beginning in youth. Bethesda, MD, National Institute of Mental Health, 2020. Available at: www.nimh.nih.gov/health/topics/ncsr-study/nimh-funded-national-comorbidity-survey-replication-ncs-r-study-mental-illness-exacts-heavy-toll-beginning-in-youth.shtml. Accessed May 19, 2020.

Ptakowski KK: Advocating for children with mental illnesses. Child Adolesc Psychiatr Clin N Am 19(1):131–138, 2010

Glossary

Term	Definition	Reference
Acculturation	Multidimensional, continuous, and dynamic process through which immigrants retain aspects of their native culture while simultaneously adopting the new society's culture, foreign attitudes, norms, values, and behaviors. Acculturation is influenced by generational differences: with each generation, there will be a greater degree of acculturation.	Bornstein 2017
Acculturative family distancing	Psychological distancing that occurs among family members due to different degrees of acculturation between parents and youth	Hwang et al. 2010
Acculturative stress	Perceived (psychological, emotional, or health) stress in relation to the process of adapting to a different community	Rothe et al. 2010
Advocacy	The act or process of supporting a cause or proposal	www.merriam-webster.com/dictionary/advocacy
Assimilation	Process in which a minority group or culture comes to resemble a dominant group or assume the values, behaviors, and beliefs of another group	
Assortativity	The propensity of similar people to be socially connected with one another more often than with their dissimilar counterparts	Child Welfare Information Gateway 2006, 2019; Lee et al. 2015

Term	Definition	Reference
Asylum seeker	An individual who is asking for international protection. In countries with individualized procedures, an asylum seeker is someone whose claim has not yet been finally decided on by the country in which the claim is submitted. Not every asylum seeker will ultimately be recognized as a refugee, but every refugee is initially an asylum seeker.	United Nations High Commissioner for Refugees 2005
Black Diaspora	The dispersion of people of African descent, language, and culture from their country of origin to various parts of the world	www.merriam-webster.com/dictionary/diaspora
Child protective services (CPS)	The system responsible for assessing suspected cases of abuse and neglect, assisting families with identifying goals of intervention, providing in-home services for families, coordinating community-based services for families, and facilitating placement of children who are removed from their home	Child Welfare Information Gateway 2006, 2019; Lee et al. 2015
Child welfare system	Provides federally mandated services to ensure safety and well-beings and strengthen the stability of families. This involves coordination of services among many organizations, including state and local social services agencies, community-based organizations, and private agencies.	Child Welfare Information Gateway 2006, 2019; Lee et al. 2015
Child welfare worker (or child protective services worker)	Professional responsible for responding to reports of neglect or abuse, determining if reports are substantiated, determining safety of current living situations, making arrangements for out-of-home placement when necessary, and supporting families throughout legal processes and engagement in social services, as needed	Child Welfare Information Gateway 2006, 2019; Lee et al. 2015
Chinese Exclusion Act of 1882	A federal law signed by President Chester Arthur in 1882 that prohibited all immigration of Chinese laborers for 10 years and deemed Chinese individuals ineligible for naturalization. The act was renewed in 1892 for another 10 years. It was the first law implemented to prevent all members of a specific ethnic or national group from immigrating.	National Archives and Records Administration 1989
Cultural competence	Ability of systems to provide care to patients with diverse values, beliefs, and behaviors, including tailoring delivery to meet patients' social, cultural, and linguistic needs	Cross et al. 1989

Term	Definition	Reference
Cultural humility	"Ability to maintain an interpersonal stance that is other-oriented (or open to the other) in relation to aspects of cultural identity that are most important to the [person]." This is a lifelong process of self-reflection and self-critique whereby the individual learns about another's culture after an examination of her or his own beliefs and cultural identities.	Hook et al. 2013, p. 2
Cultural mistrust	The tendency to distrust white individuals and the majority group culture in the United States because of direct and vicarious exposure to racism	Dean et al. 2018
Cultural psychiatry	The study and treatment of mental illness in individuals, guided by thoughtful consideration and integration of race, ethnicity, religion, and cultural backgrounds	Caracci and Mezzich 2001
Culture	"[D]istinctive patterns of norms, ideas, values, conventions, behaviors, and symbolic representations about life that are commonly held by a collection of people, persist over time, guide and regulate daily living, and constitute valued competencies that are communicated to new members of the group"	Bornstein 2013, p. 259
Cyberbullying	Bullying tactics that occur using social media and/or digital devices	
Cytochrome p450 enzymes	A group of enzymes involved in drug metabolism and found in high levels in the liver	www.cancer.gov/publications/dictionaries/cancer-terms/def/cytochrome-p450-enzyme-system
Deadname	The birth name of someone who has changed their name. The term is especially used in the LGBTQ+ community by people who are transgender and elect to go by their chosen name instead of their given name.	www.merriam-webster.com/dictionary/deadname
Digital immigrant	Term coined by Marc Prensky to refer to an individual who was not born during the digital age or was not exposed to digital technology at an early age	
Digital media	Media in which information is transmitted via the Internet through devices such as computers, tablets, gaming systems, and smartphones	

Term	Definition	Reference
Digital native	Term coined by Marc Prensky to refer to an individual who was either born during the digital age or was exposed to this form of technology at an early age. These individuals are thought to have a higher level of comfort and fluid knowledge of digital technology (computers, Internet, and social media).	
Emerging adult	Term first published in 2000 by psychologist Jeffrey Jensen Arnett to describe a discrete normal developmental phase for ages 18–25 years. The minimum age of maturity (18 vs. 21 years) for use of potentially dependence-forming substances, such as alcohol, tobacco, and cannabis, has been debated in the public health sector.	Chan et al. 2019
Ethnicity	A term that describes shared culture and national origin (e.g., Hispanic, non-Hispanic, Chinese); a large group of people who have the same national, racial, or cultural origins; or the state of belonging to such a group	https://dictionary.cambridge .org/us/dictionary/english/ ethnicity
Executive Order 9066	Presidential executive order issued in 1942 by Franklin D. Roosevelt 10 weeks after the attack on Pearl Harbor. It authorized the military to exclude "any or all persons" from any part of the United States designated as a "military area." Even though the order did not specify any group or location, the order led the way for the incarceration of Japanese Americans, German Americans, and Italian Americans in U.S. concentration camps. The order was rescinded in 1976 by President Gerald Ford.	National Archives and Records Administration 1942
Faith	An integral, centering process more expansive than religious belief yet more tangible and directive than spirituality alone. It undergirds formation of beliefs, values, and meanings that foster coherence of competing priorities, connecting these abstract concepts to shared trusts and loyalties to others and to local and global religious communities. It may connect personal and communal ties to a deity or other transcendent frames of reference. Faith facilitates dealing with concrete challenges in life, illness, suffering, and death and ties these experiences to what provides ultimate meaning in life.	Fowler and Dell 2004; Josephson and Dell 2004

Term	Definition	Reference
Familismo	Latinx cultural concept in which a family's values are held in higher esteem than the values of the individual members of the family	
Family	A group of people (often of multiple generations) who live together and are committed to each other and share their lives. They can be biologically related or together through adoption, surrogacy, marriage (stepfamilies), or refugee status, or as a "chosen" family.	Definition by Neha Sharma, D.O., and John Sargent, M.D. (authors of Chapter 9, "Diverse Families and Family Treatment")
Fictive kin	Individuals who are unrelated by either birth or marriage but have an emotionally significant relationship with each other that takes on the characteristics of a family relationship	
Filial piety	Reverence for parents considered in Chinese ethics the prime virtue and the basis of all right human relations. It is a core virtue outlined in the traditional texts of the Chinese philosopher Confucius.	www.merriam-webster.com/dictionary/filialpiety
First generation	Individuals who are foreign born; also known as immigrants	Kim et al. 2018
Forcibly displaced person	An individuals who is forced to move, within or across borders, because of armed conflict, persecution, terrorism, human rights violations and abuses, violence, the adverse effects of climate change, natural disasters, development projects, or a combination of these factors	United Nations Human Rights Office of the High Commissioner 2019
Foster care	Temporary living arrangement for children who are removed from their home setting because of concerns about their well-being. Foster care may include living with relatives or unrelated foster parents or in a group home; living in a residential care facility or emergency shelter; or supervised independent living.	Child Welfare Information Gateway 2006, 2019; Lee et al. 2015
Gentlemen's Agreement of 1907	Informal agreement between the United States and Japan in which Japan agreed not to issue passports to emigrants to the United States, except to certain categories of business and professional men. In return, U.S. President Theodore Roosevelt agreed to urge the city of San Francisco to rescind an order by which children of Japanese parents were segregated from white students in the schools.	Encyclopædia Britannica 2020

Term	Definition	Reference
Guardianship	Legal commitment to care for a child, including financial, health, and educational needs, until age 18 without formal adoption. This does not require termination of parental rights.	Child Welfare Information Gateway 2006, 2019; Lee et al. 2015
Hispanic	Refers to a common language and describes those whose ancestry comes from Spain or Spanish-speaking countries	
Honoring Children Mending the Circle (HCMC)	Culturally enhanced treatment protocols of trauma-focused cognitive-behavioral therapy (TF-CBT) developed to treat trauma in children ages 3–18. HCMC is a treatment for American Indian and Alaskan Native children and their families. TF-CBT is an evidence-based treatment for children and adolescents impacted by trauma and their parents or caregivers. It is a components-based treatment model that incorporates trauma-sensitive interventions with cognitive-behavioral, family, and humanistic principles and techniques. TF-CBT has proved successful with children and adolescents who have significant emotional problems (e.g., symptoms of PTSD, fear, anxiety, or depression) related to traumatic life events. It can be used with children and adolescents who have experienced a single trauma or multiple traumas in their lives.	www.icctc.org/ HC%20MC%20NICWA%20 2007-no%20pics.pdf
Immigration Act of 1917	A federal legislation (also known as the Literacy Act or Asiatic Barred Zone Act) that prohibited immigration from any country that was in or adjacent to Asia but "not owned by the U.S." The ban was the first to target a specific geographical region, expanding on the Chinese Exclusion Act of 1882. The act also required all immigrants older than age 16 to pass a literacy test and expanded an existing list of "undesirables" to include persons with epilepsy, alcoholics, political radicals, anarchists, criminals, people with contagious diseases or mental or physical disabilities, and the poor.	Weisberger 2017

Term	Definition	Reference
Immigration and Nationality Act of 1965	A federal legislation passed by Congress and signed into law by President Lyndon B. Johnson in 1965 to end the practice of basing immigration entry into the United States on the individual's birthplace. Also known as the Hart-Celler Act, it eliminated national origin, race, and ancestry as bases for barring immigration and opened pathways for groups such as southern and eastern Europeans, the Irish, and Asians to enter the United States for the first time since the 1920s.	Chin 2015
Infant mental health	The developing capacity of the child from birth to age 5 years to form close and secure adult and peer relationships; to experience, manage, and express a full range of emotions; and to explore the environment and learn in the context of family, community, and culture	Clinton et al. 2016
Intersectionality	"The complex, cumulative way in which the effects of multiple forms of discrimination (such as racism, sexism, and classism) combine, overlap, or intersect especially in the experiences of marginalized individuals or groups" (www.merriam-webster.com/dictionary/intersectionality). In 1989, Professor Kimberlé Crenshaw introduced the theory of intersectionality, the idea that when it comes to thinking about how inequalities persist, such categories as gender, race, and class are best understood as overlapping and mutually constitutive rather than isolated and distinct.	www.merriam-webster.com/dictionary/intersectionality
Involuntary transnational	An individual with one parent who lacks legal status and has been deported back to the country of origin	Kim et al. 2018
Kinship care	Living situation in which children within the child welfare system are placed with relatives when they cannot safely live with biological parents	Child Welfare Information Gateway 2006, 2019; Lee et al. 2015
Latinx	Gender-neutral alternative term for Latino or Latina. The term itself refers to geography, specifically describing individuals of Latin American origin.	www.merriam-webster.com/dictionary/Latinx#h1
Media	Channel or system of communication, information, or entertainment	www.merriam-webster.com/dictionary/media

Term	Definition	Reference
Microassaults	Explicit, conscious racial or derogatory actions that are intended to hurt (e.g., intentionally serving a white person before a person of color or deliberatly referring to an Asian person as "Oriental"). Most akin to conventional racism.	Nadal 2012; Sue et al. 2007
Microinsults	"Communications that convey rudeness and insensitivities and demean a person's racial heritage or identity" (Sue et al. 2007, p. 274). They may also be described as subtle snubs that convey to the person of color a hidden, insulting message of which the perpetrator often is unaware. Examples include a white teacher not calling on students of color in the classroom or a white employer avoiding eye contact with an employee of color.	Nadal 2012; Sue et al. 2007
Microinvalidation	"Communications that exclude, negate, or nullify the psychological thoughts, feelings, or experiential reality of a person of color" (Sue et al. 2007, p. 274). Examples include complimenting Asian Americans or Latinx individuals born and raised in the United States for speaking good English or repeatedly asking them where they were born. Other examples include telling a person of color "I don't see color."	Nadal 2012; Sue et al. 2007
Migrant	Any person who is moving or has moved across an international border or within a state away from his or her habitual place of residence, regardless of 1) the person's legal status, 2) whether the movement is voluntary or involuntary, 3) what the causes for the movement are, and 4) what the length of the stay is	International Organization for Migration 2020
Minority groups	Groups of people within society who lack power or representation relative to other groups within that society. Minorities are people with distinct characteristics that distinguish them from the majority with whom they are associated. They usually have less power and inferior status and often suffer discrimination.	Layton-Henry 2001

Term	Definition	Reference
Minority stress model	Theoretical framework that identifies negative societal stressors that lead to negative physical and mental health via layered cognitive, affective, interpersonal, and physiological responses. This model has been linked and studied within various cultural domains. Link and Phelan (2001) explained this phenomenon concisely through the lens of stigmatization, noting that diverse youth become "labeled" persons experiencing disapproval, rejection, exclusion, and discrimination, resulting in loss of power, status, and eventually health because of the development of affective disorders, substance use disorders, and suicidality in response to this isolation. Meyer (2003), utilizing stigma research, developed the minority stress theory in relation to these negative experiences in LGBTQ+ youth and adults, noting these experiences to be unique, chronic, and socially based.	Link and Phelan 2001; Meyer 2003
Mixed-status families	Families with some members who are undocumented and other members who have legal status	Kim et al. 2018
Parenting practices	Specific behaviors that parents use to socialize their children	Darling and Steinberg 1993
Perceived discrimination	The belief that one is being treated poorly and/or unfairly on the basis of race, ethnicity, gender, age, religion, physical appearance, sexual orientation, or other characteristics	Dean et al. 2018
Permanency	The establishment of a legally permanent home setting for children within the child welfare system. Permanent home may be with biological family, adoptive family, legal guardians, or relatives who obtain legal custody.	Child Welfare Information Gateway 2006, 2019; Lee et al. 2015
Personalismo	Latinx cultural concept that places great emphasis on personal relationships	

Term	Definition	Reference
Public Law 280	Public Law 83-280 (commonly referred to as Public Law 280 or PL-280), was originally enacted in 1953 and did two things to alter the usual allocation of criminal jurisdiction in Indian country. First, on the reservations to which it applied, it took away the federal government's authority to prosecute Indian country crimes on the basis of 18 USC 1152 (the Indian Country General Crimes Act) and 18 USC 1153 (the Major Crimes Act). Second, it authorized the states of Alaska, California, Minnesota, Nebraska, Oregon, and Wisconsin to prosecute most crimes that occurred in Indian country. Exceptions were set forth for a few topic areas and on a few reservations, but the main result of Public Law 280 is that for most reservations in the six named states, federal criminal jurisdiction became extremely limited, whereas state jurisdiction was greatly expanded.	www.justice.gov/usao-mn/ Public-Law%2083-280
Race	How one self-identifies with one or more social groups (e.g., white, Black or African American, Asian, American Indian or Alaskan Native, Native Hawaiian or other Pacific Islander); a family, tribe, people, or nation belonging to the same stock; a class or kind of people unified by shared interests, habits, or characteristics; a category of humankind that shares certain distinctive physical traits	www.merriam-webster.com/ dictionary/race
Refugee	"Any person who owing to well-founded fear of being persecuted for reasons of race, religion, nationality, membership of a particular social group or political opinion, is outside the country of his nationality and is unable or, owing to such fear, is unwilling to avail himself of the protection of that country; or who, not having a nationality and being outside the country of his former habitual residence as a result of such events, is unable or, owing to such fear, is unwilling to return to it."	United Nations High Commissioner for Refugees 1991, p, 14
Salience	Being able focus on what is important, notice what is different, or attend to what is relevant	
Second generation	Individuals who are born in the United States and have at least one foreign-born parent	Kim et al. 2018

Term	Definition	Reference
Sexual and gender minority	Having a sexual orientation and gender identity that differ from that of the mainstream population. Lesbians, gay men, bisexual men and women, and individuals who are gender fluid are defined according to their sexual orientation, sexual attraction, behavior, identity, or some combination of these dimensions. They share the fact that their sexual orientation is not exclusively heterosexual. Transgender people are defined according to their gender identity and presentation. This group encompasses individuals whose gender identity differs from the sex originally assigned to them at birth or whose gender expression varies significantly from what is traditionally associated with or typical for that sex, as well as other individuals who vary from or reject traditional cultural conceptualizations of gender in terms of the male-female dichotomy.	Institute of Medicine (U.S.) Committee on Lesbian, Gay, Bisexual, and Transgender Health Issues and Research Gaps and Opportunities 2011
Social media	Subset of digital media through which users engage in online communities to share content such as information, ideas, images, videos, and personal messages. This term is sometimes used interchangeably with the term *social networking*, although the latter is a form of the former.	
Social media influencer	A media user with a mass following or specific demographic group or audience who uses his or her influence or popularity to promote a specific lifestyle or product	
Social media platform	Means by which a specific type of media content is created, gathered, shared, and stored. Platform styles include video blogging, microblogging, video sharing, and social networking. Examples of platforms include Facebook, LinkedIn, Twitter, YouTube, Reddit, Pinterest, Instagram, Snapchat, and TikTok.	
Syndemic	"The synergistic nature of the health and social problems facing the poor and underserved"	Singer and Snipes 1992, p. 225
System transference	Positive or negative emotions a patient may experience toward the use of telecare as he or she navigates bureaucratic or organizational systems of care, teledelivery experiences, technology use, and distance care	Shore et al. 2006

Term	Definition	Reference
The Way	A translation of the Chinese word Tao or Dao, meaning path or road. In a metaphorical sense, it is the natural order of the universe that keeps life in balance and in order and a practice of living to achieve attainment and spiritual enlightenment.	https://en.wikipedia.org/wiki/Tao
Traditional Chinese medicine	A system of treatments and therapies that have been around for more than 2,500 years embracing the concepts of balance, yin and yang, and the Five Phases Theory. Practices that fall under this category include acupuncture, exercise (*qigong*), massage (*tui na*), and herbal medicine.	National Center for Complementary and Integrative Health 2020
Transitional-age youth	A term that originated with the Substance Abuse and Mental Health Services Administration (SAMHSA) to refer to youth exiting foster care by "aging out." There was an early awareness of the lack of developmentally appropriate services and support, and since 1995, SAMHSA grants have encouraged projects serving youth ages 16–25 years at risk of serious mental health conditions.	Chan et al. 2019
Transnational families	Families whose members maintain relationships across one or more countries	
Unaccompanied minor	Children who are not in the company of parents or another adult caregiver	United Nations High Commissioner for Refugees 2005
Unauthorized immigrant	A foreign national residing in a country without legal authorization. These individuals are crucial to the economic prosperity of the United States because of their work in many low-paying positions.	

References

Bornstein MH: Parenting and child mental health: a cross-cultural perspective. World Psychiatry 12(3):258–265, 2013

Bornstein MH: The specificity principle in acculturation science. Perspect Psychol Sci 12(1):3–45, 2017

Caracci G, Mezzich JE: Culture and urban mental health. Psychiatr Clin North Am 24(3):581–593, 2001

Chan V, Moore J, Derenne J, et al: Transitional age youth and college mental health. Child Adolesc Psychiatr Clin N Am 28(3):363–375, 2019

Child Welfare Information Gateway: Child Neglect: A Guide for Prevention, Assessment, and Intervention. Washington, DC, Children's Bureau, U.S. Department of Health and Human Services, 2006

Child Welfare Information Gateway: Kinship Guardianship as a Permanency Option. Washington, DC, Children's Bureau, U.S. Department of Health and Human Services, 2019

Chin G: Were the Immigration and Nationality Act Amendments of 1965 antiracist?, in The Immigration and Nationality Act of 1965: Legislating a New America. Edited by Chin G, Cuison Villazor R. Cambridge, MA, Cambridge University Press, 2015, pp 11–59

Clinton J, Feller A, Williams R: The importance of infant mental health. Paediatr Child Health 21(5):239–241, 2016

Cross TL, Bazron BJ, Dennis KW, Isaacs MR: Promoting Cultural Competence and Cultural Diversity in Early Intervention and Early Childhood Settings. Washington, DC, National Center for Cultural Competence, Georgetown University, 1989

Darling N, Steinberg L: Parenting style as context: an integrative model. Psychol Bull 113(3), 487–496, 1993

Dean KE, Long AC, Matthews RA, et al: Willingness to seek treatment among black students with anxiety or depression: the synergistic effect of sociocultural factors with symptom severity and intolerance of uncertainty. Behavior Therapy 49(5):691–701, 2018

Encyclopædia Britannica: Gentlemen's agreement, Encyclopædia Britannica, 2020. Available at: www.britannica.com/event/Gentlemens-Agreement. Accessed August 4, 2020.

Fowler JW, Dell ML: Stages of faith and identity: birth to teens. Child Adolesc Psychiatr Clin N Am 13(1):17–33, 2004

Hook JN, Davis DE, Owen J, et al: Cultural humility: measuring openness to culturally diverse clients. J Couns Psychol 60(3):353–366, 2013

Hwang WC, Wood JJ, Fujimoto K: Acculturative family distancing (AFD) and depression in Chinese American families. J Consult Clin Psychol 78(5):655–667, 2010

Institute of Medicine (U.S.) Committee on Lesbian, Gay, Bisexual, and Transgender Health Issues and Research Gaps and Opportunities: The Health of Lesbian, Gay, Bisexual, and Transgender People: Building a Foundation for Better Understanding. Washington, DC, National Academies Press, 2011, p 12

International Organization for Migration: Who is a migrant? Geneva, Switzerland, International Organization for Migration, 2020. Available at: www.iom.int/who-is-a-migrant. Accessed May 19, 2020.

Josephson AM, Dell ML: Religion and spirituality in child and adolescent psychiatry: a new frontier. Child Adolesc Psychiatr Clin N Am 13(1):1–15, 2004

Kim SY, Schwartz SJ, Perreira KM, et al: Culture's influence on stressors, parental socialization, and developmental processes in the mental health of children of immigrants. Annu Rev Clin Psychol 14:343–70, 2018

Layton-Henry Z: Minorities, in International Encyclopedia of the Social and Behavioral Sciences. Edited by Smelser NJ, Baltes PB. New York, ÜfaPergamon, 2001, pp 9894–9898

Lee T, Fouras G, Brown R: Practice parameter for the assessment and management of youth involved with the child welfare system. J Am Acad Child Adolesc Psychiatry 54(6):502–517, 2015

Link B, Phelan J: Conceptualizing stigma. Ann Rev Sociol 27(1):363–385, 2001

Meyer IH: Prejudice, social stress, and mental health in lesbian, gay, and bisexual populations: conceptual issues and research evidence. Psychol Bull 129(5):674–697, 2003

Nadal KL: Featured commentary: Trayvon, Troy, Sean: when racial biases and microaggressions kill. Washington, DC, American Psychological Association, July 2012. Available at: www.apa.org/pi/oema/resources/communique/2012/07/microaggressions. Accessed May 19, 2020.

National Archives and Records Administration: Executive Order 9066, February 19, 1942. General Records of the United States Government Record Group 11. Washington, DC, National Archives and Records Administration, 1942. Available at: www.ourdocuments.gov/document_data/document_transcripts/document_074_transcript.html. Accessed May 19, 2020.

National Archives and Records Administration: Chinese Exclusion Act (1882), in Teaching With Documents: Using Primary Sources from the National Archives. Washington, DC, National Archives and Records Administration, 1989. Available at: www.ourdocuments.gov/doc.php?flash=false&doc=47. Accessed May 19, 2020.

National Center for Complementary and Integrative Health: Traditional Chinese medicine: what you need to know. Bethesda, MD, National Center for Complementary and Integrative Health, 2020. Available at: https://nccih.nih.gov/health/whatiscam/chinesemed.htm. Accessed May 19, 2020.

Rothe EM, Tzuang D, Pumariega AJ: Acculturation, development, and adaptation. Child Adolesc Psychiatr Clin N Am 19(4):681–696, 2010

Shore JH, Savin DM, Novins D, et al: Cultural aspects of telepsychiatry. J Telemed Telecare 12(3):116–121, 2006

Singer M, Snipes C: Generations of suffering: experiences of a treatment program for substance abuse during pregnancy. J Health Care Poor Underserved 3(1):222–234, 1992

Sue DW, Capodilupo CM, Torino GC, et al: Racial microaggressions in everyday life: implications for practice. Am Psychol 62(4):271–286, 2007

United Nations High Commissioner for Refugees: Convention and protocol relating to the status of refugees. Geneva, Switzerland, United Nations High Commissioner for Refugees, 1991. Available at: https://cms.emergency.unhcr.org/documents/11982/55726/Convention+relating+to+the+Status+of+Refugees+%28signed+28+July+1951%2C+entered+into+force+22+April+1954%29+189+UNTS+150+and+Protocol+relating+to+the+Status+of+Refugees+%28signed+31+January+1967%2C+entered+into+force+4+October+1967%29+606+UNTS+267/0bf3248a-cfa8-4a60-864d-65cdfece1d47. Accessed May 19, 2020.

United Nations High Commissioner for Refugees: Glossary. Geneva, Switzerland, United Nations High Commissioner for Refugees, 2005. Available at: www.unhcr.org/449267670.pdf. Accessed May 19, 2020.

United Nations Human Rights Office of the High Commissioner: The human rights to water and sanitation of forcibly displaced persons in need of humanitarian assistance. Geneva, Switzerland, United Nations High Commissioner for Refugees, 2019. Available at: www.ohchr.org/EN/Issues/WaterAndSanitation/SRWater/Pages/ForciblyDisplacedPersons.aspx. Accessed May 19, 2020.

Weisberger M: "Immigration Act of 1917" turns 100: America's long history of immigration prejudice. Live Science, February 5, 2017. Available at: www.livescience.com/57756-1917-immigration-act-100th-anniversary.html. Accessed August 4, 2020.

APPENDIX A
DSM-5 Outline for Cultural Formulation

THE Outline for Cultural Formulation introduced in DSM-IV provided a framework for assessing information about cultural features of an individual's mental health problem and how it relates to a social and cultural context and history. DSM-5 not only includes an updated version of the Outline but also presents an approach to assessment, using the Cultural Formulation Interview (CFI), which has been field-tested for diagnostic usefulness among clinicians and for acceptability among patients.

The revised Outline for Cultural Formulation calls for systematic assessment of the following categories:

- **Cultural identity of the individual:** Describe the individual's racial, ethnic, or cultural reference groups that may influence his or her relationships with others, access to resources, and developmental and current challenges, conflicts, or predicaments. For immigrants and racial or ethnic minorities, the degree and kinds of involvement with both the culture of origin and the host culture or majority culture should be noted separately. Language abilities, preferences, and patterns of use are relevant for identifying difficulties with access to care, social integration, and the need for an interpreter. Other clinically relevant aspects of identity may include religious affiliation, socioeconomic background, personal and family places of birth and growing up, migrant status, and sexual orientation.
- **Cultural conceptualizations of distress:** Describe the cultural constructs that influence how the individual experiences, understands, and communicates his or her symptoms or problems to others. These constructs may include cultural syndromes, idioms of distress, and explanatory models or perceived causes. The level of severity and meaning of the distressing experiences should be assessed in relation to the norms of the individual's cultural reference

groups. Assessment of coping and help-seeking patterns should consider the use of professional as well as traditional, alternative, or complementary sources of care.

- **Psychosocial stressors and cultural features of vulnerability and resilience:** Identify key stressors and supports in the individual's social environment (which may include both local and distant events) and the role of religion, family, and other social networks (e.g., friends, neighbors, coworkers) in providing emotional, instrumental, and informational support. Social stressors and social supports vary with cultural interpretations of events, family structure, developmental tasks, and social context. Levels of functioning, disability, and resilience should be assessed in light of the individual's cultural reference groups.

- **Cultural features of the relationship between the individual and the clinician:** Identify differences in culture, language, and social status between an individual and clinician that may cause difficulties in communication and may influence diagnosis and treatment. Experiences of racism and discrimination in the larger society may impede establishing trust and safety in the clinical diagnostic encounter. Effects may include problems eliciting symptoms, misunderstanding of the cultural and clinical significance of symptoms and behaviors, and difficulty establishing or maintaining the rapport needed for an effective clinical alliance.

- **Overall cultural assessment:** Summarize the implications of the components of the cultural formulation identified in earlier sections of the Outline for diagnosis and other clinically relevant issues or problems as well as appropriate management and treatment intervention.

APPENDIX B
DSM-5 Cultural Formulation Interview

The Cultural Formulation Interview (CFI) is a set of 16 questions that clinicians may use to obtain information during a mental health assessment about the impact of culture on key aspects of an individual's clinical presentation and care. In the CFI, *culture* refers to

- The values, orientations, knowledge, and practices that individuals derive from membership in diverse social groups (e.g., ethnic groups, faith communities, occupational groups, veterans groups).
- Aspects of an individual's background, developmental experiences, and current social contexts that may affect his or her perspective, such as geographical origin, migration, language, religion, sexual orientation, or race/ethnicity.
- The influence of family, friends, and other community members (the individual's *social network*) on the individual's illness experience.

The CFI is a brief semistructured interview for systematically assessing cultural factors in the clinical encounter that may be used with any individual. The CFI focuses on the individual's experience and the social contexts of the clinical problem. The CFI follows a person-centered approach to cultural assessment by eliciting information from the individual about his or her own views and those of others in his or her social network. This approach is designed to avoid stereotyping, in that each individual's cultural knowledge affects how he or she interprets illness experience and guides how he or she seeks help. Because the CFI concerns the individual's personal views, there are no right or wrong answers to these questions. The interview follows and is available online at www.psychiatry.org/dsm5.

The CFI is formatted as two text columns. The left-hand column contains the instructions for administering the CFI and describes the goals for each interview domain. The questions in the right-hand column illustrate how to explore these domains, but they are not meant to be exhaustive. Follow-up questions may be needed to clarify individuals' answers. Questions may be rephrased as needed. The CFI is intended as a guide to cultural assessment and should be used flexibly to maintain a natural flow of the interview and rapport with the individual.

The CFI is best used in conjunction with demographic information obtained prior to the interview in order to tailor the CFI questions to address the individual's background and current situation. Specific demographic domains to be explored with the CFI will vary across individuals and settings. A comprehensive assessment may include place of birth, age, gender, racial/ethnic origin, marital status, family composition, education, language fluencies, sexual orientation, religious or spiritual affiliation, occupation, employment, income, and migration history.

The CFI can be used in the initial assessment of individuals in all clinical settings, regardless of the cultural background of the individual or of the clinician. Individuals and clinicians who appear to share the same cultural background may nevertheless differ in ways that are relevant to care. The CFI may be used in its entirety, or components may be incorporated into a clinical evaluation as needed. The CFI may be especially helpful when there is

- Difficulty in diagnostic assessment owing to significant differences in the cultural, religious, or socioeconomic backgrounds of clinician and the individual.
- Uncertainty about the fit between culturally distinctive symptoms and diagnostic criteria.
- Difficulty in judging illness severity or impairment.
- Disagreement between the individual and clinician on the course of care.
- Limited engagement in and adherence to treatment by the individual.

The CFI emphasizes four domains of assessment: Cultural Definition of the Problem (questions 1–3); Cultural Perceptions of Cause, Context, and Support (questions 4–10); Cultural Factors Affecting Self-Coping and Past Help Seeking (questions 11–13); and Cultural Factors Affecting Current Help Seeking (questions 14–16). Both the person-centered process of conducting the CFI and the information it elicits are intended to enhance the cultural validity of diagnostic assessment, facilitate treatment planning, and promote the individual's engagement and satisfaction. To achieve these goals, the information obtained from the CFI should be integrated with all other available clinical material into a comprehensive clinical and contextual evaluation. An Informant version of the CFI can be used to collect collateral information on the CFI domains from family members or caregivers.

Supplementary modules have been developed that expand on each domain of the CFI and guide clinicians who wish to explore these domains in greater depth. Supplementary modules have also been developed for specific populations, such as children and adolescents, elderly individuals, and immigrants and refugees. These supplementary modules are referenced in the CFI under the pertinent subheadings and are available online at www.psychiatry.org/dsm5.

Cultural Formulation Interview (CFI)

Supplementary modules used to expand each CFI subtopic are noted in parentheses.

GUIDE TO INTERVIEWER	**INSTRUCTIONS TO THE INTERVIEWER ARE *ITALICIZED.***

The following questions aim to clarify key aspects of the presenting clinical problem from the point of view of the individual and other members of the individual's social network (i.e., family, friends, or others involved in current problem). This includes the problem's meaning, potential sources of help, and expectations for services.

INTRODUCTION FOR THE INDIVIDUAL:
I would like to understand the problems that bring you here so that I can help you more effectively. I want to know about ***your*** experience and ideas. I will ask some questions about what is going on and how you are dealing with it. Please remember there are no right or wrong answers.

CULTURAL DEFINITION OF THE PROBLEM
CULTURAL DEFINITION OF THE PROBLEM

(Explanatory Model, Level of Functioning)

Elicit the individual's view of core problems and key concerns.

Focus on the individual's own way of understanding the problem.

Use the term, expression, or brief description elicited in question 1 to identify the problem in subsequent questions (e.g., "your conflict with your son").

Ask how individual frames the problem for members of the social network.

1. What brings you here today?
   IF INDIVIDUAL GIVES FEW DETAILS OR ONLY MENTIONS SYMPTOMS OR A MEDICAL DIAGNOSIS, PROBE:
   People often understand their problems in their own way, which may be similar to or different from how doctors describe the problem. How would *you* describe your problem?

2. Sometimes people have different ways of describing their problem to their family, friends, or others in their community. How would you describe your problem to them?

Focus on the aspects of the problem that matter most to the individual.

3. What troubles you most about your problem?

CULTURAL PERCEPTIONS OF CAUSE, CONTEXT, AND SUPPORT
CAUSES

(Explanatory Model, Social Network, Older Adults)

This question indicates the meaning of the condition for the individual, which may be relevant for clinical care.

Note that individuals may identify multiple causes, depending on the facet of the problem they are considering.

4. Why do you think this is happening to you? What do you think are the causes of your [PROBLEM]?
   PROMPT FURTHER IF REQUIRED:
   Some people may explain their problem as the result of bad things that happen in their life, problems with others, a physical illness, a spiritual reason, or many other causes.

Focus on the views of members of the individual's social network. These may be diverse and vary from the individual's.

5. What do others in your family, your friends, or others in your community think is causing your [PROBLEM]?

Cultural Formulation Interview (CFI) *(continued)*

Supplementary modules used to expand each CFI subtopic are noted in parentheses.

GUIDE TO INTERVIEWER

INSTRUCTIONS TO THE INTERVIEWER ARE *ITALICIZED*.

STRESSORS AND SUPPORTS

(Social Network, Caregivers, Psychosocial Stressors, Religion and Spirituality, Immigrants and Refugees, Cultural Identity, Older Adults, Coping and Help Seeking)

Elicit information on the individual's life context, focusing on resources, social supports, and resilience. May also probe other supports (e.g., from co-workers, from participation in religion or spirituality).

6. Are there any kinds of support that make your [PROBLEM] better, such as support from family, friends, or others?

Focus on stressful aspects of the individual's environment. Can also probe, e.g., relationship problems, difficulties at work or school, or discrimination.

7. Are there any kinds of stresses that make your [PROBLEM] worse, such as difficulties with money, or family problems?

ROLE OF CULTURAL IDENTITY

(Cultural Identity, Psychosocial Stressors, Religion and Spirituality, Immigrants and Refugees, Older Adults, Children and Adolescents)

Sometimes, aspects of people's background or identity can make their [PROBLEM] better or worse. By ***background*** or ***identity,*** I mean, for example, the communities you belong to, the languages you speak, where you or your family are from, your race or ethnic background, your gender or sexual orientation, or your faith or religion.

Ask the individual to reflect on the most salient elements of his or her cultural identity. Use this information to tailor questions 9–10 as needed.

8. For you, what are the most important aspects of your background or identity?

Elicit aspects of identity that make the problem better or worse.

9. Are there any aspects of your background or identity that make a difference to your [PROBLEM]?

Probe as needed (e.g., clinical worsening as a result of discrimination due to migration status, race/ethnicity, or sexual orientation).

Probe as needed (e.g., migration-related problems; conflict across generations or due to gender roles).

10. Are there any aspects of your background or identity that are causing other concerns or difficulties for you?

CULTURAL FACTORS AFFECTING SELF-COPING AND PAST HELP SEEKING

SELF-COPING

(Coping and Help Seeking, Religion and Spirituality, Older Adults, Caregivers, Psychosocial Stressors)

Clarify self-coping for the problem.

11. Sometimes people have various ways of dealing with problems like [PROBLEM]. What have you done on your own to cope with your [PROBLEM]?

Cultural Formulation Interview (CFI) *(continued)*

Supplementary modules used to expand each CFI subtopic are noted in parentheses.

GUIDE TO INTERVIEWER

INSTRUCTIONS TO THE INTERVIEWER ARE *ITALICIZED.*

PAST HELP SEEKING

(Coping and Help Seeking, Religion and Spirituality, Older Adults, Caregivers, Psychosocial Stressors, Immigrants and Refugees, Social Network, Clinician-Patient Relationship)

Elicit various sources of help (e.g., medical care, mental health treatment, support groups, work-based counseling, folk healing, religious or spiritual counseling, other forms of traditional or alternative healing).

Probe as needed (e.g., "What other sources of help have you used?").

Clarify the individual's experience and regard for previous help.

12. Often, people look for help from many different sources, including different kinds of doctors, helpers, or healers. In the past, what kinds of treatment, help, advice, or healing have you sought for your [PROBLEM]?

PROBE IF DOES NOT DESCRIBE USEFULNESS OF HELP RECEIVED:

What types of help or treatment were most useful? Not useful?

BARRIERS

(Coping and Help Seeking, Religion and Spirituality, Older Adults, Psychosocial Stressors, Immigrants and Refugees, Social Network, Clinician-Patient Relationship)

Clarify the role of social barriers to help seeking, access to care, and problems engaging in previous treatment.

Probe details as needed (e.g., "What got in the way?").

13. Has anything prevented you from getting the help you need?

PROBE AS NEEDED:

For example, money, work or family commitments, stigma or discrimination, or lack of services that understand your language or background?

CULTURAL FACTORS AFFECTING CURRENT HELP SEEKING

PREFERENCES

(Social Network, Caregivers, Religion and Spirituality, Older Adults, Coping and Help Seeking)

Clarify individual's current perceived needs and expectations of help, broadly defined.

Probe if individual lists only one source of help (e.g., "What other kinds of help would be useful to you at this time?").

Focus on the views of the social network regarding help seeking.

Now let's talk some more about the help you need.

14. What kinds of help do you think would be most useful to you at this time for your [PROBLEM]?

15. Are there other kinds of help that your family, friends, or other people have suggested would be helpful for you now?

CLINICIAN-PATIENT RELATIONSHIP

(Clinician-Patient Relationship, Older Adults)

Elicit possible concerns about the clinic or the clinician-patient relationship, including perceived racism, language barriers, or cultural differences that may undermine goodwill, communication, or care delivery.

Probe details as needed (e.g., "In what way?").

Address possible barriers to care or concerns about the clinic and the clinician-patient relationship raised previously.

Sometimes doctors and patients misunderstand each other because they come from different backgrounds or have different expectations.

16. Have you been concerned about this and is there anything that we can do to provide you with the care you need?

Cultural Formulation Interview (CFI)—Informant Version

The CFI–Informant Version collects collateral information from an informant who is knowledgeable about the clinical problems and life circumstances of the identified individual. This version can be used to supplement information obtained from the core CFI or can be used instead of the core CFI when the individual is unable to provide information—as might occur, for example, with children or adolescents, floridly psychotic individuals, or persons with cognitive impairment.

Cultural Formulation Interview (CFI)—Informant Version

GUIDE TO INTERVIEWER	INSTRUCTIONS TO THE INTERVIEWER ARE *ITALICIZED.*
The following questions aim to clarify key aspects of the presenting clinical problem from the informant's point of view. This includes the problem's meaning, potential sources of help, and expectations for services.	*INTRODUCTION FOR THE INFORMANT:* I would like to understand the problems that bring your family member/friend here so that I can help you and him/her more effectively. I want to know about **your** experience and ideas. I will ask some questions about what is going on and how you and your family member/friend are dealing with it. There are no right or wrong answers.
	RELATIONSHIP WITH THE PATIENT
Clarify the informant's relationship with the individual and/or the individual's family.	1. How would you describe your relationship to [INDIVIDUAL OR TO FAMILY]? *PROBE IF NOT CLEAR:* How often do you see [INDIVIDUAL]?
	CULTURAL DEFINITION OF THE PROBLEM
Elicit the informant's view of core problems and key concerns.	2. What brings your family member/friend here today?
Focus on the informant's way of understanding the individual's problem.	*IF INFORMANT GIVES FEW DETAILS OR ONLY MENTIONS SYMPTOMS OR A MEDICAL DIAGNOSIS, PROBE:*
Use the term, expression, or brief description elicited in question 1 to identify the problem in subsequent questions (e.g., "her conflict with her son").	People often understand problems in their own way, which may be similar or different from how doctors describe the problem. How would **you** describe [INDIVIDUAL'S] problem?
Ask how informant frames the problem for members of the social network.	3. Sometimes people have different ways of describing the problem to family, friends, or others in their community. How would **you** describe [INDIVIDUAL'S] problem to them?
Focus on the aspects of the problem that matter most to the informant.	4. What troubles you most about [INDIVIDUAL'S] problem?

Cultural Formulation Interview (CFI)—Informant Version *(continued)*

GUIDE TO INTERVIEWER	INSTRUCTIONS TO THE INTERVIEWER ARE *ITALICIZED.*

CULTURAL PERCEPTIONS OF CAUSE, CONTEXT, AND SUPPORT

CAUSES

This question indicates the meaning of the condition for the informant, which may be relevant for clinical care.

Note that informants may identify multiple causes depending on the facet of the problem they are considering.

5. Why do you think this is happening to [INDIVIDUAL]? What do you think are the causes of his/her [PROBLEM]?
PROMPT FURTHER IF REQUIRED:
Some people may explain the problem as the result of bad things that happen in their life, problems with others, a physical illness, a spiritual reason, or many other causes.

Focus on the views of members of the individual's social network. These may be diverse and vary from the informant's.

6. What do others in [INDIVIDUAL'S] family, his/her friends, or others in the community think is causing [INDIVIDUAL'S] [PROBLEM]?

STRESSORS AND SUPPORTS

Elicit information on the individual's life context, focusing on resources, social supports, and resilience. May also probe other supports (e.g., from co-workers, from participation in religion or spirituality).

7. Are there any kinds of supports that make his/her [PROBLEM] better, such as from family, friends, or others?

Focus on stressful aspects of the individual's environment. Can also probe, e.g., relationship problems, difficulties at work or school, or discrimination.

8. Are there any kinds of stresses that make his/her [PROBLEM] worse, such as difficulties with money, or family problems?

ROLE OF CULTURAL IDENTITY

Sometimes, aspects of people's background or identity can make the [PROBLEM] better or worse. By **background** or **identity,** I mean, for example, the communities you belong to, the languages you speak, where you or your family are from, your race or ethnic background, your gender or sexual orientation, and your faith or religion.

Ask the informant to reflect on the most salient elements of the individual's cultural identity. Use this information to tailor questions 10–11 as needed.

9. For you, what are the most important aspects of [INDIVIDUAL'S] background or identity?

Elicit aspects of identity that make the problem better or worse.

Probe as needed (e.g., clinical worsening as a result of discrimination due to migration status, race/ethnicity, or sexual orientation).

10. Are there any aspects of [INDIVIDUAL'S] background or identity that make a difference to his/her [PROBLEM]?

Probe as needed (e.g., migration-related problems; conflict across generations or due to gender roles).

11. Are there any aspects of [INDIVIDUAL'S] background or identity that are causing other concerns or difficulties for him/her?

Cultural Formulation Interview (CFI)—Informant Version *(continued)*

GUIDE TO INTERVIEWER	INSTRUCTIONS TO THE INTERVIEWER ARE *ITALICIZED*.

CULTURAL FACTORS AFFECTING SELF-COPING AND PAST HELP SEEKING

SELF-COPING

Clarify individual's self-coping for the problem.

12. Sometimes people have various ways of dealing with problems like [PROBLEM]. What has [INDIVIDUAL] done on his/her own to cope with his/her [PROBLEM]?

PAST HELP SEEKING

Elicit various sources of help (e.g., medical care, mental health treatment, support groups, work-based counseling, folk healing, religious or spiritual counseling, other alternative healing).

Probe as needed (e.g., "What other sources of help has he/she used?").

Clarify the individual's experience and regard for previous help.

13. Often, people also look for help from many different sources, including different kinds of doctors, helpers, or healers. In the past, what kinds of treatment, help, advice, or healing has [INDIVIDUAL] sought for his/her [PROBLEM]?

PROBE IF DOES NOT DESCRIBE USEFULNESS OF HELP RECEIVED:
What types of help or treatment were most useful? Not useful?

BARRIERS

Clarify the role of social barriers to help-seeking, access to care, and problems engaging in previous treatment.

Probe details as needed (e.g., "What got in the way?").

14. Has anything prevented [INDIVIDUAL] from getting the help he/she needs?

PROBE AS NEEDED:
For example, money, work or family commitments, stigma or discrimination, or lack of services that understand his/her language or background?

CULTURAL FACTORS AFFECTING CURRENT HELP SEEKING

PREFERENCES

Clarify individual's current perceived needs and expectations of help, broadly defined, from the point of view of the informant.

Probe if informant lists only one source of help (e.g., "What other kinds of help would be useful to [INDIVIDUAL] at this time?").

Now let's talk about the help [INDIVIDUAL] needs.

15. What kinds of help would be most useful to him/her at this time for his/her [PROBLEM]?

Focus on the views of the social network regarding help seeking.

16. Are there other kinds of help that [INDIVIDUAL'S] family, friends, or other people have suggested would be helpful for him/her now?

Cultural Formulation Interview (CFI)—Informant Version *(continued)*

GUIDE TO INTERVIEWER	INSTRUCTIONS TO THE INTERVIEWER ARE *ITALICIZED.*

CLINICIAN-PATIENT RELATIONSHIP

Elicit possible concerns about the clinic or the clinician-patient relationship, including perceived racism, language barriers, or cultural differences that may undermine goodwill, communication, or care delivery.	Sometimes doctors and patients misunderstand each other because they come from different backgrounds or have different expectations.
Probe details as needed (e.g., "In what way?").	17. Have you been concerned about this, and is there anything that we can do to provide [INDIVIDUAL] with the care he/she needs?
Address possible barriers to care or concerns about the clinic and the clinician-patient relationship raised previously.	

Supplementary Modules to the Core Cultural Formulation Interview (CFI)

Guidelines for Implementing the CFI Supplementary Modules

These modules supplement the core Cultural Formulation Interview and can help clinicians conduct a more comprehensive cultural assessment. The first eight supplementary modules explore the domains of the core CFI in greater depth. The next three modules focus on populations with specific needs, such as children and adolescents, older adults, and immigrants and refugees. The last module explores the experiences and views of individuals who perform caregiving functions, in order to clarify the nature and cultural context of caregiving and how they affect social support in the immediate environment of the individual receiving care. In addition to these supplementary modules, an Informant version of the core CFI collects collateral information on the CFI domains from family members or caregivers.

Clinicians may use these supplementary modules in two ways:

- As adjuncts to the core CFI for additional information about various aspects of illness affecting diverse populations. The core CFI refers to pertinent modules under each subheading to facilitate such use of the modules.
- As tools for in-depth cultural assessment independent of the core CFI. Clinicians may administer one, several, or all modules depending on what areas of an individual's problems they would like to elaborate.

Clinicians should note that a few questions in the modules duplicate questions in the core CFI (indicated by an asterisk [*]) or in other modules. This makes it possible to administer each module independently. Clinicians who use the modules as an adjunct to the core CFI or who administer the modules independently may skip redundant questions.

As with the core CFI, follow-up questions may be needed to clarify the individual's answers. Questions may be rephrased as needed. The modules are intended as a guide to cultural assessment and should be used flexibly to maintain a natural flow of the interview and rapport with the individual. In situations where the individual cannot answer these questions (e.g., due to cognitive impairment or severe psychosis) these questions can be administered to the identified caregiver. The caregiver's own perspective can also be ascertained using the module for caregivers.

In every module, instructions to the interviewer are in italics. The modules may be administered during the initial clinical evaluation, at a later point in care, or several times over the course of treatment. Multiple administrations may reveal additional information as rapport develops, especially when assessing the patient-clinician relationship.

Please refer to DSM-5 Section III, chapter "Cultural Formulation," section "Outline for Cultural Formulation," for additional suggestions regarding this type of interview.

1. Explanatory Model

Related Core CFI Questions: 1, 2, 3, 4, 5   Some of the core CFI questions are repeated below and are marked with an asterisk (*). The CFI question that is repeated is indicated in brackets.

GUIDE TO INTERVIEWER: This module aims to clarify the individual's understanding of the problem based on his or her ideas about cause and mechanism (explanatory models) and past experiences of, or knowing someone with, a similar problem (illness prototypes). The individual may identify the problem as a symptom, a specific term or expression (e.g., "nerves," "being on edge"), a situation (e.g., loss of a job), or a relationship (e.g., conflict with others). In the examples below, the individual's own words should be used to replace "[PROBLEM]". If there are multiple problems, each relevant problem can be explored. The following questions may be used to elicit the individual's understanding and experience of that problem or predicament.

INTRODUCTION FOR THE INDIVIDUAL BEING INTERVIEWED: I would like to understand the problems that bring you here so that I can help you more effectively. I will be asking you some questions to learn more about your own ideas about the causes of your problems and the way they affect your daily life.

General understanding of the problem

1. *Can you tell me more about how you understand your [PROBLEM]? [RELATED TO CFI Q#1–2.]
2. What did you know about your [PROBLEM] before it affected you?

Illness prototypes

3. Had you ever had anything like your [PROBLEM] before? Please tell me about that.
4. Do you know anyone else, or heard of anyone else, with this [PROBLEM]? If so, please describe that person's [PROBLEM] and how it affected that person. Do you think this will happen to you too?
5. Have you seen on television, heard on the radio, read in a magazine, or found on the internet anything about your [PROBLEM]? Please tell me about it.

Causal explanations

6. *Can you tell me what you think caused your [PROBLEM]? (*PROBE AS NEEDED:* Is there more than one cause that may explain it?] [RELATED TO CFI Q#4.)

7. Have your ideas about the cause of the [PROBLEM] changed? How? What changed your ideas about the cause?

8. *What do people in your family, friends, or others in your community think caused the [PROBLEM]? (*PROBE AS NEEDED:* Are their ideas about it different from yours? How so?) [RELATED TO CFI Q#5.]

9. How do you think your [PROBLEM] affects your body? Your mind? Your spiritual well-being?

Course of illness

10. What usually happens to people who have this [PROBLEM]? In your own case, what do you think is likely to happen?

11. Do you consider your [PROBLEM] to be serious? Why? What is the worst that could happen?

12. How concerned are other people in your family, friends or community about your having this [PROBLEM]? Please tell me about that.

Help seeking and treatment expectations

13. What do you think is the best way to deal with this kind of problem?

14. What do your family, friends, or others in your community think is the best way of dealing with this kind of problem?

2. Level of Functioning

Related Core CFI Question: 3

GUIDE TO INTERVIEWER: The following questions aim to clarify the individual's level of functioning in relation to his or her own priorities and those of the cultural reference group. The interview begins with a general question about everyday activities that are important for the individual. Questions follow about domains important for positive health (social relations, work/school, economic viability, and resilience). Questions should be kept relatively broad and open to elicit the individual's own priorities and perspective. For a more detailed evaluation of specific domains of functioning, a standard instrument such as the WHO-DAS II may be used together with this interview.

INTRODUCTION FOR THE INDIVIDUAL BEING INTERVIEWED: I would like to know about the daily activities that are most important to you. I would like to better understand how your [PROBLEM] has affected your ability to perform these activities, and how your family and other people around you have reacted to this.

1. How has your [PROBLEM] affected your ability to do the things you need to do each day, that is, your daily activities and responsibilities?

2. How has your [PROBLEM] affected your ability to interact with your family and other people in your life?

3. How has your [PROBLEM] affected your ability to work?
4. How has your [PROBLEM] affected your financial situation?
5. How has your [PROBLEM] affected your ability to take part in community and social activities?
6. How has your [PROBLEM] affected your ability to enjoy everyday life?
7. Which of these concerns are most troubling to you?
8. Which of these concerns are most troubling to your family and to other people in your life?

3. Social Network

Related Core CFI Questions: 5, 6, 12, 15

   GUIDE TO INTERVIEWER: The following questions identify the influences of the informal social network on the individual's problem. **Informal social network** *refers to family, friends and other social contacts through work, places of prayer/worship or other activities and affiliations. Question #1 identifies important people in the individual's social network, and the clinician should tailor subsequent questions accordingly. These questions aim to elicit the social network's response, the individual's interpretation of how this would impact on the problem, and the individual's preferences for involving members of the social network in care.*

   INTRODUCTION FOR THE INDIVIDUAL BEING INTERVIEWED: I would like to know more about how your family, friends, colleagues, co-workers, and other important people in your life have had an impact on your [PROBLEM].

Composition of the individual's social network

1. Who are the most important people in your life at present?
2. Is there anyone in particular whom you trust and can talk with about your [PROBLEM]? Who? Anyone else?

Social network understanding of problem

3. Which of your family members, friends, or other important people in your life know about your [PROBLEM]?
4. What ideas do your family and friends have about the nature of your [PROBLEM]? How do they understand your [PROBLEM]?
5. Are there people who do not know about your [PROBLEM]? Why do they not know about your [PROBLEM]?

Social network response to problem

6. What advice have family members and friends given you about your [PROBLEM]?
7. Do your family, friends, and other people in your life treat you differently because of your [PROBLEM]? How do they treat you differently? Why do they treat you differently?
8. (IF HAS NOT TOLD FAMILY OR FRIENDS ABOUT PROBLEM): Can you tell me more about why you have chosen not to tell family or friends about the [PROBLEM]? How do you think they would respond if they knew about your [PROBLEM]?

Social network as a stress/buffer

9. What have your family, friends, and other people in your life done to make your [PROBLEM] better or easier for you to deal with? (*IF UNCLEAR:* How has that made your [PROBLEM] better?)

10. What kinds of help or support were you expecting from family or friends?
11. What have your family, friends, and other people in your life done to make your [PROBLEM] worse or harder for you to deal with? (*IF UNCLEAR:* How has that made your [PROBLEM] worse?)

Social network in treatment

12. Have any family members or friends helped you get treatment for your [PROBLEM]?
13. What would your family and friends think about your coming here to receive treatment?
14. Would you like your family, friends, or others to be part of your treatment? If so, who would you like to be involved and how?
15. How would involving family or friends make a difference in your treatment?

4. Psychosocial Stressors

Related Core CFI Questions: 7, 9, 10, 12

GUIDE TO INTERVIEWER: The aim of these questions is to further clarify the stressors that have aggravated the problem or otherwise affected the health of the individual. (Stressors that initially caused the problem are covered in the module on Explanatory Models.) In the examples below, the individual's own words should be used to replace "[STRESSORS]". If there are multiple stressors, each relevant stressor can be explored.

INTRODUCTION FOR THE INDIVIDUAL BEING INTERVIEWED: You have told me about some things that make your [PROBLEM] worse. I would like to learn more about that.

1. Are there things going on that have made your [PROBLEM] worse, for example, difficulties with family, work, money, or something else? Tell me more about that.
2. How are the people around you affected by these [STRESSORS]?
3. How do you cope with these [STRESSORS]?
4. What have other people suggested about coping with these [STRESSORS]?
5. What else could be done about these [STRESSORS]?

GUIDE TO INTERVIEWER: Patients may be reluctant to discuss areas of their life they consider sensitive, which may vary across cultural groups. Asking specific questions may help the patient discuss these stressors. Insert questions about relevant stressors here. For example:

1. Have you experienced discrimination or been treated badly as a result of your background or identity? By background or identity I mean, for example, the communities you belong to, the languages you speak, where you or your family are from, your racial or ethnic background, your gender or sexual orientation, and your faith or religion. Have these experiences had an impact on [STRESSORS] or your [PROBLEM]?

5. Spirituality, Religion, and Moral Traditions

Related Core CFI Questions: 6, 7, 8, 9, 10, 11, 12, 14, 15

GUIDE TO INTERVIEWER: The following questions aim to clarify the influence of spirituality, religion, and other moral or philosophical traditions on the individual's problems and related stresses. People may have multiple spiritual, moral, and religious affiliations or practices. If the individual reports having specific beliefs or practices, inquire about the level of involvement in that tradition and its impact on coping with the clinical problem. In the examples below, the individual's own words should be used to replace "[NAME(S) OF SPIRITUAL, RELIGIOUS OR MORAL TRADITION(S)]". If the individual identifies more than one tradition, each can be explored. If the individual does not describe a specific tradition, use the phrase "spirituality, religion or other moral traditions" instead of the specific name of a tradition (e.g., Q5: "What role do spirituality, religion or other moral traditions play in your everyday life?")

INTRODUCTION FOR THE INDIVIDUAL BEING INTERVIEWED: To help you more effectively, I would like to ask you some questions about the role that spirituality, religion or other moral traditions play in your life and how they may have influenced your dealing with the problems that bring you here.

Spiritual, religious, and moral identity

1. Do you identify with any particular spiritual, religious or moral tradition? Can you tell me more about that?
2. Do you belong to a congregation or community associated with that tradition?
3. What are the spiritual, religious or moral tradition backgrounds of your family members?
4. Sometimes people participate in several traditions. Are there any other spiritual, religious or moral traditions that you identify with or take part in?

Role of spirituality, religion, and moral traditions

5. What role does [NAME(S) OF SPIRITUAL, RELIGIOUS OR MORAL TRADITION(S)] play in your everyday life?
6. What role does [NAME(S) OF SPIRITUAL, RELIGIOUS OR MORAL TRADITION(S)] play in your family, for example, family celebrations or choices in marriage or schooling?
7. What activities related to [NAME(S) OF SPIRITUAL, RELIGIOUS OR MORAL TRADITION(S)] do you carry out <u>in the home</u>, for example, prayers, meditation, or special dietary laws? How often do you carry out these activities? How important are these activities in your life?
8. What activities do you engage in <u>outside the home</u> related to [NAME(S) OF SPIRITUAL, RELIGIOUS OR MORAL TRADITION(S)], for example, attending ceremonies or participating in a [CHURCH, TEMPLE OR MOSQUE]? How often do you attend? How important are these activities in your life?

Relationship to the [PROBLEM]

9. How has [NAME(S) OF SPIRITUAL, RELIGIOUS OR MORAL TRADITION(S)] helped you cope with your [PROBLEM]?

10. Have you talked to a leader, teacher or others in your [NAME(S) OF SPIRITUAL, RELIGIOUS OR MORAL TRADITION(S)] community, about your [PROBLEM]? How have you found that helpful?

11. Have you found reading or studying [BOOK(S) OF SPIRITUAL, RELIGIOUS OR MORAL TRADITION(S), (e.g., BIBLE, KORAN)], or listening to programs related to [NAME(S) OF SPIRITUAL, RELIGIOUS OR MORAL TRADITION(S)] on TV, radio, the Internet or other media [e.g., DVD, tape] to be helpful? In what way?

12. Have you found any practices related to [NAME(S) OF SPIRITUAL, RELIGIOUS OR MORAL TRADITION(S)], like prayer, meditation, rituals, or pilgrimages to be helpful to you in dealing with [PROBLEM]? In what way?

Potential stresses or conflicts related to spirituality, religion, and moral traditions

13. Have any issues related to [NAME(S) OF SPIRITUAL, RELIGIOUS OR MORAL TRADITION(S)] contributed to [PROBLEM]?

14. Have you experienced any personal challenges or distress in relation to your [NAME(S) OF SPIRITUAL, RELIGIOUS OR MORAL TRADITION(S)] identity or practices?

15. Have you experienced any discrimination due to your [NAME(S) OF SPIRITUAL, RELIGIOUS OR MORAL TRADITION(S)] identity or practices?

16. Have you been in conflict with others over spiritual, religious or moral issues?

6. Cultural Identity

Related Core CFI Questions: 6, 7, 8, 9, 10   Some of the core CFI questions are repeated below and are marked with an asterisk (*). The CFI question that is repeated is indicated in brackets.

GUIDE TO INTERVIEWER: This module aims to further clarify the individual's cultural identity and how this has influenced the individual's health and well being. The following questions explore the individual's cultural identity and how this may have shaped his or her current problem. We use the word **culture** *broadly to refer to all the ways the individual understands his or her identity and experience in terms of groups, communities or other collectivities, including national or geographic origin, ethnic community, racialized categories, gender, sexual orientation, social class, religion/spirituality, and language.*

INTRODUCTION FOR THE INDIVIDUAL BEING INTERVIEWED: Sometimes peoples' background or identity influences their experience of illness and the type of care they receive. In order to better help you, I would like to understand your own background or identity. By background or identity I mean, for example, the communities you belong to, the languages you speak, where you or your family are from, your racial or ethnic background, your gender or sexual orientation, and your faith or religion.

National, Ethnic, Racial Background

1. Where were you born?

2. Where were your parents and grandparents born?

3. How would you describe your family's national, ethnic, and/or racial background?

4. In terms of your background, how do you usually describe yourself to people outside your community? Sometimes people describe themselves somewhat differently to members of their own community. How do you describe yourself to them?

5. Which part of your background do you feel closest to? Sometimes this varies, depending on what aspect of your life we are talking about. What about at home? Or at work? Or with friends?

6. Do you experience any difficulties related to your background, such as discrimination, stereotyping, or being misunderstood?

7. *Is there anything about your background that might impact on your [PROBLEM] or impact on your health or health care more generally? [RELATED TO CFI Q#9.]

Language

8. What languages do you speak fluently?
9. What languages did you speak growing up?
10. What languages are spoken at home? Which of these do you speak?
11. What languages do you use at work or school?
12. What language would you prefer to use in getting health care?
13. What languages do you read? Write?

Migration

GUIDE TO INTERVIEWER: *If the individual was born in another country, ask questions 1–7. [For refugees, refer to the module on Immigrants and Refugees to obtain more detailed migration history.]*

14. When did you come to this country?
15. What made you decide to leave your country of origin?
16. How has your life changed since coming here?
17. What do you miss about the place or community you came from?
18. What are your concerns for your own and your family's future here?
19. What is your current status in this country (e.g., refugee claimant, citizen, student visa, work permit)? *Be aware this may be a sensitive or confidential issue for the individual, if they have precarious status.*
20. How has migration influenced your health or that of your family?
21. Is there anything about your migration experience or current status in this country that has made a difference to your [PROBLEM]?
22. Is there anything about your migration experience or current status that might influence your ability to get the right kind of help for your [PROBLEM]?

Spirituality, Religion, and Moral Traditions

23. Do you identify with any particular religious, moral or spiritual tradition?

GUIDE TO INTERVIEWER: *In the next question, the individual's own words should be used to replace "[NAME(S) OF SPIRITUAL, RELIGIOUS OR MORAL TRADITION(S)]".*

24. What role does [NAME(S) OF SPIRITUAL, RELIGIOUS OR MORAL TRADITION(S)] play in your everyday life?
25. Do your family members share your spiritual, religious or moral traditions? Can you tell me more about that?

Gender Identity

INTRODUCTION FOR THE INDIVIDUAL BEING INTERVIEWED: Some individuals feel that their gender [e.g., the social roles and expectations they have related to being male, female, transgender, genderqueer, or intersex] influences their health and the kind of health care they need.

GUIDE TO INTERVIEWER: In the examples below, the individual's own words should be used to replace "[GENDER]". The interviewer may need to exemplify or explain the term 'GENDER" with relevant wording (e.g., "being a man," "being a transgender woman").

26. Do you feel that your [GENDER] has influenced <u>your [PROBLEM] or your health</u> more generally?
27. Do you feel that your [GENDER] has influenced <u>your ability to get the kind of health care</u> you need?
28. Do you feel that health care providers have certain assumptions or attitudes about you or your [PROBLEM] because of your [GENDER]?

Sexual Orientation Identity

INTRODUCTION FOR THE INDIVIDUAL BEING INTERVIEWED: Sexual orientation may also be important to individuals and their comfort in seeking health care. I would like to ask you some questions about your sexual orientation. Are you comfortable answering questions about your sexual orientation?

29. How would you describe your sexual orientation (e.g., heterosexual, gay, lesbian, bisexual, queer, pansexual, asexual)?
30. Do you feel that your sexual orientation has influenced <u>your [PROBLEM] or your health</u> more generally?
31. Do you feel that your sexual orientation influences <u>your ability to get the kind of health care</u> you need for your [PROBLEM]?
32. Do you feel that health care providers have assumptions or attitudes about you or your [PROBLEM] that are related to your sexual orientation?

Summary

33. You have told me about different aspects of your background and identity and how this has influenced your health and well being. Are there other aspects of your identity I should know about to better understand your health care needs?
34. What are the most important aspects of your background or identity in relation to [PROBLEM]?

7. Coping and Help-Seeking

Related Core CFI Questions: 6, 11, 12, 14, 15   Some of the core CFI question are repeated below and are marked with an asterisk (*). The CFI question that is repeated is indicated in brackets.

GUIDE TO INTERVIEWER: This module aims to clarify the individual's ways of coping with the current problem. The individual may have identified the problem as a symptom or men-

tioned a term or expression (e.g., "nerves," "being on edge," spirit possession), or a situation (e.g., loss of a job), or a relationship (e.g., conflict with others). In the examples below, the individual's own words should be used to replace "[PROBLEM]". If there are multiple problems, each relevant problem can be explored. The following questions may be used to learn more about the individual's understanding and experiencing of that problem.

INTRODUCTION FOR THE INDIVIDUAL BEING INTERVIEWED: I would like to understand the problems that bring you here so that I can help you more effectively. I will be asking you questions about how you have tried to cope with your problems and get help for them.

Self-coping

1. *Can you tell me more about how you are trying to cope with [PROBLEM] at this time? Has that way of coping with it been helpful? If so, how? [RELATED TO CFI Q#11.]

2. *Can you tell me more about how you tried to cope with the [PROBLEM] or with similar problems in the past? Was that way of coping with it helpful? If so, how? [RELATED TO CFI Q#11.]

3. Have you sought help for your [PROBLEM] on the internet, by reading books, by viewing television shows, or by listening to audiotapes, videos or other sources? If so, which of these? What did you learn? Was it helpful?

4. Do you engage by yourself in practices related to a spiritual, religious or moral tradition to help you cope with your [PROBLEM]? For example, prayer, meditation, or other practices that you carry out by yourself?

5. Have you sought help for your [PROBLEM] from natural remedies or medications that you take without a doctor's prescription, such as over-the-counter medicines? If so, which natural remedies or medications? Were they helpful?

Social network

6. *Have you told a family member about your [PROBLEM]? Have family members helped you cope with the [PROBLEM]? If so, how? What did they suggest you do to cope with the [PROBLEM]? Was it helpful? [RELATED TO CFI Q#15.]

7. *Have you told a friend or co-worker about your [PROBLEM]? Have friends or co-workers helped you cope with the [PROBLEM]? If so, how? What did they suggest you do to cope with the [PROBLEM]? Was it helpful? [RELATED TO CFI Q#15.]

Help- and treatment-seeking beyond social network

8. Are you involved in activities that involve other people related to a spiritual, religious or moral tradition? For example, do you go to worship or religious gatherings, speak with other people in your religious group or speak with the religious or spiritual leader? Have any of these been helpful in coping with [PROBLEM]? In what way?

9. Have you ever tried to get help for your [PROBLEM] from your general doctor? If so, who and when? What treatment did they give? Was it helpful?

10. Have you ever tried to get help for your [PROBLEM] from a mental health clinician, such as a counselor, psychologist, social worker, psychiatrist, or other professional? If so, who and when? What treatment did they give? Was it helpful?

11. Have you sought help from <u>any other kind of helper</u> to cope with your [PROBLEM] other than going to the doctor, for example, a chiropractor, acupuncturist, homeopath, or other kind of healer? What kind of treatment did they recommend to resolve the problem? Was it helpful?

Current treatment episode

12. What were the circumstances that led to your coming here for treatment for your [PROBLEM]? Did anyone suggest you come here for treatment? If so, who, and why did he or she suggest you come here?

13. What help are you hoping to get here [at this clinic] for your [PROBLEM]?

8. Patient-Clinician Relationship

Related Core CFI Question: 16   Some of the core CFI questions are repeated below and are marked with an asterisk (*). The CFI question that is repeated is indicated in brackets.

GUIDE TO INTERVIEWER: *The following questions address the role of culture in the patient-clinician relationship with respect to the individual's presenting concerns and to the clinician's evaluation of the individual's problem. We use the word* **culture** *broadly to refer to all the ways the individual understands his or her identity and experience in terms of groups, communities or other collectivities, including national or geographic origin, ethnic community, racialized categories, gender, sexual orientation, social class, religion/spirituality, and language.*

The first set of questions evaluates four domains in the clinician-patient relationship from the point of view of the patient: experiences, expectations, communication, and possibility of collaboration with the clinician. The second set of questions is directed to the clinician to guide reflection on the role of cultural factors in the clinical relationship, the assessment, and treatment planning.

INTRODUCTION FOR THE PATIENT: I would like to learn about how it has been for you to talk with me and other clinicians about your [PROBLEM] and your health more generally. I will ask some questions about your views, concerns, and expectations.

QUESTIONS FOR THE PATIENT:

1. What kind of experiences have you had with clinicians in the past? What was most helpful to you?

2. Have you had difficulties with clinicians in the past? What did you find difficult or unhelpful?

3. Now let's talk about the help that you would like to get here. Some people prefer clinicians of a similar background (for example, age, race, religion, or some other characteristic) because they think it may be easier to understand each other. Do you have any preference or ideas about what kind of clinician might understand you best?

4. *Sometimes differences among patients and clinicians make it difficult for them to understand each other. Do you have any concerns about this? If so, in what way? [RELATED TO CFI Q#16.]

GUIDE TO INTERVIEWER: *Question #5 addresses the patient-clinician relationship moving forward in treatment. It elicits the patient's expectations of the clinician and may be used to start a discussion on how the two of them can collaborate in the individual's care.*

5. What patients expect from their clinicians is important. As we move forward in your care, how can we best work together?

QUESTIONS FOR THE CLINICIAN AFTER THE INTERVIEW:

1. How did you feel about your relationship with the patient? Did cultural similarities and differences influence your relationship? In what way?
2. What was the quality of communication with the patient? Did cultural similarities and differences influence your communication? In what way?
3. If you used an interpreter, how did the presence of an interpreter or his/her way of interpreting influence your relationship or your communication with the patient and the information you received?
4. How do the patient's cultural background or identity, life situation, and/or social context influence your understanding of his/her problem and your diagnostic assessment?
5. How do the patient's cultural background or identity, life situation, and/or social context influence your treatment plan or recommendations?
6. Did the clinical encounter confirm or call into question any of your prior ideas about the cultural background or identity of the patient? If so, in what way?
7. Are there aspects of your own identity that may influence your attitudes toward this patient?

9. School-Age Children and Adolescents

Related Core CFI Questions: 8, 9, 10

   GUIDE TO INTERVIEWER: This supplement is directed to adolescents and mature school-age children. It should be used in conjunction with standard child mental health assessments that evaluate family relations (including intergenerational issues), peer relations, and the school environment. The aim of these questions is to identify, from the perspective of the child/ youth, the role of age-related cultural expectations, the possible cultural divergences between school, home, and the peer group, and whether these issues impact on the situation or problem that brought the youth for care. The questions indirectly explore cultural challenges, stressors and resilience, and issues of cultural hybridity, mixed ethnicity or multiple ethnic identifications. Peer group belonging is important to children and adolescents, and questions exploring ethnicity, religious identity, racism or gender difference should be included following the child's lead. Some children may not be able to answer all questions; clinicians should select and adapt questions to ensure they are developmentally appropriate for the individual. Children should not be used as informants to provide socio-demographic information on the family or an explicit analysis of the cultural dimensions of their problems. An Addendum lists cultural aspects of development and parenting that can be evaluated during parents' interviews.

   INTRODUCTION FOR THE CHILD/YOUTH: We have talked about the concerns of your family. Now I would like to know more about how you feel about being ___ years old.

Feelings of age appropriateness in different settings

1. Do you feel you are like other children/youth your age? In what way?
2. Do you sometimes feel different from other children/youth your age? In what way?
3. *IF THE CHILD/YOUTH ACKNOWLEDGES SOMETIMES FEELING DIFFERENT:* Does this feeling of being different happen more at home, at school, at work, and/or some other place?
4. Do you feel your family is different from other families?
5. Do you use different languages? With whom and when?
6. Does your name have any special meaning for you? Your family? Your community?
7. Is there something special about you that you like or that you are proud of?

Age-related stressors and supports

8. What <u>do</u> you like about being a child/youth at home? At school? With friends?
9. What <u>don't</u> you like about being a child/youth at home? At school? With friends?
10. Who is there to support you when you feel you need it? At home? At school? Among your friends?

Age-related expectations

GUIDE TO INTERVIEWER: *Concepts of childhood and age-appropriate behavior vary significantly across cultures. The aim of these questions is to elicit the normative frame(s) of the child/family and how this may be different from other cultural environments.*

11. What do your <u>parents or grandparents</u> expect from a child/youth your age? (*CLARIFY:* For example, chores, schoolwork, play, religious observance.)
12. What do your <u>school teachers</u> expect from a child/youth your age?
13. *IF INDIVIDUAL HAS SIBLINGS:* What do your <u>siblings</u> expect from a child/youth your age? (*CLARIFY:* For example, babysitting, help with homework, dating, dress.)
14. What do other <u>children/youth your age</u> expect from a child/youth your age?

Transition to adulthood/maturity (FOR ADOLESCENTS ONLY)

15. Are there any important celebrations or events in your community to recognize reaching a certain age or growing up?
16. When is a youth considered ready to become an adult <u>in your family or community</u>?
17. When is a youth considered ready to become an adult <u>according to your school teachers</u>?
18. What is good or difficult about becoming a young woman or a young man in your family? In your school? In your community?
19. How do you feel about "growing up" or becoming an adult?
20. In what ways are your life and responsibilities different from the life and responsibilities of your parents?

ADDENDUM FOR PARENTS' INTERVIEW

GUIDE TO INTERVIEWER: *Information on cultural influences on development and parenting is best obtained by interviewing the child's parents or caretakers. In addition to issues directly related to presenting problems, it is useful to inquire about:*

- The child's particular place in the family (e.g., oldest boy, only girl)
- The process of naming the child (Who chose the name? Does it have special meaning? Who else is called like this?)
- Developmental milestones in the culture of origin of the mother (and father): expected age for weaning, walking, toilet training, speaking. Vision of normal autonomy/dependency, appropriate disciplining and so on
- Perceptions of age-appropriate behaviors (e.g., age for staying home alone, participation in chores, religious observance, play)
- Child-adult relations (e.g., expression of respect, eye contact, physical contact)
- Gender relations (expectations around appropriate girl-boy behavior, dress code)
- Languages spoken at home, in daycare, at school
- The importance of religion, spirituality, and community in family life and related expectations for the child.

10. Older Adults

Related Core CFI Questions: 5, 6, 7, 8, 9, 10, 12, 13, 15, 16

GUIDE TO INTERVIEWER: The following questions are directed to older adults. The goal of these questions is to identify the role of cultural conceptions of aging and age-related transitions on the illness episode.

INTRODUCTION FOR THE INDIVIDUAL BEING INTERVIEWED: I would like to ask some questions to better understand your problem and how we can help you with it, taking into account your age and specific experiences.

Conceptions of aging and cultural identity

1. How would you describe a person of your age?
2. How does your experience of aging compare to that of your friends and relatives who are of a similar age?
3. Is there anything about being your age that helps you cope with your current life situation?

Conceptions of aging in relationship to illness attributions and coping

4. How does being older influence your [PROBLEM]? Would it have affected you differently when you were younger?
5. Are there ways that being older influences how you deal with your [PROBLEM]? Would you have dealt with it differently when you were younger?

Influence of comorbid medical problems and treatments on illness

6. Have you had health problems due to your age?
7. How have your health conditions or the treatments for your health conditions affected your [PROBLEM]?
8. Are there any ways that your health conditions or treatments influence how you deal with your [PROBLEM]?
9. Are there things that are important to you that you are unable to do because of your health or age?

Quality and nature of social supports and caregiving

10. Who do you rely on for help or support in your daily life in general? Has this changed now that you are going through [PROBLEM]?
11. How has [PROBLEM] affected your relationships with family and friends?
12. Are you receiving the amount and kind of support you expected?
13. Do the people you rely on share your view of your [PROBLEM]?

Additional age-related transitions

14. Are there other changes you are going through related to aging that are important for us to know about in order to help you with your [PROBLEM]?

Positive and negative attitudes towards aging and clinician–patient relationship

15. How has your age affected how health providers treat you?
16. Have any people, including health care providers, discriminated against you or treated you poorly because of your age? Can you tell me more about that? How has this experience affected your [PROBLEM] or how you deal with it?
17. *[IF THERE IS A SIGNIFICANT AGE DIFFERENCE BETWEEN PROVIDER AND PATIENT:]* Do you think that the difference in our ages will influence our work in any way? If so, how?

11. Immigrants and Refugees

Related Core CFI Questions: 7, 8, 9, 10, 13

GUIDE TO INTERVIEWER: The following questions aim to collect information from refugees and immigrants about their experiences of migration and resettlement. Many refugees have experienced stressful interviews with officials or health professionals in their home country, during the migration process (which may involve prolonged stays in refugee camps or other precarious situations), and in the receiving country, so it may take longer than usual for the interviewee to feel comfortable with and trust the interview process. When patient and clinician do not share a high level of fluency in a common language, accurate language translation is essential.

INTRODUCTION FOR THE INDIVIDUAL BEING INTERVIEWED: Leaving one's country of origin and resettling elsewhere can have a great impact on people's lives and health. To better understand your situation, I would like to ask you some questions related to your journey here from your country of origin.

Background information

1. What is your country of origin?
2. How long have you been living here in _____ (HOST COUNTRY)?
3. When and with whom did you leave _____ (COUNTRY OF ORIGIN)?
4. Why did you leave _____ (COUNTRY OF ORIGIN)?

Pre-migration difficulties

5. Prior to arriving in _____ (HOST COUNTRY), were there any challenges in your country of origin that you or your family found especially difficult?

6. Some people experience hardship, persecution, or even violence before leaving their country of origin. Has this been the case for you or members of your family? Can you tell me something about your experiences?

Migration-related losses and challenges

7. Of the persons important/close to you, who stayed behind?

8. Often people leaving a country experience losses. Did you or any of your family members experience losses upon leaving the country? If so, what are they?

9. Were there any challenges on your journey to _____ (HOST COUNTRY) that you or your family found especially difficult?

10. Do you or your family miss anything about your way of life in (COUNTRY OF ORIGIN)?

Ongoing relationship with country of origin

11. Do you have concerns about relatives that remain in (COUNTRY OF ORIGIN)?

12. Do relatives in (COUNTRY OF ORIGIN) have any expectations of you?

Resettlement and new life

13. Have you or your family experienced any difficulties related to your visa, citizenship, or refugee status here in _____ (HOST COUNTRY)?

14. Are there any (other) challenges or problems you or others in your family are facing related to your resettlement here?

15. Has coming to [HOST COUNTRY] resulted in something positive for you or your family? Can you tell me more about that?

Relationship with problem

16. Is there anything about your migration experience or current status in this country that has made a difference to your [PROBLEM]?

17. Is there anything about your migration experience or current status that might make it easier or harder to get help for your [PROBLEM]?

Future expectations

18. What hopes and plans do you have for you and your family in the coming years?

12. Caregivers

Related Core CFI Questions: 6, 12, 14

GUIDE TO INTERVIEWER: This module is designed to be administered to individuals who provide caregiving for the individual being assessed with the CFI. This module aims to explore the nature and cultural context of caregiving, and the social support and stresses in the immediate environment of the individual receiving care, from the perspective of the caregiver.

INTRODUCTION FOR THE CAREGIVER: People like yourself who take care of the needs of patients are very important participants in the treatment process. I would like to understand your relationship with [INDIVIDUAL RECEIVING CARE] and how you help him/her with his/her problems and concerns. By *help*, I mean support in the home, community, or clinic. Knowing more about that will help us plan his/her care more effectively.

Nature of relationship

1. How long have you been taking care of [INDIVIDUAL RECEIVING CARE]? How did this role for you start?
2. How are you connected to [INDIVIDUAL RECEIVING CARE]?

Caregiving activities and cultural perceptions of caregiving

3. How do you help him/her with the [PROBLEM] or with day-to-day activities?
4. What is most rewarding about helping him/her?
5. What is most challenging about helping him/her?
6. How, if at all, has his/her [PROBLEM] changed your relationship?

Sometimes caregivers like yourself are influenced in doing what they do by cultural traditions of helping others, such as beliefs and practices in your family or community. By cultural traditions I mean, for example, what is done in the communities you belong to, where you or your family are from, or among people who speak your language or who share your race or ethnic background, your gender or sexual orientation, or your faith or religion.

7. Are there any cultural traditions that influence how you approach helping [INDIVIDUAL RECEIVING CARE]?
8. Is the amount or kind of help you are giving him/her different in any way from what would be expected in the community that you come from or the one he/she comes from? Is it different from what society in general would expect?

Social context of caregiving

9. *[IF CAREGIVER IS A FAMILY MEMBER:]* How do you, as a family, cope with this [PROBLEM]?
10. Are there others, such as family members, friends, or neighbors, who also help him/her with the [PROBLEM]? If so, what do they do?
11. How do you feel about how much or how little others are helping with his/her [PROBLEM]?

Clinical support for caregiving

12. How do you see yourself helping to provide care to [INDIVIDUAL RECEIVING CARE] now and in the future?
13. *[IF UNCLEAR:]* How do you see yourself helping with the care that he/she receives in this clinic?
14. How can we make it easier for you to be able to help [INDIVIDUAL RECEIVING CARE] with the [PROBLEM]?

APPENDIX C
DSM-5 Glossary of Cultural Concepts of Distress

Ataque de nervios

Ataque de nervios ("attack of nerves") is a syndrome among individuals of Latino descent, characterized by symptoms of intense emotional upset, including acute anxiety, anger, or grief; screaming and shouting uncontrollably; attacks of crying; trembling; heat in the chest rising into the head; and becoming verbally and physically aggressive. Dissociative experiences (e.g., depersonalization, derealization, amnesia), seizure-like or fainting episodes, and suicidal gestures are prominent in some *ataques* but absent in others. A general feature of an *ataque de nervios* is a sense of being out of control. Attacks frequently occur as a direct result of a stressful event relating to the family, such as news of the death of a close relative, conflicts with a spouse or children, or witnessing an accident involving a family member. For a minority of individuals, no particular social event triggers their *ataques;* instead, their vulnerability to losing control comes from the accumulated experience of suffering (Guarnaccia et al. 1993; Guarnaccia et al. 1996; Lewis-Fernández et al. 2010).

No one-to-one relationship has been found between *ataque* and any specific psychiatric disorder, although several disorders, including panic disorder, other specified or unspecified dissociative disorder, and conversion disorder, have symptomatic overlap with *ataque* (Brown and Lewis-Fernández 2011; Guarnaccia et al. 1993; Lewis-Fernández et al. 2002a; Lewis-Fernández et al. 2002b).

In community samples, *ataque* is associated with suicidal ideation, disability, and outpatient psychiatric utilization, after adjustment for psychiatric diagnoses, traumatic exposure, and other covariates (Lewis-Fernández et al. 2009). However, some *ataques* represent normative expressions of acute distress (e.g., at a funeral) without clinical sequelae. The term *ataque de nervios* may also refer to an idiom of distress that includes any "fit"-like paroxysm of emotionality (e.g., hysterical laughing) and may be used to indicate an episode of loss of control in response to an intense stressor.

Related conditions in other cultural contexts: Indisposition in Haiti, blacking out in the Southern United States, and falling out in the West Indies (Weidman 1979).

Related conditions in DSM-5: Panic attack, panic disorder, other specified or unspecified dissociative disorder, conversion (functional neurologic symptom) disorder, intermittent explosive disorder, other specified or unspecified anxiety disorder, other specified or unspecified trauma and stressor-related disorder.

References

Brown RJ, Lewis-Fernández R: Culture and conversion disorder: implications for DSM-5. Psychiatry 74(3):187–206, 2011 21916627

Guarnaccia PJ, Canino G, Rubio-Stipec M, Bravo M: The prevalence of ataques de nervios in the Puerto Rico disaster study: the role of culture in psychiatric epidemiology. J Nerv Ment Dis 181(3):157–165, 1993 8445374

Guarnaccia PJ, Rivera M, Franco F, Neighbors C: The experiences of ataques de nervios: towards an anthropology of emotions in Puerto Rico. Cult Med Psychiatry 20(3):343–367, 1996 8899285

Lewis-Fernández R, Garrido-Castillo P, Bennasar MC, et al: Dissociation, childhood trauma, and ataque de nervios among Puerto Rican psychiatric outpatients. Am J Psychiatry 159(9):1603–1605, 2002a 12202287

Lewis-Fernández R, Guarnaccia PJ, Martínez IE, et al: Comparative phenomenology of ataques de nervios, panic attacks, and panic disorder. Cult Med Psychiatry 26(2):199–223, 2002b 12211325

Lewis-Fernández R, Horvitz-Lennon M, Blanco C, et al: Significance of endorsement of psychotic symptoms by US Latinos. J Nerv Ment Dis 197(5):337–347, 2009 19440107

Lewis-Fernández R, Gorritz M, Raggio GA, et al: Association of trauma-related disorders and dissociation with four idioms of distress among Latino psychiatric outpatients. Cult Med Psychiatry 34(2):219–243, 2010 20414799

Weidman HH: Falling-out: a diagnostic and treatment problem viewed from a transcultural perspective. Soc Sci Med Med Anthropol 13B(2):95–112, 1979 505060

Dhat syndrome

Dhat syndrome is a term that was coined in South Asia little more than half a century ago to account for common clinical presentations of young male patients who attributed their various symptoms to semen loss. Despite the name, it is not a discrete syndrome but rather a cultural explanation of distress for patients who refer to diverse symptoms, such as anxiety, fatigue, weakness, weight loss, impotence, other multiple somatic complaints, and depressive mood. The cardinal feature is anxiety and distress about the loss of *dhat* in the absence of any identifiable physiological dysfunction (Gautham et al. 2008). *Dhat* was identified by patients as a white discharge that was noted on defecation or urination (Murthy and Wig 2002). Ideas about this substance are related to the concept of *dhatu* (semen) described in the Hindu system of medicine, Ayurveda, as one of seven essential bodily fluids whose balance is necessary to maintain health (Jadhav 2004; Raguram et al. 1994).

Although *dhat syndrome* was formulated as a cultural guide to local clinical practice, related ideas about the harmful effects of semen loss have been shown to be widespread in the general population (Malhotra and Wig 1975), suggesting a cultural disposition for explaining health problems and symptoms with reference to *dhat syndrome*. Research in health care settings has yielded diverse estimates of the syndrome's prevalence (e.g., 64% of men attending psychiatric clinics in India for sexual complaints; 30% of men attending general medical clinics in Pakistan) (Bhatia and Malik 1991; Mumford 1996). Although *dhat syndrome* is most commonly identified with young men from lower socioeconomic backgrounds, middle-aged men may also be affected (Khan 2005). Comparable concerns about white vaginal discharge (leukorrhea) have been associated with a variant of the concept for women (Trollope-Kumar 2001).

Related conditions in other cultural contexts: *koro* in Southeast Asia, particularly Singapore and *shen-k'uei* ("kidney deficiency") in China (Sumathipala et al. 2004).

Related conditions in DSM-5: Major depressive disorder, persistent depressive disorder (dysthymia), generalized anxiety disorder, somatic symptom disorder, illness anxiety disorder, erectile disorder, early (premature) ejaculation, other specified or unspecified sexual dysfunction, academic problem.

References

Bhatia MS, Malik SC: Dhat syndrome—a useful diagnostic entity in Indian culture. Br J Psychiatry 159:691–695, 1991 1756347

Gautham M, Singh R, Weiss H, et al: Socio-cultural, psychosexual and biomedical factors associated with genital symptoms experienced by men in rural India. Trop Med Int Health 13(3):384–395, 2008 18298609

Jadhav S: Dhat syndrome: a re-evaluation. Psychiatry 3(8):14–16, 2004

Khan N: Dhat syndrome in relation to demographic characteristics. Indian J Psychiatry 47(1): 54–57, 2005

Malhotra HK, Wig NN: Dhat syndrome: a culture-bound sex neurosis of the orient. Arch Sex Behav 4(5):519–528, 1975 1191004

Mumford DB: The 'Dhat syndrome': a culturally determined symptom of depression? Acta Psychiatr Scand 94(3):163–167, 1996 8891081

Murthy RS, Wig NN: Psychiatric diagnosis and classification in developing countries, in Psychiatric Diagnosis and Classification. Edited by Maj M, Gaebel W, López-Ibor JJ, Sartorius N. Chichester, UK, Wiley, 2002, pp 249–279

Raguram R, Jadhav S, Weiss MG: Historical perspectives on Dhat syndrome. NIMHANS Journal 12(2):117–124, 1994

Sumathipala A, Siribaddana SH, Bhugra D: Culture-bound syndromes: the story of dhat syndrome. Br J Psychiatry 184:200–209, 2004 14990517

Trollope-Kumar K: Cultural and biomedical meanings of the complaint of leukorrhea in South Asian women. Trop Med Int Health 6(4):260–266, 2001 11348516

Khyâl cap

"*Khyâl* attacks" (*khyâl cap*), or "wind attacks," is a syndrome found among Cambodians in the United States and Cambodia (Hinton et al. 2001; Hinton et al. 2010; Hinton et al. 2012). Common symptoms include those of panic attacks, such as dizziness, palpitations, shortness of breath, and cold extremities, as well as other symptoms of anxiety and autonomic arousal (e.g., tinnitus and neck soreness). *Khyâl* attacks include catastrophic cognitions centered on the concern that *khyâl* (a windlike substance) may rise in the body—along with blood—and cause a range of serious effects (e.g., compressing the lungs to cause shortness of breath and asphyxia; entering the cranium to cause tinnitus, dizziness, blurry vision, and a fatal syncope). *Khyâl* attacks may occur without warning, but are frequently brought about by triggers such as worrisome thoughts, standing up (i.e., orthostasis), specific odors with negative associations, and agoraphobic-type cues like going to crowded spaces or riding in a car. *Khyâl* attacks usually meet panic attack criteria and may shape the experience of other anxiety and trauma- and stressor-related disorders. *Khyâl* attacks may be associated with considerable disability.

Related conditions in other cultural contexts: Laos (*pen lom*), Tibet (*srog rlung gi nad*), Sri Lanka (*vata*), and Korea (*hwa byung*) (Hinton and Good 2009).

Related conditions in DSM-5: Panic attack, panic disorder, generalized anxiety disorder, agoraphobia, posttraumatic stress disorder, illness anxiety disorder.

References

Hinton DE, Good BJ (eds): Culture and Panic Disorder. Palo Alto, CA, Stanford University Press, 2009

Hinton DE, Um K, Ba P: Kyol goeu ("wind overload"), part I: a cultural syndrome of orthostatic panic among Khmer refugees. Transcult Psychiatry 38(4):403–432, 2001 20852723

Hinton DE, Pich V, Marques L, et al: Khyâl attacks: a key idiom of distress among traumatized Cambodia refugees. Cult Med Psychiatry 34(2):244–278, 2010 20407813

Hinton DE, Hinton AL, Eng KT, Choung S: PTSD and key somatic complaints and cultural syndromes among rural Cambodians: the results of a needs assessment survey. Med Anthropol Q 26(3):383–407, 2012 23259349

Kufungisisa

Kufungisisa ("thinking too much" in Shona) is an idiom of distress and a cultural explanation among the Shona of Zimbabwe. As an explanation, it is considered to be causative of anxiety, depression, and somatic problems (e.g., "my heart is painful because I think too much"). As an idiom of psychosocial distress, it is indicative of interpersonal and social difficulties (e.g., marital problems, having no money to take care of children) (Patel et al. 1995a; Patel et al. 1995b). *Kufungisisa* involves ruminating on upsetting thoughts, particularly worries (Abas and Broadhead 1997).

Kufungisisa is associated with a range of psychopathology, including anxiety symptoms, excessive worry, panic attacks, depressive symptoms, and irritability (Patel et al. 1995b). In a study of a random community sample, two-thirds of the cases identified by a general psychopathology measure were of this complaint (Abas and Broadhead 1997).

In many cultures, "thinking too much" is considered to be damaging to the mind and body (Hinton et al. 2012; van der Ham et al. 2011; Yarris 2011) and to cause specific symptoms like headache and dizziness. "Thinking too much" may also be a key component of cultural syndromes such as "brain fag" in Nigeria (Ola and Igbokwe 2011; Ola et al. 2009). In the case of brain fag, "thinking too much" is primarily attributed to excessive study, which is considered to damage the brain in particular, with symptoms including feelings of heat or crawling sensations in the head.

Related conditions in other cultural contexts: "Thinking too much" is a common idiom of distress and cultural explanation across many countries and ethnic groups. It has been described in Africa (Avotri and Walters 1999; Patel et al. 1995a; Patel et al. 1995b), the Caribbean and Latin America (Bolton et al. 2012; Keys et al. 2012; Yarris 2011), and among East Asian (Frye and D'Avanzo 1994; van der Ham et al. 2011; Westermeyer and Wintrob 1979; Yang et al. 2010) and Native American groups (Kirmayer et al. 1997).

Related conditions in DSM-5: Major depressive disorder, persistent depressive disorder (dysthymia), generalized anxiety disorder, posttraumatic stress disorder, obsessive-compulsive disorder, persistent complex bereavement disorder (see "Conditions for Further Study").

References

Abas MA, Broadhead JC: Depression and anxiety among women in an urban setting in Zimbabwe. Psychol Med 27(1):59–71, 1997 9122309

Avotri JY, Walters V: "You just look at our work and see if you have any freedom on earth": Ghanaian women's accounts of their work and their health. Soc Sci Med 48(9):1123–1133, 1999 10220014

Bolton P, Surkan PJ, Gray AE, Desmousseaux M: The mental health and psychosocial effects of organized violence: a qualitative study in northern Haiti. Transcult Psychiatry 49(3–4):590–612, 2012 22228786

Frye BA, D'Avanzo C: Themes in managing culturally defined illness in the Cambodian refugee family. J Community Health Nurs 11(2):89–98, 1994 8021721

Hinton DE, Hinton AL, Eng KT, Choung S: PTSD and key somatic complaints and cultural syndromes among rural Cambodians: the results of a needs assessment survey. Medical Anthropology Quarterly 26:383–407, 2012 10.1111/j.1548-1387.2012.01224.x

Keys HM, Kaiser BN, Kohrt BA, et al: Idioms of distress, ethnopsychology, and the clinical encounter in Haiti's Central Plateau. Soc Sci Med 75(3):555–564, 2012 22595073

Kirmayer LJ, Fletcher CM, Boothroyd LJ: Inuit attitudes toward deviant behavior: a vignette study. J Nerv Ment Dis 185(2):78–86, 1997 9048699

Ola BA, Igbokwe DO: Factorial validation and reliability analysis of the Brain Fag Syndrome Scale. Afr Health Sci 11(3):334–340, 2011 22275921

Ola BA, Morakinyo O, Adewuya AO: Brain fag syndrome—a myth or a reality. Afr J Psychiatry (Johannesbg) 12(2):135–143, 2009 19582315

Patel V, Gwanzura F, Simunyu E, et al: The phenomenology and explanatory models of common mental disorder: a study in primary care in Harare, Zimbabwe. Psychol Med 25(6):1191–1199, 1995a 8637949

Patel V, Simunyu E, Gwanzura F: Kufungisisa (thinking too much): a Shona idiom for non-psychotic mental illness. Cent Afr J Med 41(7):209–215, 1995b 7553793

van der Ham L, Wright P, Van TV, et al: Perceptions of mental health and help-seeking behavior in an urban community in Vietnam: an explorative study. Community Ment Health J 47(5):574–582, 2011 21409418

Westermeyer J, Wintrob R: "Folk" explanations of mental illness in rural Laos. Am J Psychiatry 136(7):901–905, 1979 453350

Yang LH, Phillips MR, Lo G, et al: "Excessive thinking" as explanatory model for schizophrenia: impacts on stigma and "moral" status in Mainland China. Schizophr Bull 36(4):836–845, 2010 19193742

Yarris KE: The pain of "thinking too much": dolor de cerebro and the embodiment of social hardship among Nicaraguan women. Ethos 39(2):226–248, 2011 10.1111/j.1548-1352.2011.01186.x

Maladi moun

Maladi moun (literally "humanly caused illness," also referred to as "sent sickness") is a cultural explanation in Haitian communities for diverse medical and psychiatric disorders. In this explanatory model, interpersonal envy and malice cause people to harm their enemies by sending illnesses such as psychosis (Brodwin 1996), depression (Nicolas et al. 2007), social or academic failure, and inability to perform activities of daily living (Desrosiers and St. Fleurose 2002). The etiological model assumes that illness may be caused by others' envy and hatred, provoked by the victim's economic success as evidenced by a new job or expensive purchase (Farmer 1990). One person's gain is assumed to produce another person's loss, so visible success makes one vulnerable to attack (Vonars and Vodou 2007). Assigning the label of sent sickness depends on mode of onset and social status more than presenting symptoms. The acute onset of new symptoms or an abrupt behavioral change raises suspicions of a spiritual attack. Someone who is attractive, intelligent, or wealthy is perceived as especially vulnerable, and even young healthy children are at risk (DeSantis and Thomas 1990).

Related conditions in other cultural contexts: Concerns about illness (typically, physical illness) caused by envy or social conflict are common across cultures and often expressed in the form of "evil eye" (e.g., in Spanish, *mal de ojo*; in Italian, *mal'occhiu*) (Al-Sughayir 1996; Migliore and Mal'occhiu 1997; Risser and Mazur 1995).

Related conditions in DSM-5: Delusional disorder, persecutory type; schizophrenia with paranoid features.

References

Al-Sughayir MA: Public view of the "evil eye" and its role in psychiatry: a study in Saudi society. Arab Journal of Psychiatry 7(2):152–160, 1996

Brodwin P: Medicine and Morality in Haiti: The Contest for Healing Power (Cambridge Studies in Medical Anthropology series). Cambridge, UK, Cambridge University Press, 1996

DeSantis L, Thomas JT: The immigrant Haitian mother: transcultural nursing perspective on preventive health care for children. J Transcult Nurs 2(1):2–15, 1990 2264938

Desrosiers A, St. Fleurose S: Treating Haitian patients: key cultural aspects. Am J Psychother 56(4):508–521, 2002 12520887

Farmer P: Sending sickness: sorcery, politics, and changing concepts of AIDS in rural Haiti. Medical Anthropology Quarterly 4(1):6–27, 1990 10.1525/maq.1990.4.1.02a00020

Migliore S: Mal'occhiu: Ambiguity, Evil Eye, and the Language of Distress. Toronto, ON, University of Toronto Press, 1997

Nicolas G, Desilva AM, Subrebost KL, et al: Expression and treatment of depression among Haitian immigrant women in the United States: clinical observations. Am J Psychother 61(1):83–98, 2007 17503679

Risser AL, Mazur LJ: Use of folk remedies in a Hispanic population. Arch Pediatr Adolesc Med 149(9):978–981, 1995 7655602

Vonarx N: Vodou: Illness and models in Haiti: from local meanings to broader relations of domination. Anthropology in Action 14(3):18–29, 2007

Nervios

Nervios ("nerves") is a common idiom of distress among Latinos in the United States and Latin America. *Nervios* refers to a general state of vulnerability to stressful life experiences and to difficult life circumstances (Baer et al. 2003; Finkler 2001; Guarnaccia and Farias 1988; Guarnaccia et al. 2003; Lewis-Fernández et al. 2010; Low 1981; Weller et al. 2008). The term *nervios* includes a wide range of symptoms of emotional distress, somatic disturbance, and inability to function (Salgado de Snyder et al. 2000). The most common symptoms attributed to *nervios* include headaches and "brain aches" (occipital neck tension), irritability, stomach disturbances, sleep difficulties, nervousness, easy tearfulness, inability to concentrate, trembling, tingling sensations, and *mareos* (dizziness with occasional vertigo-like exacerbations) (Baer et al. 2003; Guarnaccia et al. 2003). *Nervios* is a broad idiom of distress that spans the range of severity from cases with no mental disorder to presentations resembling adjustment, anxiety, depressive, dissociative, somatic symptom, or psychotic disorders. "Being nervous since childhood" appears to be more of a trait and may precede social anxiety disorder, while "being ill with nerves" is more related than other forms of *nervios* to psychiatric problems, especially dissociation (Lewis-Fernández et al. 2010) and depression (Weller et al. 2008).

Related conditions in other cultural contexts: *Nevra* among Greeks in North America (Dunk 1989), *nierbi* among Sicilians in North America (Migliore 2001), and *nerves* among whites in Appalachia (Van Schaik 1989) and Newfoundland (Davis 1989).

Related conditions in DSM-5: Major depressive disorder, persistent depressive disorder (dysthymia), generalized anxiety disorder, social anxiety disorder, other specified or unspecified dissociative disorder, somatic symptom disorder, schizophrenia.

References

Baer RD, Weller SC, de Alba Garcia JG, et al: A cross-cultural approach to the study of the folk illness nervios. Cult Med Psychiatry 27(3):315–337, 2003 14510097

Davis DL: The variable character of nerves in a Newfoundland fishing village. Med Anthropol 11(1):63–78, 1989 2725214

Dunk P: Greek women and broken nerves in Montreal. Med Anthropol 11(1):29–45, 1989 2725212

Finkler K: Physicians at Work, Patients in Pain: Biomedical Practice and Patient Response in Mexico, 2nd Edition. Durham, NC, Carolina Academic Press, 2001

Guarnaccia PJ, Farias P: The social meanings of nervios: a case study of a Central American woman. Soc Sci Med 26(12):1223–1231, 1988 3206244

Guarnaccia PJ, Lewis-Fernández R, Marano MR: Toward a Puerto Rican popular nosology: nervios and ataque de nervios. Cult Med Psychiatry 27(3):339–366, 2003 14510098

Lewis-Fernández R, Gorritz M, Raggio GA, et al: Association of trauma-related disorders and dissociation with four idioms of distress among Latino psychiatric outpatients. Cult Med Psychiatry 34(2):219–243, 2010 20414799

Low SM: The meaning of nervios: a sociocultural analysis of symptom presentation in San Jose, Costa Rica. Cult Med Psychiatry 5(1):25–47, 1981 7249673

Migliore S: From illness narratives to social commentary: a Pirandellian approach to "nerves." Med Anthropol Q 15(1):100–125, 2001 11288611

Salgado de Snyder VN, Diaz-Perez MJ, Ojeda VD: The prevalence of nervios and associated symptomatology among inhabitants of Mexican rural communities. Cult Med Psychiatry 24(4):453–470, 2000 11128627

Van Schaik E: Paradigms underlying the study of nerves as a popular illness term in eastern Kentucky. Med Anthropol 11(1):15–28, 1989 2725211

Weller SC, Baer RD, Garcia de Alba Garcia J, Salcedo Rocha AL: Susto and nervios: expressions for stress and depression. Cult Med Psychiatry 32(3):406–420, 2008 18535889

Shenjing shuairuo

Shenjing shuairuo ("weakness of the nervous system" in Mandarin Chinese) is a cultural syndrome that integrates conceptual categories of traditional Chinese medicine with the Western diagnosis of neurasthenia. In the second, revised edition of the *Chinese Classification of Mental*

Disorders (CCMD-2-R), *shenjing shuairuo* is defined as a syndrome composed of three out of five nonhierarchical symptom clusters: weakness (e.g., mental fatigue), emotions (e.g., feeling vexed), excitement (e.g., increased recollections), nervous pain (e.g., headache), and sleep (e.g., insomnia) (Lee 1994). *Fan nao* (feeling vexed) is a form of irritability mixed with worry and distress over conflicting thoughts and unfulfilled desires. The third edition of the CCMD (Chinese Society of Psychiatry 2001) retains *shenjing shuairuo* as a somatoform diagnosis of exclusion (Lee and Kleinman 2007). Salient precipitants of *shenjing shuairuo* include work- or family-related stressors, loss of face (*mianzi, lianzi*), and an acute sense of failure (e.g., in academic performance) (Kleinman 1986; Lewis-Fernández et al. 2009). *Shenjing shuairuo* is related to traditional concepts of weakness (*xu*) and health imbalances related to deficiencies of a vital essence (e.g., the depletion of *qi* [vital energy] following overstraining or stagnation of *qi* due to excessive worry) (Lee and Kleinman 2007). In the traditional interpretation, *shenjing shuairuo* results when bodily channels (*jing*) conveying vital forces (*shen*) become dysregulated as a result of various social and interpersonal stressors, such as the inability to change a chronically frustrating and distressing situation (Lee 1994; Lin 1989). Various psychiatric disorders are associated with *shenjing shuairuo,* notably mood, anxiety, and somatic symptom disorders. In medical clinics in China, however, up to 45% of patients with *shenjing shuairuo* do not meet criteria for any DSM-IV disorder (Chang et al. 2005).

Related conditions in other cultural contexts: Neurasthenia-spectrum idioms and syndromes are present in India (*ashaktapanna*) (Paralikar et al. 2011) and Japan (*shinkei-suijaku*) (Lin 1989), among other settings. Other conditions, such as brain fag syndrome (Ola and Igbokwe 2011), burnout syndrome (Leone et al. 2011), and chronic fatigue syndrome (Fukuda et al. 1994), are also closely related.

Related conditions in DSM-5: Major depressive disorder, persistent depressive disorder (dysthymia), generalized anxiety disorder, somatic symptom disorder, social anxiety disorder, specific phobia, posttraumatic stress disorder.

References

Chang DF, Myers HF, Yeung A, et al: Shenjing shuairuo and the DSM-IV: diagnosis, distress, and disability in a Chinese primary care setting. Transcult Psychiatry 42(2):204–218, 2005 16114583

Chinese Medical Association and Nanjing Medical University: Chinese Classification of Mental Disorders, 2nd Edition, Revised (CCMD-2-R). Nanjing, Dong Nan University Press, 1995

Chinese Society of Psychiatry: The Chinese Classification and Diagnostic Criteria of Mental Disorders, Version 3 (CCMD-3). Ginan, China, Chinese Society of Psychiatry, 2001

Fukuda K, Straus SE, Hickie I, et al: The chronic fatigue syndrome: a comprehensive approach to its definition and study. International Chronic Fatigue Syndrome Study Group. Ann Intern Med 121(12):953–959, 1994 7978722

Kleinman A: Social Origins of Distress and Disease: Depression, Neurasthenia, and Pain in Modern China. New Haven, CT, Yale University Press, 1986

Lee S: The vicissitudes of Neurasthenia in Chinese societies: where will it go from the ICD-10? Transcultural Psychiatry 31(2):153–172, 1994 10.1177/136346159403100205

Lee S, Kleinman A: Are somatoform disorders changing with time? The case of neurasthenia in China. Psychosom Med 69(9):846–849, 2007 18040092

Leone SS, Wessely S, Huibers MJ, et al: Two sides of the same coin? On the history and phenomenology of chronic fatigue and burnout. Psychol Health 26(4):449–464, 2011 20437294

Lewis-Fernández R, Guarnaccia PJ, Ruiz P: Culture-bound syndromes, in Kaplan and Sadock's Comprehensive Textbook of Psychiatry, 9th Edition. Edited by Sadock VJ, Sadock VA, Ruiz P. Philadelphia, PA, Lippincott Williams & Wilkins, 2009, pp 2519–2538

Lin TY: Neurasthenia revisited: its place in modern psychiatry. Cult Med Psychiatry 13(2):105–129, 1989 2766788

Ola BA, Igbokwe DO: Factorial validation and reliability analysis of the Brain Fag Syndrome Scale. Afr Health Sci 11(3):334–340, 2011 22275921

Paralikar V, Agashe M, Sarmukaddam S, et al: Cultural epidemiology of neurasthenia spectrum disorders in four general hospital outpatient clinics of urban Pune, India. Transcult Psychiatry 48(3):257–283, 2011 21742952

Susto

Susto ("fright") is a cultural explanation for distress and misfortune prevalent among some Latinos in the United States and among people in Mexico, Central America, and South America. It is not recognized as an illness category among Latinos from the Caribbean (Weller et al. 2002). *Susto* is an illness attributed to a frightening event that causes the soul to leave the body and results in unhappiness and sickness, as well as difficulties functioning in key social roles (Rubel et al. 1984; Villaseñor-Bayardo 2008). Symptoms may appear any time from days to years after the fright is experienced. In extreme cases, *susto* may result in death. There are no specific defining symptoms for *susto* (Zolla 2005); however, symptoms that are often reported by people with *susto* include appetite disturbances, inadequate or excessive sleep, troubled sleep or dreams, feelings of sadness, low self-worth or dirtiness, interpersonal sensitivity, and lack of motivation to do anything. Somatic symptoms accompanying *susto* may include muscle aches and pains, cold in the extremities, pallor, headache, stomachache, and diarrhea. Precipitating events are diverse, and include natural phenomena, animals, interpersonal situations, and supernatural agents, among others (Ruiz Velasco 2010).

Three syndromic types of *susto* (referred to as *cibih* in the local Zapotec language) have been identified, each having different relationships with psychiatric diagnoses (Taub 1992). An interpersonal *susto* characterized by feelings of loss, abandonment, and not being loved by family, with accompanying symptoms of sadness, poor self-image, and suicidal ideation, seemed to be closely related to major depressive disorder. When *susto* resulted from a traumatic event that played a major role in shaping symptoms and in emotional processing of the experience, the diagnosis of posttraumatic stress disorder appeared more appropriate. *Susto* characterized by various recurrent somatic symptoms—for which the person sought health care from several practitioners—was thought to resemble a somatic symptom disorder.

Related conditions in other cultural contexts: Similar etiological concepts and symptom configurations are found globally (Simons 1985). In the Andean region, *susto* is referred to as *espanto* (Tousignant 1979).

Related conditions in DSM-5: Major depressive disorder, posttraumatic stress disorder, other specified or unspecified trauma and stressor-related disorder, somatic symptom disorders.

References

Rubel AJ, O'Nell CW, Collado-Ardón R: Susto: A Folk Illness. Berkeley, University of California Press, 1984

Ruíz Velasco ME: La cosmovisión de la salud y los "peligros del alma" en la zona de los Altos de Chiapas [The worldview of health and the "perils of the soul" in the Chiapas Highlands]. Atopos 10:83–100, 2010 Available at: http://www.atopos.es/pdf_10/5_La%20cosmovisi%C3%B3n%20de%20la%20salud%20y%20los%20peligros%20del%20alma.pdf. Accessed December 14, 2012.

Simons RC: Introduction: the fright illness taxon, in The Culture-Bound Syndromes: Folk Illnesses of Psychiatric and Anthropological Interest. Edited by Simons RC, Hughes CC. Dordrecht, Holland, D Reidel, 1985, pp 329–331

Taub B: Calling the soul back to the heart: soul loss, depression and healing among indigenous Mexicans. Unpublished doctoral dissertation, University of California, Los Angeles, 1992

TousignantM : Espanto: a dialogue with the gods. Cult Med Psychiatry 3(4):347–361, 1979 535409

Villaseñor-Bayardo S: Apuntes para una Etnopsiquiatría mexicana. Guadalajara, Mexico, Universidad de Guadalajara, 2008

Weller SC, Baer RD, de Alba Garcia JG, et al: Regional variation in Latino descriptions of susto. Cult Med Psychiatry 26(4):449–472, 2002 12572769

Weller SC, Baer RD, Garcia de Alba Garcia J, Salcedo Rocha AL: Susto and nervios: expressions for stress and depression. Cult Med Psychiatry 32(3):406–420, 2008 18535889

Zolla C: La medicina tradicional indígena en el México actual [Traditional indigenous medicine in Mexico today]. Arqueología Mexicana 13(74):62–68, 2005 Available at: http://www.arqueomex.com/S2N2 SUMARIO74.html. Accessed December 14, 2012.

Taijin kyofusho

Taijin kyofusho ("interpersonal fear disorder" in Japanese) is a cultural syndrome characterized by anxiety about and avoidance of interpersonal situations due to the thought, feeling, or conviction that one's appearance and actions in social interactions are inadequate or offensive to others (Nakamura et al. 2002; Tarumi et al. 2004). In the United States, the variant involves having an offensive body odor and is termed *olfactory reference syndrome.* Individuals with *taijin kyofusho* tend to focus on the impact of their symptoms and behaviors on others (Kinoshita et al. 2008). Variants include major concerns about facial blushing (erythrophobia), having an offensive body odor (olfactory reference syndrome), inappropriate gaze (too much or too little eye contact), stiff or awkward facial expression or bodily movements (e.g., stiffening, trembling), or body deformity (Takahashi 1989).

Taijin kyofusho is a broader construct than social anxiety disorder in DSM-5 (Tarumi et al. 2004). In addition to performance anxiety, *taijin kyofusho* includes two culture-related forms: a "sensitive type," with extreme social sensitivity and anxiety about interpersonal interactions, and an "offensive type," in which the major concern is offending others. As a category, *taijin kyofusho* thus includes syndromes with features of body dysmorphic disorder as well as delusional disorder. Concerns may have a delusional quality, responding poorly to simple reassurance or counterexample.

The distinctive symptoms of *taijin kyofusho* occur in specific cultural contexts and, to some extent, with more severe social anxiety across cultures (Choy et al. 2008; Kim et al. 2008). Similar syndromes are found in Korea and other societies that place a strong emphasis on the self-conscious maintenance of appropriate social behavior in hierarchical interpersonal relationships. *Taijin kyofusho*–like symptoms have also been described in other cultural contexts, including the United States, Australia, and New Zealand.

Related conditions in other cultural contexts: *Taein kong po* in Korea (Choy et al. 2008).

Related conditions in DSM-5: Social anxiety disorder, body dysmorphic disorder, delusional disorder, obsessive-compulsive disorder, olfactory reference syndrome (a type of other specified obsessive-compulsive and related disorder). Olfactory reference syndrome is related specifically to the *jikoshu-kyofu* variant of *taijin kyofusho,* whose core symptom is the concern that the person emits an offensive body odor (Suzuki et al. 2004). This presentation is seen in various cultures outside Japan.

References

Choy Y, Schneier FR, Heimberg RG, et al: Features of the offensive subtype of Taijin-Kyofu-Sho in US and Korean patients with DSM-IV social anxiety disorder. Depress Anxiety 25(3):230–240, 2008 17340609

Kim J, Rapee RM, Gaston JE: Symptoms of offensive type Taijin-Kyofusho among Australian social phobics. Depress Anxiety 25(7):601–608, 2008 17607747

Kinoshita Y, Chen J, Rapee RM, et al: Cross-cultural study of conviction subtype Taijin Kyofu: proposal and reliability of Nagoya-Osaka diagnostic criteria for social anxiety disorder. J Nerv Ment Dis 196(4):307–313, 2008 18414125

Nakamura K, Kitanishi K, Miyake Y, et al: The neurotic versus delusional subtype of taijin-kyofu-sho: their DSM diagnoses. Psychiatry Clin Neurosci 56(6):595–601, 2002 12485300

Suzuki K, Takei N, Iwata Y, et al: Do olfactory reference syndrome and jiko-shu-kyofu (a subtype of taijin-kyofu) share a common entity? Acta Psychiatr Scand 109(2):150–155, 2004 14725599

Takahashi T: Social phobia syndrome in Japan. Compr Psychiatry 30(1):45–52, 1989 2647401

Tarumi S, Ichimiya A, Yamada S, et al: Taijin Kyofusho in university students: patterns of fear and predispositions to the offensive variant. Transcult Psychiatry 41(4):533–546, 2004 15709650

Index

Page numbers printed in **boldface** type refer to tables or figures.